Autism and Child Psychopathology Series

Series Editor
Johnny L. Matson
Baton Rouge, Louisiana, USA

More information about this series at
http://www.springer.com/series/8665

Johnny L. Matson
Editor

Comorbid Conditions Among Children with Autism Spectrum Disorders

Springer

Editor
Johnny L. Matson
Department of Psychology
Louisiana State University
Baton Rouge
Louisiana
USA

ISSN 2192-922X ISSN 2192-9238 (electonic)
Autism and Child Psychopathology Series
ISBN 978-3-319-37154-2 ISBN 978-3-319-19183-6 (eBook)
DOI 10.1007/978-3-319-19183-6

Springer Cham Heidelberg New York Dordrecht London

Softcover re-print of the Hardcover 1st edition 2016

Printed on acid-free paper

Springer International Publishing AG Switzerland is part of Springer Science+Business Media (www.springer.com)

Contents

About the Editor

Johnny L. Matson PhD is a professor and distin[illegible] research master in the Department of Psychology a[illegible] Louisiana State University, Baton Rouge, LA, USA. He has also previously held a professorship in psychiatry and clinical psychology at the University of Pittsburgh. He is the author of more than 800 publications including 41 books. He also serves as founding editor-in-chief of three journals: *Research in Developmental Disabilities* (Elsevier), *Research in Autism Spectrum Disorders* (Elsevier), *and Review Journal of Autism and Developmental Disorders* (Springer).

Contributors

Fahad Alresheed Department of Special Education and Clinical Sciences, University of Oregon, Eugene, OR, USA

Casey M. Breslin Temple University, Philadelphia, PA, USA

John Cairney Department of Psychiatry and Behavioral Neuroscience Family Medicine, Kinesiology and CanChild, Center for Childhood Disability Research, McMaster University, Hamilton, ON, Canada

Amarie Carnett Victoria University of Wellington, Wellington, New Zealand

Paige Cervantes Department of Psychology, Louisiana State University, Baton Rouge, LA, USA

Robert Didden Behavioural Science Institute, Radboud University, Nijmegen, HE, The Netherlands

Sayed ElGarhy Fayoum University, Al Fayoum, Faiyum Governorate, Egypt

Jill C. Fodstad Department of Psychiatry, Indiana University School of Medicine, Indianapolis, IN, USA

Christopher Gillberg Research Department, National Center for Young People with Epilepsy, Lingfield, Surrey, UK

Jina Jang Department of Psychology, Louisiana State University, Baton Rouge, LA, USA

Sara King-Dowling Department of Kinesiology, McMaster University, Hamilton, ON, Canada

Christen Knowles Department of Special Education and Clinical Sciences, University of Oregon, Eugene, OR, USA

Russell Lang College of Education, Texas State University, San Marcos, TX, USA

Geraldine Leader Irish Centre for Autism and Neurodevelopmental Research, School of Psychology, National University of Ireland, Galway, Galway, Ireland

Ting Liu Department of Health and Human Performance, Texas State University, San Marcos, TX, USA

Wendy Machalicek Department of Special Education and Clinical Sciences, University of Oregon, Eugene, OR, USA

Caroline I. Magyar Department of Pediatrics, University of Rochester Medical Center, Rochester, NY, USA

Arlene Mannion Irish Centre for Autism and Neurodevelopmental Research, National University of Ireland, Galway, Galway, Ireland

Susan D. Mayes Department of Psychiatry, Penn State College of Medicine, Hershey, PA, USA

Micah O. Mazurek University of Missouri-Columbia, Columbia, MO, USA

Iain McClure NHS Lothian, Musselburgh, UK

Sandra McCourt Department of Psychiatry, Indiana University School of Medicine, Indianapolis, IN, USA

Karen McKenzie Northumbria University, Newcastle upon Tyne, UK

Lisa R. Minor Department of Psychiatry, Indiana University School of Medicine, Indianapolis, IN, USA

Noha F. Minshawi Department of Psychiatry, Indiana University School of Medicine, Indianapolis, IN, USA

Vincent Pandolfi Psychology Department, Rochester Institute of Technology, Rochester, NY, USA

Amanda M. Pearl Department of Psychiatry, Penn State College of Medicine, Hershey, PA, USA

Nienke Peters-Scheffer Behavioural Science Institute, Radboud University, Nijmegen, HE, The Netherlands

Tracy Raulston Department of Special Education and Clinical Sciences, University of Oregon, Eugene, OR, USA

Colin Reilly Research Department, National Center for Young People with Epilepsy, Lingfield, Surrey, UK

Traci Ruppert Department of Special Education and Clinical Sciences, University of Oregon, Eugene, OR, USA

Halina Rzepecka NHS Tayside, Dundee, UK

John F. Strang Center for Autism Spectrum Disorders, Children's National Medical Center, Washington, D.C., USA

Despite the importance of the problem, comorbidity has received relatively little specific attention in autism research until recent years. This chapter explores historical perspectives on comorbidity in autism, and considers how changes over time in diagnostic practices have affected the study of co-occurring conditions.

History of Diagnosis

The term "autistic" was first used in the early 20th century by Dr. Eugen Bleuler (1911) to describe particular patterns of thought. The term was used to describe the tendency to detach oneself from external reality, with inner life predominating, and was also used to characterize individuals with schizophrenia. The term "autistic" was later employed in the first and second editions of the *Diagnostic and Statistical Manual of Mental Disorders* (DSM) in reference to schizophrenia. In the first edition of the DSM, the diagnosis of schizophrenic reaction, paranoid type was described as being "characterized by autistic, unrealistic thinking" (American Psychiatric Association 1952). Similarly, in both the first and second editions of the DSM, schizophrenic reaction, childhood type was described as being "manifested by autistic, atypical and withdrawn behavior" (American Psychiatric Association 1968).

The first clinical account of autism as condition distinct from schizophrenia was offered by Leo Kanner (1943) in his description of 11 children described as having "autistic disturbances of affective contact." In his descriptions, Kanner chose the term "autistic" to characterize an observed pattern of detachment from the social world, or "extreme autistic aloneness" (p. 242). During the same period of time, yet independently, Hans Asperger (1944) also used the term "autism" to describe deficits in social relatedness in four children he observed (Asperger 1944; Asperger and Frith 1991). In the decades immediately following these initial clinical accounts, the syndrome (primarily as described by Kanner) received considerable scientific and clinical attention. Foremost to the scientific debate were the issues of how best to characterize the disorder and whether and how it could be differentiated from other childhood conditions.

Despite this active and continued discourse, autism was not included as a separate diagnosis until 1980 in the third edition of the DSM (DSM-III, American Psychiatric Association 1980). At that time, separate diagnostic categories of infantile autism and childhood onset pervasive developmental disorder were offered. However, the criteria for the two disorders were qualitatively and quantitatively different. For example, the criteria for infantile autism included an age of onset prior to 30 months, pervasive lack of responsiveness to other people, deficits in language impairment, peculiar speech patterns (if speech was present), and bizarre responses to the environment. In contrast, the criteria for childhood onset pervasive developmental disorder were more detailed, and included later age of onset, impairment in social relationships, and at least three of seven bizarre responses to the environment (i.e., sudden excessive anxiety, constricted or inappropriate affect, resistance to change/rituals, oddities of motor movement, abnormalities of speech, hyper- or hyposensitivity to sensory stimuli, and self-mutilation).

Since its initial introduction into the DSM, additional changes to autism diagnostic classification have occurred with each major revision. In DSM-III-R, the diagnostic categories were revised to include autistic disorder and pervasive developmental disorder not otherwise specified (PDD NOS). The criteria for autistic disorder were changed to represent a triadic approach to symptom structure (i.e., deficits in social interaction, deficits in communication, and restricted activities and interests) (American Psychiatric Association 1987). In DSM-IV, the number of diagnostic categories was expanded to include Asperger's disorder, childhood disintegrative disorder, and Rett disorder in addition to the previous categories of autistic disorder and PDD NOS. Importantly, the addition of the Asperger's disorder diagnosis was intended to provide a classification for individuals with later age of onset, lack of language impairment, and average or above IQ (American Psychiatric Association 1994). However, evidence from empirical studies and clinical practice revealed problems with the use of the subcategories of Asperger's disorder and PDD NOS (Frith 2004; Miller and Ozonoff 2000; Ozonoff 2012a, b). Notably, in a large multi-site study using a consistent standardized battery, clinical distinctions across autism spectrum subcategories were not found to be reliable (Lord et al. 2012).

In response to this mounting evidence, the most recent edition (DSM-5) adopted even more significant changes to autism classification (American Psychiatric Association 2013). The new criteria included a shift from the previous triadic grouping of symptoms to a more parsimonious grouping of only two domains: (1) social communication/social interaction and (2) restricted, repetitive behaviors and interests. More notably, DSM-5 criteria collapsed four previous subcategories into a single diagnostic category:ASD.

Diagnostic Classification and Comorbidity

In addition to numerous revisions to the classification of primary autism symptoms, the classification of associated features and comorbid conditions has also been a subject to substantial change over time. Despite longstanding recognition of the complexity and heterogeneity of the disorder, comorbidity has received relatively little attention in its own right until recent years. Although the reasons for this are likely to be manifold, diagnostic overshadowing bias is one of the contributors.

Diagnostic overshadowing biases occur when symptoms or behaviors are attributed to one disorder without consideration of an additional comorbid diagnosis. This term has been used primarily in reference to the tendency to overlook mental health problems in individuals with intellectual disabilities (Levitan and Reiss 1983; Reiss and Szyszko 1983); however, it also applies to the recognition of co-occurring conditions in individuals with other disabilities (Garner et al. 1994) including autism (Rosenberg et al. 2011). As an example, the diagnostic overshadowing bias may occur when all behavioral symptoms are attributed to a previously diagnosed genetic disorder rather than considering an additional autism diagnosis. Alternatively, an autism diagnosis may overshadow the possibility of other comorbid diagnoses even when such diagnoses would be warranted. For example, anxiety symptoms may be misinterpreted as a manifestation of repetitive behaviors, rather than as evidence of an additional comorbid anxiety disorder.

The diagnostic classification system itself has presented an additional barrier to both research and clinical practice focused on comorbidities. Over time, the DSM criteria for autism have varied significantly in the extent to which they have permitted concurrent diagnoses. This has been particularly true with regard to psychiatric comorbidities. For example, DSM-III criteria specified that attention-deficit/hyperactivity disorder (ADHD), pica, separation anxiety, or overanxious disorder could not be diagnosed if a pervasive developmental disorder was present (American Psychiatric Association 1987). The prevailing belief was that these symptoms occurred so frequently alongside other symptoms of autism that they were characteristic of the primary disorder, thereby preempting additional diagnoses. This approach was maintained in DSM-IV (American Psychiatric Association 1994) and DSM-IV-TR (American Psychiatric Association 2000). In both editions, an autism spectrum diagnosis precluded additional diagnoses of ADHD, separation anxiety disorder, or generalized anxiety disorder. New exclusions were also added in DSM-IV, such that autism spectrum diagnoses also precluded additional diagnoses of selective mutism and social phobia, while a comorbid diagnosis of pica was permitted if the symptoms were severe enough to warrant clinical attention (American Psychiatric Association 1994).

With the publication of the new DSM-5 criteria for ASD, exclusionary criteria for co-occurring diagnoses have been removed and the possibility and frequency of comorbid diagnoses are now specifically discussed (American Psychiatric Association 2013, pp. 58–59). Regarding intellectual disability, DSM-5 criteria specify that symptoms of ASD should not be better explained by intellectual disability; noting, however, that a comorbid "diagnosis of autism spectrum disorder in an individual with intellectual disability is appropriate when social communication and interaction are significantly impaired relative to … developmental level" (p. 58). In addition, the criteria allow for the characterization of cognitive, language, medical, and behavioral comorbidities, as follows:

> With or without accompanying intellectual impairment
> With or without accompanying language impairment
> Associated with a known medical or genetic condition or environmental factor
> Associated with another neurodevelopmental, mental, or behavioral disorder
> With catatonia (American Psychiatric Association 2013, p. 51)

The intention behind these coding changes in DSM-5 is to maintain specificity of autism diagnoses, while also allowing for characterization of additional features and comorbid conditions that are not specific to autism. In the future, these changes to diagnostic practice are expected to foster a better understanding of potential subtypes of autism, which may be characterized by both variations in core symptoms as well as comorbid conditions (Grzadzinski et al. 2013).

Historical Perspectives on Comorbid Conditions

Since the very early accounts of autism, there has been a long-standing recognition of the medical, cognitive, and behavioral complexities that occur in at least a subset of children with the disorder. However, specific interest in studying comorbidity in autism has burgeoned only in recent years. The following discussion will review historical perspectives across different types of comorbid conditions, with an emphasis on the historical roots of current investigations.

One of the first barriers to recognizing comorbid conditions in autism was the psychogenic theory. This predominant view asserted that childhood autism was a consequence of lack of parental warmth, and was not biologically or genetically determined (Eisenberg and Kanner 1956). This early theory arose from Kanner's observations that children with autism were essentially healthy with little evidence of underlying medical etiologies (Eisenberg and Kanner 1956; Kanner 1943, 1949), leading to a belief that the underlying causes and characteristics were not primarily biological in nature, but rather the results of "emotionally frigid" parenting (Eisenberg and Kanner 1956; Kanner 1949, 1954). However, this belief was eventually replaced by a growing recognition of the medical and behavioral complexity associated with the disorder, and of the probable neurobiological underpinnings of autism (Gillberg 1988; Schain and Yannet 1960; Van Krevelen 1958).

As this recognition emerged, clinical researchers began to debate the most appropriate classification of children with and without obvious neurological conditions. Early in the history of the diagnosis, investigators expressed differing views about how to classify children with clear neurological difficulties who also shared common core symptoms of autism. Some argued that "true" autism cases (as described by Kanner) were distinct from cases that were attributable to brain dysfunction. Others advocated for the distinction between "primary" and "secondary" autism as a way to characterize the presence or absence of comorbid medical conditions (Chess et al. 1978). From this standpoint, individuals with a clear genetically determined syndrome, such as fragile X syndrome or tuberous sclerosis (TS), or another known etiology, such as congenital rubella, were characterized as having "secondary autism." In contrast, individuals for whom there was no known genetic syndrome were characterized as having "primary" or "idiopathic" autism (Chess 1971; Chess et al. 1978; Rutter et al. 1994). However, research over the past decade has revealed an increasingly complex etiological picture (Abrahams and Geschwind 2008; State and Šestan 2012), with even greater numbers of identifiable genetic and neurobiological abnormalities associated with autism.

Comorbid Intellectual Impairment

The historical debate regarding comorbid intellectual impairment in autism provides a clear illustration of the changes over time in understanding and classifying comorbid conditions. In Kanner's (1943) first description of the syndrome, he observed that the children he studied were of generally normal intelligence, and that neurological conditions or signs were not apparent. As a result, one prevailing diagnostic view of that time was that intellectual impairment and classic Kannerian autism were mutually exclusive (Douglas and Sanders 1968; Eisenberg 1966). In contrast, other classifications of the disorder permitted the inclusion of intellectual impairment. For example, the work of Creak (working group chairman) and colleagues (1961, 1964) included the following in their key characteristics of the disorder: "a background of serious retardation in which islets of normal, near normal, or exceptional intellectual function or skill may appear" (Creak 1961, p. 890). Others also advocated for the recognition that autism and intellectual impairment could co-occur (Rutter et al. 1969), and that their co-occurrence may be indicative of "organic" versus "nonorganic" etiology (Goldfarb 1961; Rutter 1970). In their comparison of children with autism with and without intellectual impairment, Bartak and Rutter (1976) found that the primary features of autism were present in children with both high and low intellectual functioning, providing support for the notion that intellectual disability and autism are separate conditions that may co-occur.

In the years following Creak's (1961) paper, additional studies reported a high rate of co-occurrence of autism and intellectual impairment (Gillies 1965; Lockyer and Rutter 1970), with a majority of studies in the 1960s reporting high rates of intellectual impairment across samples (Gillies 1965; Lockyer and Rutter 1970). For example, Gittelman and Birch (1967) found that the majority (58 %) of their sample of 97 children obtained IQ scores below 70. Similarly, Lotter (1966b) found that 69 % of their small sample of 32 children with autism obtained IQ scores below 55 or were not testable. In a larger sample of 63 children with autism, Rutter and Lockyer (1967) reported that 71 % had IQ of 70 or below, and 16 % of the sample could not be tested. Shortly thereafter, Alpern and Kimberlin (1970) found that IQ scores ranged from 4 to 78 in a small sample of 32 children with autism, and that IQ scores were highly correlated with clinical ratings of abilities. Follow-up studies also showed relative stability in IQ and persistent impairment over time. For example, DeMyer et al. (1974) found that 74 % of preschool-aged children had IQ below 52, and that most children continued to score within the impaired range at 5-year follow-up.

Despite these high rates of impairment, several investigators also remarked on the uneven patterns of intellectual functioning in individuals with autism (Bartak and Rutter 1976; DeMyer et al. 1974; DeMyer 1975), suggesting that full-scale IQ estimates may not adequately represent the abilities of individuals with autism. Similarly, it has long been noted that in many cases standardized testing may not provide valid estimates of true abilities due to difficulties with cooperation and attention to task demands (Gillies 1965; Hermelin and O'Connor 1964; Hingtgen and Bryson 1972; Whittam et al. 1966).

Following the publication of Wing's 1981 paper describing the clinical features of a series of cases with Asperger syndrome, there was a growing interest in the study of individuals with autism and higher cognitive abilities. Along with this, came increasing recognition of autism as a spectrum that encompasses wide variation in both symptoms and cognitive ability (Wing 1991). With the English translation of Asperger's 1944 paper (Asperger and Frith 1991), and particularly after the inclusion of Asperger's disorder as a discrete diagnosis in DSM-IV (American Psychiatric Association 1994), there was a corresponding increase in research on high-functioning individuals with autism (Ehlers et al. 1997). In fact, over the past decade, the shift in focus toward examination of higher functioning individuals has been marked. Despite the fact that intellectual disability commonly co-occurs in a large percentage of the autism population, a substantial proportion of recent research studies have specifically excluded individuals with low IQ. Notably, in a review of all studies published in the *Journal of Autism and Neurodevelopmental Disorders* in 2008, Dykens and Lense (2011) found that 77 % of the studies of children and 90 % of the studies of adults with autism included participants with high IQ only. This trend is concerning, as it highlights the potential lack of generalizability of findings to the broader population of individuals with autism.

From this brief historical overview, it is clear that intellectual functioning will continue to be an important area of inquiry for future research among individuals with autism (Matson and Shoemaker 2009), particularly as it may relate to distinct phenotypic subtypes and etiologies (Charman et al. 2011; Munson et al. 2008). However, efforts are needed in future research to ensure that samples include the full range of intellectual ability, including those with low IQ.

Medical Comorbidities

Scientific and clinical awareness of co-occurring medical conditions in individuals with autism has also shifted significantly over time. Although Kanner and others initially asserted that children with autism were generally healthy and unaffected by medical problems (Kanner 1949), subsequent research has led to the current understanding that autism is frequently accompanied by medical comorbidities (Bauman 2010). Of these, seizure disorders, gastrointestinal (GI) problems, and sleep problems are among the most prevalent. As will be discussed, the timing of historical recognition of these co-occurring conditions has varied significantly across specific problem types.

Seizures

Seizure disorders are among the most widely recognized medical comorbidities in individuals with autism (Tuchman and Cuccaro 2011; Tuchman et al. 2013), and have been recognized since the very early accounts of the disorder. Although he asserted that the majority of his patients had no major medical conditions, Kanner (1943) reported that at least one patient in his initial sample and one patient in a larger clinical sample (1954) had a history of seizures.

Subsequent research published throughout the 1960s documented much higher rates of seizures among children with autism, although prevalence varied substantially across studies. In a long-term follow-up study of children presenting to Maudsley Hospital Children's Department between 1950 and 1958, Rutter and colleagues found that 3 % of the children with autism had a prior history of seizures, and 16 % developed seizures during the follow-up period. An additional 16 % demonstrated some evidence of abnormalities on EEG (Rutter et al. 1967; Rutter and Lockyer 1967). Across other studies from this time period, the prevalence of seizure history ranged from as low as 12 % (Creak 1963) to as high as 42 % (Schain and Yannet 1960). Even higher rates of EEG abnormalities were observed, ranging from 58 to 83 % of the children with autism across samples described during this period (Creak and Pampiglione 1969; Hinton 1963; White et al. 1964).

In the following decades, additional case studies increasingly remarked on the co-occurrence of seizures and autism (Mnukhin et al. 1975; Taft and Cohen 1971), leading many to conclude that epilepsy may indicate an "organic neurological basis" for the syndrome (Mnukhin et al. 1975). Deykin and MacMahon (1979) reported that the incidence of seizures among individuals with autism was between 3 and 28 times that of the typical population. In a sample of 183 children with autism, the prevalence of seizures was 12.6 %, and the cumulative risk of developing seizures before 18 years of age was 23 %. In a population-based study, Olsson et al. (1988) found a 27 % prevalence of epilepsy among 52 young children with autism. More recently, Volkmar and Nelson (1990) found similar prevalence rates in a large sample referred for specialized developmental assessment over an 8-year period. The prevalence of seizure disorder was reported to be 21 % among their sample of 192 individuals with autism, and evidence of abnormal EEG was found in 24 % of the sample without diagnosed seizure disorder.

These earlier findings have led to continued research into the co-occurrence of seizures and autism from the 1990s to the present. This has led to a much better understanding of the prevalence of co-occurring seizure disorders across a wide range of age and autism severity (Bolton et al. 2011; Canitano 2007; Danielsson et al. 2005) and a better characterization of risk factors and correlates of this comorbidity (Amiet et al. 2008; Spence and Schneider 2009; Viscidi et al. 2013). As a result, a priority for current and future research will be to uncover potential risk factors and mechanisms giving rise to both (Gilby and O'Brien 2013; Tuchman et al. 2009).

Gastrointestinal Problems

Although seizure disorders have arguably received the most attention, other medical comorbidities in individuals with autism have been increasingly identified in recent years. As a case in point, high rates of GI problems among children with autism have received growing attention in the scientific literature (Coury et al. 2012). However, there is some evidence that these problems have been observed anecdotally for some time by clinicians and clinical investigators (Buhrmann 1966; Colbert and Koegler 1958; Fish 1959; Goodwin et al. 1971; Nichtern 1965). For example, Nichtern (1965) noted that children with autism "have an unusually high incidence of histories of colic, vomiting, nonspecific diarrhea, constipation, obstipation and soiling" (p. 190). However, these observations were not carefully documented or systematically examined until recently.

A few studies began to report on GI problems in children with autism during the 1990s. For example, Dalrymple and Ruble (1992) reported a high rate of parent-reported constipation (41 %) in their sample of 100 individuals with autism. D'Eufemia et al. (1996) were also among the first to specifically report on intestinal problems in a small sample of 21 children with autism, and Horvath et al. (1998) provided a case report of three patients with chronic diarrhea. Shortly thereafter, Horvath et al. (1999) also reported on a larger sample of 36 children with autism who were referred for GI symptoms. The study found high rates of reflux esophagitis (69 %), chronic gastritis (42 %) and chronic duodenitis (67 %) among this clinically referred group. Although some additional studies were conducted in the years following (see (Erickson et al. 2005; Horvath and Perman 2002), a more concerted effort to study the prevalence of these problems was not undertaken until the past decade. Since that time, there has been a growing interest in examining the nature and treatment of this comorbid condition. Even so, a number of unanswered questions remain, particularly with regard to accurate prevalence estimates and the underlying nature and etiology of GI dysfunction in this population (Buie et al. 2010; Coury et al., 2012).

Sleep Problems

Sleep problems are another common medical problem in individuals with autism (Couturier et al. 2005; Krakowiak et al. 2008; Miano et al. 2007; Souders et al. 2009), yet specific research into this comorbidity is also relatively recent. Although earlier clinical accounts mentioned sleep disturbance as being a common problem in children with autism (Gillberg 1989; Rapin 1991; Vorster 1960; Wing 1976), specific studies of this co-occurrence were not conducted until the mid-1980s and early 1990s. In one of the first such studies, Hoshino et al. (1984) examined patterns of sleep disturbance among 75 children with autism and found that 65 % experienced sleep problems. In a sample of 39 children with autism, Richdale and Prior (1995) also found that sleep problems were very common, often severe in nature, and much more likely than among children without autism.

These initial studies were followed by several subsequent studies examining the prevalence of sleep problems in the autism population (Patzold et al. 1998; Richdale 1999; Stores and Wiggs 1998). These studies also revealed a high prevalence of sleep disturbance among children with autism, leading to increased interest in understanding and addressing the problem. As a result, the past decade has seen a proliferation of research on the nature, treatment, and potential causal mechanisms of sleep problems among children with autism (Johnson and Malow 2008; Malow et al. 2006; Malow and McGrew 2008). Continued research into the pathophysiology of sleep problems in individuals with autism may also offer information about the relationship between these and other co-occurring medical and behavioral problems.

Comorbid Psychopathology

In contrast to the study of medical and neurological conditions in autism, the specific study of comorbid psychiatric disorders and symptoms in individuals with autism is much more recent (de Bruin et al. 2007; Leyfer et al. 2006; Matson and Cervantes 2014; Matson and Williams 2014; Simonoff et al. 2008). However, even the earliest descriptions of children with autism referred to many symptoms that are representative of both internalizing symptoms and disruptive behaviors.

Anxiety

Kanner's (1943) initial descriptions of patients with autism included clearly documented symptoms of anxiety. For example, specific phobias (i.e., tricycles and swings, egg beaters and elevators, wind and large animals, running water, gas burners, mechanical objects) were observed in 6 of 11 patients and frequent "worrying" was noted in one patient. In later publications, Kanner characterized some of the core behavioral features of autism as being marked by "an anxious obsessive desire for the maintenance of sameness" (Eisenberg and Kanner 1956, p. 557), and noted that some of the restricted and repetitive behaviors were marked by "fear of new patterns." However, other types of fears and worries were not mentioned (Eisenberg and Kanner 1956). Other early discussions of autism, such as those of the 1953 Childhood Schizophrenia Roundtable, emphasized "catastrophic anxiety" as a frequent and notable feature of the disorder (Herskovitz 1954, p. 489).

The work of Creak and colleagues resulted in a list of nine key features that were thought to be characteristics of the disorder. In addition to the symptoms that continue to be considered as "core features" (e.g., impairment in social relatedness, communication impairment, and restricted and repetitive behaviors) this working group also included "excessive and seemingly illogical anxiety" as a primary feature of autism (Creak 1961). However, this criterion disappeared in later diagnostic conceptualizations, whereas ritualized behavior and insistence on sameness continued to be regarded as primary symptoms (e.g., Lotter 1966a).

This lack of consensus regarding anxiety's role in autism persisted over time and may have hindered ongoing research on the topic. Despite this, some investigators continued to report high rates of anxiety when characterizing their samples. For example, Rutter et al. (1967) found evidence of anxiety and fears in a majority (63 %) of the children with autism who were admitted to Maudsley Hospital between 1950 and 1958. More recently, in an investigation of 14 adults with a history of early childhood autism diagnoses, 50 % were reported to have symptoms of generalized anxiety, 14 % had symptoms of separation anxiety, and 7 % had phobic symptoms. However, the authors concluded that these symptoms were "residuals of early autism" rather than evidence of a separate anxiety disorder diagnosis (Rumsey et al. 1985, p. 469). This conclusion has been echoed by many others, which may explain the lack of specific emphasis on anxiety as a clinical feature warranting separate investigation.

Aside from these early observations, specific studies of anxiety in individuals with autism were not published until the 1990s. In the first such study, Matson and Love (1990) found that a greater percentage of children with autism were reported by parents to have specific fears than children without autism. In one of the first studies to examine prevalence of co-occurring anxiety, Muris et al. (1998) found that 84 % of their sample of 44 children with autism also met the criteria for at least one anxiety disorder diagnosis. In the years following, a number of subsequent studies of anxiety in children with autism have been published, with consistently high rates of both anxiety disorder diagnoses (Bellini 2004; Kim et al. 2000; Sukhodolsky et al. 2008) and co-occurring anxiety symptoms (Gillott et al. 2001; Russell and Sofronoff 2005; Tonge et al. 1999; Weisbrot et al. 2005). Since the early 2000s, the literature on anxiety in individuals with autism has increased rapidly, with a focus on both assessment (Grondhuis and Aman 2012; Hallett et al. 2013; Lecavalier et al. 2014) and treatment (Lang et al. 2010; Nadeau et al. 2011; Rudy et al. 2013) of this co-occurring condition.

Despite ever growing research on the topic, investigators continue to grapple with distinguishing anxiety from core autism symptoms. As an example, social anxiety and social disinterest are both characterized behaviorally by social avoidance, making differentiation difficult without careful consideration and assessment of underlying processes (Wood and Gadow 2010). Similarly, distinguishing sensory over-responsivity from anxiety is also difficult, given the overlapping symptoms and associated behavioral responses (Green and Ben-Sasson 2010). Among the primary difficulties are a lack of consensus guidelines, lack of reliable and valid measurement tools for the autism population, and difficulties with self-report. Although multiple modalities and informants are generally recommended for assessing anxiety in children with autism (MacNeil et al. 2009; White et al. 2009; Wood and Gadow 2010), self-report is not always feasible due to communication barriers and difficulties with emotional insight (Losh and Capps 2006; Russell and Sofronoff 2005). Thus, future research will benefit from a continued emphasis on the development of psychometrically sound measurement tools and the development of consensus guidelines for assessment of anxiety in this population. Additional research is also needed to explore the underlying mechanisms of anxiety in individuals with autism as well as how it might relate to other symptoms and associated conditions.

Mood Problems

While anxiety symptoms in individuals with autism have been noted anecdotally for some time, the identification of co-occurring depression and mood difficulties has been quite recent. The early literature on depression in autism consisted of only a handful of case reports. For example, Wing reported a high prevalence of affective problems (30 %) in a series of adults with Asperger's disorder (Wing 1981). A few additional case studies also published in the 1980s documented cases of comorbid mood difficulties. These included symptoms of depression (Clarke et al. 1989; Ghaziuddin and Tsai 1991; Gillberg and Steffenburg 1987; Komoto et al. 1984) and symptoms consistent with bipolar disorder (Gillberg 1985; Komoto et al. 1984).

Ghaziuddin et al. (1992) were the first to specifically report on the prevalence of co-occurring psychiatric disorders in a larger group of children with autism. The results revealed that mood disorder was the most common comorbid diagnosis. Ghaziuddin et al. (1998) continued to examine this co-occurrence among individuals with autism and Asperger's disorder, and since that time, there has been relatively more interest in examining depression and other mood difficulties among individuals with autism (e.g., Ghaziuddin et al. 2002; Lainhart and Folstein 1994; Mayes et al. 2011; Mazefsky et al. 2008; Sterling et al. 2008; Stewart et al. 2006). On the whole, though, mood problems are a markedly understudied type of comorbidity in individuals with autism. It is likely that many of the same measurement issues that have posed problems for the study of anxiety in autism also present barriers for the study of depression and other mood difficulties.

Disruptive Behaviors

Co-occurring disruptive behaviors, including aggression, challenging behavior, and impulsivity/hyperactivity have received some attention in the literature; however, the majority of historical research on these problems has focused on treatment rather than characterizing their prevalence or correlates (see for review Horner et al. 2002; Machalicek et al. 2007; Matson 2009).

Disruptive behaviors have been noted since the early writings on autism. For example, Kanner (1943) described disruptive behaviors (i.e., temper tantrums) in one of his initial 11 patients with autism, and Asperger (1944) also reported significant disruptive behaviors (i.e., hyperactivity, impulsivity, property destruction, aggression) among 3 of the 4 children he characterized. Rutter and Lockyer (1967) also found evidence of significant behavioral disturbance in their early sample of children with autism, including aggression (43 %) and temper tantrums (78 %). Other case studies also documented frequent aggressive behaviors, often in response to interruption of repetitive behaviors or rituals (Eveloff 1960; Loomis 1960).

A number of early autism treatment studies focused on addressing aggression and challenging behaviors. These were comprised largely of case studies and single-subject designs focused on the treatment of aggression and self-injury (Jensen and Womack 1967; Lehman et al. 1957; Lovaas 1967; Risley 1968; Wetzel et al. 1966). These studies provided the basis for a rich body of clinical research on behavioral approaches for assessing the functions of problem behavior and for addressing and reducing problem behavior (see (Matson 2009; Matson et al. 1996).

However, large-scale studies to examine the prevalence and nature of disruptive behaviors across the autism population were not published during this time period.

In more recent years, there has been a growing interest in characterizing the nature and scope of the problem in children with autism. An increasing number of studies have shown high rates of co-occurring disruptive behavior problems among larger samples of individuals with autism across ages and functional level (Brereton et al. 2006; Eisenhower et al. 2005; Hartley et al. 2008; Kanne and Mazurek 2011; Lecavalier 2006; Mazurek et al. 2013). Along with the changes to nomenclature in DSM-5, which now permit concurrent diagnoses of ASD and ADHD (American Psychiatric Association 2013), the development of valid measures for assessing disruptive behaviors in the autism population (Farmer and Aman 2011; Matson et al. 2008; Matson and Nebel-Schwalm 2007) will likely enhance continued research and clinical practice in this area. Future research is needed to further characterize the nature and type of disruptive behaviors demonstrated by individuals with autism, and to determine the extent to which they relate to other clusters of symptoms. In addition, understanding the neurobiological underpinnings of these disruptive behaviors may offer insights into potential treatments.

Conclusions

As illustrated by this historical overview, much progress has been made over the past several decades in understanding and characterizing the nature of the conditions that often co-occur with autism. Changes over time in diagnostic classification have affected trends in the study of these co-occurring conditions, and continued research in this area will be essential. It is now widely recognized that autism is not a single disorder with a single cause, but a phenotypic expression of multiple underlying genetic etiologies (Abrahams and Geschwind 2008; Betancur 2011). As such, comorbidity has important implications for both etiology and treatment of autism. A better characterization of these co-occurring sets of symptoms may lead to the identification of etiologically distinct subtypes of autism. Co-occurrence patterns may reflect distinct etiologies with distinct genetic underpinnings and brain mechanisms. In addition, understanding and characterizing comorbid symptoms have direct implications for targeted treatments.

Future research should include continued emphasis on careful characterization of the full range of co-occurring symptoms and conditions in individuals with autism. Rather than simply controlling for these conditions through exclusionary criteria or in statistical analyses, investigators should seek to better understand potential differences in subpopulations of individuals based on their symptom clusters and profiles. Given the heterogeneity of the disorder and the identification of increasingly greater numbers of genetic abnormalities across the autism spectrum (Abrahams and Geschwind 2008; Betancur 2011), this approach may hold promise for identifying subtype-specific etiological mechanisms, outcomes, and treatments. Overall, the field has made significant progress in appreciating the wide variety of comorbid conditions experienced by individuals with autism. Current and future research on comorbidity promises to provide important clues regarding the pathophysiology of autism.

References

Abrahams, B. S., & Geschwind, D. H. (2008). Advances in autism genetics: On the threshold of a new neurobiology. *Nature Reviews Genetics, 9,* 341–355.

Alpern, G. D., & Kimberlin, C. C. (1970). Short intelligence test ranging from infancy levels through childhood levels for use with the retarded. *American Journal of Mental Deficiency, 75*(1), 65–71.

American Psychiatric Association. (1952). *Diagnostic and statistical manual of mental disorders.* Washington, DC: American Psychiatric Association.

American Psychiatric Association. (1968). *Diagnostic and statistical manual of mental disorders—second edition (DSM-II).* Washington, DC: American Psychiatric Association.

American Psychiatric Association. (1980). *Diagnostic and statistical manual of mental disorders—third edition (DSM-III).* Washington, DC: American Psychiatric Association.

American Psychiatric Association. (1987). *Diagnostic and statistical manual of mental disorders, third edition revised (DSM-III-R).* Washington, DC.

American Psychiatric Association. (1994). *Diagnostic and statistical manual of mental disorders* (4th edn.). Washington, DC: American Psychiatric Publishing.

American Psychiatric Association. (2000). *Diagnostic and statistical manual of mental disorders—fourth edition, text revision.* Washington, DC: American Psychiatric Association.

American Psychiatric Association. (2013). *Diagnostic and statistical manual of mental disorders, fifth edition (DSM-5).* Washington, DC: American Psychiatric Association.

Amiet, C., Gourfinkel-An, I., Bouzamondo, A., Tordjman, S., Baulac, M., Lechat, P., et al. (2008). Epilepsy in autism is associated with intellectual disability and gender: Evidence from a meta-analysis. *Biological Psychiatry, 64*(7), 577–582. doi:10.1016/j.biopsych.2008.04.030.

Asperger, H. (1944). Die 'Autistischen Psychopathen' im Kindesalter. *Archiv fur Psychiatrie und Nervenkrankheiten, 117*(1), 76–136.

Asperger, H., & Frith, U. (1991). *'Autistic psychopathy' in childhood Autism and Asperger syndrome* (pp. 37–92). New York: Cambridge University Press.

Bartak, L., & Rutter, M. (1976). Differences between mentally retarded and normally intelligent autistic children. *Journal of Autism and Childhood Schizophrenia, 6*(2), 109–120.

Bauman, M. (2010). Medical comorbidities in autism: Challenges to diagnosis and treatment. *Neurotherapeutics, 7*(3), 320–327. doi:10.1016/j.nurt.2010.06.001.

Bellini, S. (2004). Social skill deficits and anxiety in high-functioning adolescents with autism spectrum disorders. *Focus on Autism and Other Developmental Disabilities, 19*(2), 78–86. doi:10.1177/10883576040190020201.

Benson, P. R., & Karlof, K. L. (2008). Child, parent, and family predictors of latter adjustment in siblings of children with autism. *Research in Autism Spectrum Disorders, 2*(4), 583–600.

Betancur, C. (2011). Etiological heterogeneity in autism spectrum disorders: More than 100 genetic and genomic disorders and still counting. *Brain Research, 1380*(0), 42–77. doi:10.1016/j.brainres.2010.11.078.

Bleuler, E. (1911). Dementia praecox oder Gruppe der Schizophrenien. In G. Aschaffenburg (Ed.), *Handbuch der Psychiatrie. Spezieller Teil. 4. Abteilung, 1. Hälfte.* Leipzig und Wien: Franz Deuticke.

Blumberg, S. J., Bramlett, M. D., Kogan, M. D., et al. (2013). Changes in prevalence of parentreported autism spectrum disorder in school-aged U.S. children: 2007 to 2011–2012. *National health statistics reports;* No. 65. Hyattsville,: MD National Center for Health Statistics.

Bolton, P. F., Carcani-Rathwell, I., Hutton, J., Goode, S., Howlin, P., & Rutter, M. (2011). Epilepsy in autism: Features and correlates. *The British Journal of Psychiatry, 198*(4), 289–294. doi:10.1192/bjp.bp.109.076877.

Brereton, A. V., Tonge, B. J., & Einfeld, S. L. (2006). Psychopathology in children and adolescents with autism compared to young people with intellectual disability. *Journal of Autism and Developmental Disorders, 36*(7), 863–870. doi:10.1007/s10803-006-0125-y.

Bromley, B. E., & Blacher, J. (1991). Parental reasons for out-of-home placement of children with severe handicaps. *Mental Retardation, 29,* 275–280.

de Bruin, E., Ferdinand, R., Meester, S., de Nijs, P., & Verheij, F. (2007). High rates of psychiatric co-morbidity in PDD-NOS. *Journal of Autism and Developmental Disorders, 37*(5), 877–886.

Buhrmann, M. B. (1966). Childhood schizophrenia. *South African Medical Journal, 40*(38), 920–923.

Buie, T., Campbell, D. B., Fuchs, G. J., Furuta, G. T., Levy, J., VandeWater, J., et al. (2010). Evaluation, diagnosis, and treatment of gastrointestinal disorders in individuals with ASDs: A consensus report. *Pediatrics, 125*(Suppl. 1), S1-S18. doi:10.1542/peds.2009-1878C.

Canitano, R. (2007). Epilepsy in autism spectrum disorders. *European Child and Adolescent Psychiatry, 16*(1), 61–66.

Carr, E. G., Taylor, J. C., & Robinson, S. (1991). The effects of severe behavior problems in children on the teaching behavior of adults. *Journal of Applied Behavior Analysis, 24*(3), 523–535. doi:10.1901/jaba.1991.24–523.

Charman, T., Jones, C. R. G., Pickles, A., Simonoff, E., Baird, G., & Happé, F. (2011). Defining the cognitive phenotype of autism. *Brain Research, 1380*(0), 10–21. doi:10.1016/j.brainres.2010.10.075.

Chess, S. (1971). Autism in children with congenital rubella. *Journal of Autism and Childhood Schizophrenia, 1*(1), 33–47. doi:10.1007/BF01537741.

Chess, S., Fernandez, P. B., & Korn, S. J. (1978). Behavioral consequences of congenital rubella. *Journal of Pediatrics, 93,* 699–703.

Clarke, D. J., LittleJohns, C. S., Corbett, J. A., & Joseph, S. (1989). Pervasive developmental disorders and psychoses in adult life. *The British Journal of Psychiatry, 155*(5), 692–699. doi:10.1192/bjp.155.5.692.

Colbert, E. G., & Koegler, R. R. (1958). Diagnosis of schizophrenia in young children. *California Medicine, 89*(3), 215–216.

Coury, D. L., Ashwood, P., Fasano, A., Fuchs, G., Geraghty, M., Kaul, A., et al. (2012). Gastrointestinal conditions in children with autism spectrum disorder: Developing a research agenda. *Pediatrics, 130*(Suppl. 2), S160-S168. doi:10.1542/peds.2012-0900N.

Couturier, J. L., Speechley, K. N., Steele, M., Norman, R., Stringer, B., & Nicolson, R. (2005). Parental perception of sleep problems in children of normal intelligence with pervasive developmental disorders: Prevalence, severity, and pattern. *Journal of the American Academy of Child and Adolescent Psychiatry, 44*(8), 815–822.

Creak, E. M. (1961). Schizophrenic syndrome in childhood. *British Medical Journal, 2,* 889–890.

Creak, E. M. (1963). Childhood psychosis: A review of 100 cases. *The British Journal of Psychiatry, 109*(458), 84–89. doi:10.1192/bjp.109.458.84.

Creak, E. M. (1964). Schizophrenic Syndrome in Childhood: Further Progress Report of a Working Party (April, 1964). *Developmental medicine and child neurology, 6,* 530–535.

Creak, M., & Pampiglione, G. (1969). Clinical and EEG studies on a group of 35 psychotic children. *Developmental Medicine and Child Neurology, 11*(2), 218–227.

Dalrymple, N., & Ruble, L. (1992). Toilet training and behaviors of people with autism: Parent views. *Journal of Autism and Developmental Disorders, 22*(2), 265–275. doi:10.1007/BF01058155.

Danielsson, S., Gillberg, I. C., Billstedt, E., Gillberg, C., & Olsson, I. (2005). Epilepsy in young adults with autism: A prospective population-based follow-up study of 120 individuals diagnosed in childhood. *Epilepsia, 46*(6), 918–923. doi:10.1111/j.1528–1167.2005.57504.x.

DeMyer, M. K. (1975). The nature of the neuropsychological disability in autistic children. *Journal of Autism and Childhood Schizophrenia, 5*(2), 109–128. doi:10.1007/BF01537928.

DeMyer, M., Barton, S., Alpern, G., Kimberlin, C., Allen, J., Yang, E., et al. (1974). The measured intelligence of autistic children. *Journal of Autism and Childhood Schizophrenia, 4*(1), 42–60.

D'Eufemia, P., Celli, M., Finocchiaro, R., Pacifico, L., Viozzi, L., Zaccagnini, M., et al. (1996). Abnormal intestinal permeability in children with autism. *Acta Paediatrica, 85*(9), 1076–1079. doi:10.1111/j.1651–2227.1996.tb14220.x.

Deykin, E. Y., & MacMahon, B. (1979). The incidence of seizures among children with autistic symptoms. *The American Journal of Psychiatry, 136*(10), 1310–1312.

Douglas, V., & Sanders, F. A. (1968). A pilot study of Rimland's diagnostic check list with autistic and mentally retarded children. *Journal of Child Psychology and Psychiatry, 9*(2), 105–109.

Dykens, E., & Lense, M. (2011). Intellectual disabilities and autism spectrum disorder: a cautionary note. In D. G. Amaral, G. Dawson, & D. H. Geschwind (Eds.), *Autism spectrum disorders* (pp. 261–269). New York, NY: Oxford University Press.

Ehlers, S., Nydén, A., Gillberg, C., Sandberg, A. D., Dahlgren, S.-O., Hjelmquist, E., et al. (1997). Asperger syndrome, autism and attention disorders: A comparative study of the cognitive profiles of 120 children. *Journal of Child Psychology and Psychiatry, 38*(2), 207–217. doi:10.1111/j.1469–7610.1997.tb01855.x.

Eisenberg, L. (1966). The classification of the psychotic disorders in childhood. In L. D. Eron (Ed.), *Classification of behavior disorders* (pp. 87–122). Chicago: Aldine Publishing Company.

Eisenberg, L., & Kanner, L. (1956). Childhood schizophrenia: Symposium, 1955: 6. Early infantile autism, 1943–55. *American Journal of Orthopsychiatry, 26*(3), 556–566. doi:10.1111/j.1939-0025.1956.tb06202.x.

Eisenhower, A. S., Baker, B. L., & Blacher, J. (2005). Preschool children with intellectual disability: Syndrome specificity, behaviour problems, and maternal well-being. *Journal of Intellectual Disability Research, 49*(9), 657–671. doi:10.1111/j.1365-2788.2005.00699.x.

Erickson, C., Stigler, K., Corkins, M., Posey, D., Fitzgerald, J., & McDougle, C. (2005). Gastrointestinal factors in autistic disorder: A critical review. *Journal of Autism and Developmental Disorders, 35*(6), 713–727. doi:10.1007/s10803-005-0019-4.

Estes, A., Munson, J., Dawson, G., Koehler, E., Zhou, X. H., & Abbott, R. (2009). Parenting stress and psychological functioning among mothers of preschool children with autism and developmental delay. *Autism: the international journal of research and practice, 13*(4), 375–387.

Eveloff, H. H. (1960). The autistic child. *Archives of General Psychiatry, 3*(1), 66–81. doi:10.1001/archpsyc.1960.01710010068010.

Farmer, C. A., & Aman, M. G. (2011). Aggressive behavior in a sample of children with autism spectrum disorders. *Research in Autism Spectrum Disorders, 5*(1), 317–323.

Fish, B. (1959). Longitudinal observations of biological deviations in a schizophrenic infant. *The American Journal of Psychiatry, 116*, 25–31.

Fombonne, E. (2009). Epidemiology of pervasive developmental disorders. *Pediatric research, 65*(6), 591–598. doi:10.1203/PDR.0b013e31819e7203.

Frith, U. (2004). Emanuel Miller lecture: Confusions and controversies about Asperger syndrome. *Journal of Child Psychology and Psychiatry, 45*(4), 672–686. doi:10.1111/j.1469-7610.2004.00262.x.

Ganz, M. L. (2007). The lifetime distribution of the incremental societal costs of autism. *Archives of Pediatrics and Adolescent Medicine, 161*(4), 343–349. doi:10.1001/archpedi.161.4.343.

Garner, W. A., Strohmer, D. C., Langford, C. A., & Boas, G. J. (1994). Diagnostic and treatment overshadowing bias across disabilities: Are rehabilitation professionals immune? *Journal of Applied Rehabilitation Counseling, 25*(2), 33–37.

Ghaziuddin, M., & Tsai, L. (1991). Depression in autistic disorder. *The British Journal of Psychiatry, 159*(5), 721–723. doi:10.1192/bjp.159.5.721.

Ghaziuddin, M., Tsai, L., & Ghaziuddin, N. (1992). Comorbidity of autistic disorder in children and adolescents. *European Child and Adolescent Psychiatry, 1*(4), 209–213. doi:10.1007/BF02094180.

Ghaziuddin, M., Weidmer-Mikhail, E., & Ghaziuddin, N. (1998). Comorbidity of Asperger syndrome: A preliminary report. *Journal of Intellectual Disability Research, 42*(4), 279–283.

Ghaziuddin, M., Ghaziuddin, N., & Greden, J. (2002). Depression in persons with autism: Implications for research and clinical care. *Journal of Autism and Developmental Disorders, 32*(4), 299–306.

Gilby, K. L., & O'Brien, T. J. (2013). Epilepsy, autism, and neurodevelopment: Kindling a shared vulnerability? *Epilepsy and Behavior, 26*(3), 370–374. doi:10.1016/j.yebeh.2012.11.002.

Gillberg, C. (1985). Asperger's syndrome and recurrent psychosis—A case study. *Journal of Autism and Developmental Disorders, 15*(4), 389–397. doi:10.1007/BF01531783.

Gillberg, C. (1988). The neurobiology of infantile autism. *Journal of Child Psychology and Psychiatry, 29*(3), 257–266.

Gillberg, C. (1989). Early symptoms in autism. In C. Gillberg (Ed.), *Diagnosis and treatment of autism* (pp. 23–32). New York: Plenum Press.

Gillberg, C., & Steffenburg, S. (1987). Outcome and prognostic factors in infantile autism and similar conditions: A population-based study of 46 cases followed through puberty. *Journal of Autism and Developmental Disorders, 17*(2), 273–287.

Gillies, S. (1965). Some abilities of psychotic children and subnormal controls. *Journal of Intellectual Disability Research, 9*(2), 89–101.

Gillott, A., Furniss, F., & Walter, A. (2001). Anxiety in high-functioning children with autism. *Autism: the international journal of research and practice, 5*(3), 277–286. doi:10.1177/1362361301005003005.

Gittelman, M., & Birch, H. G. (1967). Childhood schizophrenia: Intellect, neurologic status, perinatal risk, prognosis, and family pathology. *Archives of General Psychiatry, 17*(1), 16–25.

Goldfarb, W. (1961). *Childhood Schizophrenia*. Cambridge: Harvard University Press.

Goodwin, M., Goodwin, T. C., & Cowen, M. (1971). Malabsorption and cerebral dysfunction: A multivariate and comparative study of autistic children. *Journal of Autism and Childhood Schizophrenia, 1*(1), 48–62. doi:10.1007/BF01537742.

Green, S., & Ben-Sasson, A. (2010). Anxiety disorders and sensory over-responsivity in children with autism spectrum disorders: Is there a causal relationship? *Journal of Autism and Developmental Disorders, 40*(12), 1495–1504.

Grondhuis, S. N., & Aman, M. G. (2012). Assessment of anxiety in children and adolescents with autism spectrum disorders. *Research in Autism Spectrum Disorders, 6*(4), 1345–1365. doi:10.1016/j.rasd.2012.04.006.

Grzadzinski, R., Huerta, M., & Lord, C. (2013). DSM-5 and autism spectrum disorders (ASDs): An opportunity for identifying ASD subtypes. *Molecular Autism, 4*(12), 1–6.

Hallett, V., Lecavalier, L., Sukhodolsky, D., Cipriano, N., Aman, M., McCracken, J., et al. (2013). Exploring the manifestations of anxiety in children with autism spectrum disorders. *Journal of Autism and Developmental Disorders, 43*(10), 2341–2352. doi:10.1007/s10803-013-1775-1.

Hartley, S. L., Sikora, D. M., & McCoy, R. (2008). Prevalence and risk factors of maladaptive behaviour in young children with Autistic Disorder. *Journal of Intellectual Disability Research, 52*(10), 819–829.

Hastings, R. P., & Brown, T. (2002). Coping strategies and the impact of challenging behaviors on special educators' burnout. *Mental Retardation, 40*(2), 148–156. doi:10.1352/0047-6765(2002)040<0148:CSATIO>2.0.CO;2.

Hermelin, B., & O'Connor, N. (1964). Crossmodal transfer in normal, subnormal and autistic children. *Neuropsychologia, 2*(3), 229–235.

Herskovitz, H. H. (1954). Childhood Schizophrenia Round Table, 1953. *American Journal of Orthopsychiatry, 24*(3), 484–528.

Hingtgen, J. N., & Bryson, C. Q. (1972). Recent developments in the study of early childhood psychoses. *Schizophrenia Bulletin, 1*(5), 8–54.

Hinton, G. G. (1963). Childhood psychosis or mental retardation: A diagnostic dilemma II. Pediatric and neurological aspects. *Canadian Medical Association Journal, 89*, 1020–1024.

Horner, R., Carr, E., Strain, P., Todd, A., & Reed, H. (2002). Problem behavior interventions for young children with autism: A research synthesis. *Journal of Autism and Developmental Disorders, 32*(5), 423–446. doi:10.1023/A:1020593922901.

Horvath, K., & Perman, J. A. (2002). Autism and gastrointestinal symptoms. *Current Gastroenterology Reports, 4*(3), 251–258.

Horvath, K., Stefanatos, G., Sokolski, K. N., Wachtel, R., Nabors, L., & Tildon, J. T. (1998). Improved social and language skills after secretin administration in patients with autistic spectrum disorders. *Journal of the Association for Academic Minority Physicians: The official publication of the Association for Academic Minority Physicians, 9*(1), 9–15.

Horvath, K., Papadimitriou, J. C., Rabsztyn, A., Drachenberg, C., & Tildon, J. T. (1999). Gastrointestinal abnormalities in children with autistic disorder. *The Journal of Pediatrics, 135*(5), 559–563.

Hoshino, Y., Watanabe, H., Yashima, Y., Kaneko, M., & Kumashiro, H. (1984). An investigation on sleep disturbance of autistic children. *Psychiatry and Clinical Neurosciences, 38*(1), 45–51. doi:10.1111/j.1440-1819.1984.tb00353.x.

Jensen, G. D., & Womack, M. G. (1967). Operant conditioning techniques applied in the treatment of an autistic child. *American Journal of Orthopsychiatry, 37*(1), 30–34. doi:10.1111/j.1939-0025.1967.tb01064.x.

Johnson, K., & Malow, B. (2008). Sleep in children with autism spectrum disorders. *Current Treatment Options in Neurology, 10*(5), 350–359.

Kanne, S., & Mazurek, M. (2011). Aggression in children and adolescents with ASD: Prevalence and risk factors. *Journal of Autism and Developmental Disorders, 41*(7), 926–937.

Kanner, L. (1943). Autistic disturbances of affective contact. *Nervous Child, 2,* 217–253.

Kanner, L. (1949). Problems of nosology and psychodynamics of early infantile autism. *American Journal of Orthopsychiatry, 19*(3), 416–426.

Kanner, L. (1954). To what extent is early infantile autism determined by constitutional inadequacies? *Research Publications—Association for Research in Nervous and Mental Disease, 33,* 378–385.

Kim, J. A., Szatmari, P., Bryson, S. E., Streiner, D. L., & Wilson, F. J. (2000). The prevalence of anxiety and mood problems among children with autism and Asperger syndrome. *Autism: the international journal of research and practice, 4*(2), 117–132. doi:10.1177/1362361300004002002.

Kogan, M. D., Strickland, B. B., Blumberg, S. J., Singh, G. K., Perrin, J. M., & van Dyck, P. C. (2008). A national profile of the health care experiences and family impact of autism spectrum disorder among children in the United States, 2005–2006. *Pediatrics, 122*(6), e1149–e1158. doi:10.1542/peds.2008-1057.

Kogan, M. D., Blumberg, S. J., Schieve, L. A., Boyle, C. A., Perrin, J. M., Ghandour, R. M., et al. (2009). Prevalence of the Autism Spectrum Disorders in multiple areas of the United States, surveillance years 2000 and 2002 Prevalence of parent-reported diagnosis of autism spectrum disorder among children in the US, 2007. *Pediatrics, 124,* 1395–1403.

Komoto, J., Usui, S., & Hirata, J. (1984). Infantile autism and affective disorder. *Journal of Autism and Developmental Disorders, 14*(1), 81–84. doi:10.1007/BF02408557.

Krakowiak, P., Goodlin-Jones, B., Hertz-Picciotto, I., Croen, L. A., & Hansen, R. L. (2008). Sleep problems in children with autism spectrum disorders, developmental delays, and typical development: A population-based study. *Journal of Sleep Research, 17*(2), 197–206.

Van Krevelen, A. (1958). Problematlk des Autisms. *Prax. Kinderpsychol, 7,* 4.

Lainhart, J. E., & Folstein, S. E. (1994). Affective disorders in people with autism: A review of published cases. *Journal of Autism and Developmental Disorders, 24*(5), 587–601.

Lakin, K. C. (1983). New admissions and readmissions to a national sample of public residential facilities. *American Journal of Mental Deficiency, 88*(1), 13–20.

Lang, R., Regester, A., Lauderdale, S., Ashbaugh, K., & Haring, A. (2010). Treatment of anxiety in autism spectrum disorders using cognitive behaviour therapy: A systematic review. *Developmental Neurorehabilitation, 13*(1), 53–63. doi:10.3109/17518420903236288.

Lecavalier, L. (2006). Behavioral and emotional problems in young people with pervasive developmental disorders: Relative prevalence, effects of subject characteristics, and empirical classification. *Journal of Autism and Developmental Disorders, 36*(8), 1101–1114.

Lecavalier, L., Leone, S., & Wiltz, J. (2006). The impact of behaviour problems on caregiver stress in young people with autism spectrum disorders. *Journal of Intellectual Disability Research: JIDR, 50*(Pt 3), 172–183.

Lecavalier, L., Wood, J. J., Halladay, A. K., Jones, N. E., Aman, M. G., Cook, E., et al. (2014). Measuring anxiety as a treatment endpoint in youth with autism spectrum disorder. *Journal of Autism and Developmental Disorders, 44*(5), 1128–1143. doi:10.1007/s10803-013-1974-9.

Lehman, E., Haber, J., & Lesser, S. (1957). The use of reserpine in autistic children. *The Journal of Nervous and Mental Disease, 125*(3), 351–356.
Levitan, G. W., & Reiss, S. (1983). Generality of diagnostic overshadowing across disciplines. *Applied Research in Mental Retardation, 4*(1), 59–64.
Leyfer, O. T., Folstein, S. E., Bacalman, S., Davis, N. O., Dinh, E., Morgan, J., et al. (2006). Comorbid psychiatric disorders in children with autism: Interview development and rates of disorders. *Journal of Autism and Developmental Disorders, 36*(7), 849–861.
Liptak, G. S., Stuart, T., & Auinger, P. (2006). Health care utilization and expenditures for children with autism: Data from U.S. national samples. *Journal of Autism and Developmental Disorders, 36*(7), 871–879.
Lockyer, L., & Rutter, M. (1970). A five- to fifteen-year follow-up study of infantile psychosis. IV: Patterns of cognitive ability. *British Journal of Social and Clinical Psychology and Health, 9*(152–163).
Loomis, E. A. Jr. (1960). Autistic and symbiotic syndromes in children. *Monographs of the Society for Research in Child Development, 25*(3), 39–48. doi:10.2307/1165634.
Lord, C., Petkova, E., Hus, V., Gan, W., Lu, F., Martin, D., et al. (2012). A multisite study of the clinical diagnosis of different autism spectrum disorders. *Archives of General Psychiatry, 69*(3), 306–313.
Losh, M., & Capps, L. (2006). Understanding of emotional experience in autism: Insights from the personal accounts of high-functioning children with autism. *Developmental Psychology, 42*(5), 809–818.
Lotter, V. (1966a). Epidemiology of autistic conditions in young children. *Social Psychiatry, 1,* 124–137.
Lotter, V. (1966b). Services for a group of autistic children in Middlesex. In J. K. Wing (Ed.), *Early childhood autism: clinical, educational, and social aspects*. London: Pergamon Press.
Lovaas, O. I. (1967). *A behavior therapy approach to the treatment of childhood schizophrenia.* Paper presented at the Minnesota symposia on child psychology.
Machalicek, W., O'Reilly, M. F., Beretvas, N., Sigafoos, J., & Lancioni, G. E. (2007). A review of interventions to reduce challenging behavior in school settings for students with autism spectrum disorders. *Research in Autism Spectrum Disorders, 1*(3), 229–246. doi:10.1016/j.rasd.2006.10.005.
MacNeil, B. M., Lopes, V. A., & Minnes, P. M. (2009). Anxiety in children and adolescents with autism spectrum disorders. *Research in Autism Spectrum Disorders, 3*(1), 1–21.
Malow, B. A., & McGrew, S. G. (2008). Sleep disturbances and autism. *Sleep Medicine Clinics, 3*(3), 479–488.
Malow, B. A., Marzec, M. L., McGrew, S. G., Wang, L., Henderson, L. M., & Stone, W. L. (2006). Characterizing sleep in children with autism spectrum disorders: A multidimensional approach. *Sleep, 29,* 1563–1571.
Matson, J. (2009). Aggression and tantrums in children with autism: A Review of behavioral treatments and maintaining variables. *Journal of Mental Health Research in Intellectual Disabilities, 2*(3), 169–187. doi:10.1080/19315860902725875.
Matson, J. L., & Cervantes, P. E. (2014). Commonly studied comorbid psychopathologies among persons with autism spectrum disorder. *Research in Developmental Disabilities, 35*(5), 952–962. doi:10.1016/j.ridd.2014.02.012.
Matson, J. L., & Kozlowski, A. M. (2011). The increasing prevalence of autism spectrum disorders. *Research in Autism Spectrum Disorders, 5*(1), 418–425.
Matson, J. L., & Love, S. R. (1990). A comparison of parent-reported fear for autistic and non-handicapped age-matched children and youth. *Journal of Intellectual and Developmental Disability, 16*(4), 349–357. doi:10.1080/07263869000034161.
Matson, J. L., & Nebel-Schwalm, M. (2007). Assessing challenging behaviors in children with autism spectrum disorders: A review. *Research in Developmental Disabilities, 28*(6), 567–579.
Matson, J. L., & Shoemaker, M. (2009). Intellectual disability and its relationship to autism spectrum disorders. *Research in Developmental Disabilities, 30*(6), 1107–1114. doi:10.1016/j.ridd.2009.06.003.

Matson, J. L., & Williams, L. W. (2014). The making of a field: The development of comorbid psychopathology research for persons with intellectual disabilities and autism. *Research in Developmental Disabilities, 35*(1), 234–238. doi:10.1016/j.ridd.2013.09.043.

Matson, J. L., Benavidez, D. A., Stabinsky Compton, L., Paclawskyj, T., & Baglio, C. (1996). Behavioral treatment of autistic persons: A review of research from 1980 to the present. *Research in Developmental Disabilities, 17*(6), 433–465. doi:10.1016/S0891-4222(96)00030-3.

Matson, J. L., Gonzalez, M. L., & Rivet, T. T. (2008). Reliability of the Autism Spectrum Disorder-Behavior Problems for Children (ASD-BPC). *Research in Autism Spectrum Disorders, 2*(4), 696–706.

Mayes, S. D., Calhoun, S. L., Murray, M. J., & Zahid, J. (2011). Variables associated with anxiety and depression in children with autism. *Journal of Developmental and Physical Disabilities, 23*(4), 325–337.

Mazefsky, C. A., Folstein, S. E., & Lainhart, J. E. (2008). Overrepresentation of mood and anxiety disorders in adults with autism and their first-degree relatives: What does it mean? *Autism Research, 1*(3), 193–197.

Mazurek, M. O., Kanne, S. M., & Wodka, E. (2013). Physical aggression in children and adolescents with autism spectrum disorders. *Research in Autism Spectrum Disorders, 7*(3), 455–465.

Miano, S., Bruni, O., Elia, M., Trovato, A., Smerieri, A., Verrillo, E., et al. (2007). Sleep in children with autistic spectrum disorder: A questionnaire and polysomnographic study. *Sleep Medicine, 9*(1), 64–70.

Miller, J. N., & Ozonoff, S. (2000). The external validity of Asperger disorder: Lack of evidence from the domain of neuropsychology. *Journal of Abnormal Psychology, 109*(2), 227–238. doi:10.1037/0021-843X.109.2.227.

Mnukhin, S. S., Isaev, D. N., & O'Tuama, L. (1975). On the organic nature of some forms of schizoid or autistic psychopathy. *Journal of Autism and Childhood Schizophrenia, 5*(2), 99–108.

Munson, J., Dawson, G., Sterling, L., Beauchaine, T., Zhou, A., Koehler, E., et al. (2008). Evidence for latent classes of IQ in young children with autism spectrum disorder. *American Journal on Mental Retardation, 113*(6), 439–452. doi:10.1352/2008.113:439-452.

Muris, P., Steerneman, P., Merckelbach, H., Holdrinet, I., & Meesters, C. (1998). Comorbid anxiety symptoms in children with pervasive developmental disorders. *Journal of Anxiety Disorders, 12*(4), 387–393.

Myers, S. M., & Johnson, C. P. (2007). Management of children with autism spectrum disorders. *Pediatrics, 120*(5), 1162–1182. doi:10.1542/peds.2007-2362.

Nadeau, J., Sulkowski, M. L., Ung, D., Wood, J. J., Lewin, A. B., Murphy, T. K., et al. (2011). Treatment of comorbid anxiety and autism spectrum disorders. *Neuropsychiatry, 1*(6), 567–578. doi:10.2217/npy.11.62.

Nichtern, S. (1965). Developmental disturbances in childhood schizophrenia. *Psychosomatics, 6*(4), 189–191.

Office of Autism Research Coordination (OARC). (2012a). 2010 IACC autism spectrum disorder research portfolio analysis report. U.S. Department of health and human services interagency autism coordinating committee website. http://iacc.hhs.gov/portfolio-analysis/2010/index.shtml: National Institute of Mental Health, Interagency Autism Coordinating Committee (IACC).

Office of Autism Research Coordination (OARC). (2012b). IACC/OARC autism spectrum disorder research publications analysis report: The global landscape of autism research. Department of health and human services interagency autism coordinating committee website. http://iacc.hhs.gov/publications-analysis/july2012/index.shtml.

Olsson, I., Steffenburg, S., & Gillberg, C. (1988). Epilepsy in autism and autisticlike conditions A population-based study. *Archives of Neurology, 45*(6), 666–668.

Ozonoff, S. (2012a). Editorial perspective: Autism spectrum disorders in DSM-5– An historical perspective and the need for change. *Journal of Child Psychology and Psychiatry, 53*(10), 1092–1094. doi:10.1111/j.1469-7610.2012.02614.x.

Ozonoff, S. (2012b). Editorial: DSM-5 and autism spectrum disorders—two decades of perspectives from the JCPP. *Journal of Child Psychology and Psychiatry, 53*(9), e4–e6. doi:10.1111/j.1469-7610.2012.02587.x.

Patzold, L. M., Richdale, A. L., & Tonge, B. J. (1998). An investigation into sleep characteristics of children with autism and Asperger's Disorder. *Journal of Paediatrics and Child Health, 34*(6), 528–533. doi:10.1046/j.1440-1754.1998.00291.x.

Rapin, I. (1991). Autistic children: Diagnosis and clinical features. *Pediatrics, 87*(5), 751–760.

Reiss, S., & Szyszko, J. (1983). Diagnostic overshadowing and professional experience with mentally retarded persons. *American Journal of Mental Deficiency, 87*(4), 396–402.

Rice, C., Nicholas, J., Baio, J., Pettygrove, S., Lee, L.-C., Van Naarden Braun, K., et al. (2010). Changes in autism spectrum disorder prevalence in 4 areas of the United States. *Disability and Health Journal, 3*(3), 186–201. doi:10.1016/j.dhjo.2009.10.008.

Richdale, A. L. (1999). Sleep problems in autism: Prevalence, cause, and intervention. *Developmental Medicine and Child Neurology, 41*(1), 60–66.

Richdale, A., & Prior, M. (1995). The sleep/wake rhythm in children with autism. *European Child and Adolescent Psychiatry, 4*(3), 175–186. doi:10.1007/BF01980456.

Risley, T. R. (1968). The effects and side effects of punishing the autistic behavior of a deviant child. *Journal of applied behavior analysis, 1*(1), 21–34. doi:10.1901/jaba.1968.1–21.

Rosenberg, R. E., Kaufmann, W. E., Law, J. K., & Law, P. A. (2011). Parent report of community psychiatric comorbid diagnoses in autism spectrum disorders. *Autism Research and Treatment, 2011,* 10. doi:10.1155/2011/405849.

Rudy, B. M., Lewin, A. B., & Storch, E. A. (2013). Managing anxiety comorbidity in youth with autism spectrum disorders. *Neuropsychiatry, 3*(4), 411–421. doi:10.2217/npy.13.53.

Rumsey, J. M., Rapoport, J. L., & Sceery, W. R. (1985). Autistic children as adults: Psychiatric, social, and behavioral outcomes. *Journal of the American Academy of Child Psychiatry, 42*(4), 465–473.

Russell, E., & Sofronoff, K. (2005). Anxiety and social worries in children with Asperger syndrome. *Australian and New Zealand Journal of Psychiatry, 39*(7), 633–638.

Rutter, M. (1970). Autistic children: Infancy to adulthood. *Seminars in Psychiatry, 2,* 435–450.

Rutter, M., & Lockyer, L. (1967). A five to fifteen year follow-up study of infantile psychosis: I. Description of sample. *The British Journal of Psychiatry, 113*(504), 1169–1182. doi:10.1192/bjp.113.504.1169.

Rutter, M., Greenfeld, D., & Lockyer, L. (1967). A five to fifteen year follow-up study of infantile psychosis: II. Social and behavioural outcome. *The British Journal of Psychiatry, 113*(504), 1183–1199. doi: 10.1192/bjp.113.504.1183.

Rutter, M., Lebovici, S., Eisenberg, L., Sneznevskij, A. V., Sadoun, R., Brooke, E., et al. (1969). A tri-axial classification of mental disorders in childhood: An international study. *Journal of Child Psychology and Psychiatry, 10,* 41–61.

Rutter, M., Bailey, A., Bolton, P., & Le Couteur, A. (1994). Autism and known medical conditions: Myth and substance. *Journal of Child Psychology and Psychiatry, 35*(2), 311–322. doi:10.1111/j.1469–7610.1994.tb01164.x.

Schain, R. J., & Yannet, H. (1960). Infantile autism: An analysis of 50 cases and a consideration of certain relevant neurophysiologic concepts. *The Journal of Pediatrics, 57*(4), 560–567.

Shoham-Vardi, I., Davidson, P. W., Cain, N. N., Sloane-Reeves, J. E., Giesow, V. E., Quijano, L. E., et al. (1996). Factors predicting re-referral following crisis intervention for community-based persons with developmental disabilities and behavioral and psychiatric disorders. *American Journal on Mental Retardation, 101*(2), 109–117.

Simonoff, E. M., Pickles, A. P., Charman, T. P., Chandler, S. P., Loucas, T. O. M. P., & Baird, G. F. (2008). Psychiatric disorders in children with autism spectrum disorders: Prevalence, comorbidity, and associated factors in a population-derived sample. *Journal of the American Academy of Child & Adolescent Psychiatry, 47*(8), 921–929.

Souders, M. C., Mason, T. B. A., Valladares, O., Bucan, M., Levy, S. E., Mandell, D. S., et al. (2009). Sleep behaviors and sleep quality in children with autism spectrum disorders. *Sleep, 32*(12), 1566–1578.

Spence, S. J., & Schneider, M. T. (2009). The role of epilepsy and epileptiform EEGs in autism spectrum disorders. *Pediatric Research, 65*(6), 599–606.

State, M. W., & Šestan, N. (2012). The emerging biology of autism spectrum disorders. *Science, 337*(6100), 1301–1303. doi:10.1126/science.1224989.

Sterling, L., Dawson, G., Estes, A., & Greenson, J. (2008). Characteristics associated with presence of depressive symptoms in adults with autism spectrum disorder. *Journal of Autism and Developmental Disorders, 38*(6), 1011–1018.

Stewart, M. E., Barnard, L., Pearson, J., Hasan, R., & O'Brien, G. (2006). Presentation of depression in autism and Asperger syndrome: A review. *Autism: the international journal of research and practice, 10*(1), 103–116. doi:10.1177/1362361306062013.

Stores, G., & Wiggs, L. (1998). Abnormal sleep patterns associated with autism: A brief review of research findings, assessment methods and treatment strategies. *Autism: The International Journal of Research and Practice, 2*(2), 157–169. doi:10.1177/1362361398022004.

Sukhodolsky, D., Scahill, L., Gadow, K., Arnold, L., Aman, M., McDougle, C., et al. (2008). Parent-rated anxiety symptoms in children with pervasive developmental disorders: Frequency and association with core autism symptoms and cognitive functioning. *Journal of Abnormal Child Psychology, 36*(1), 117–128.

Taft, L., & Cohen, H. (1971). Hypsarrhythmia and infantile autism: A clinical report. *Journal of Autism and Childhood Schizophrenia, 1*(3), 327–336.

Tonge, B. J., Brereton, A. V., Gray, K. M., & Einfeld, S. L. (1999). Behavioural and emotional disturbance in high-functioning autism and Asperger syndrome. *Autism: The International Journal of Research and Practice, 3*(2), 117–130. doi:10.1177/1362361399003002003.

Tuchman, R., & Cuccaro, M. (2011). Epilepsy and autism: Neurodevelopmental perspective. *Current Neurology and Neuroscience Reports, 11*(4), 428–434. doi:10.1007/s11910-011-0195-x.

Tuchman, R., Moshé, S. L., & Rapin, I. (2009). Convulsing toward the pathophysiology of autism. *Brain Dev, 31*(2), 95–103.

Tuchman, R., Hirtz, D., & Mamounas, L. A. (2013). NINDS epilepsy and autism spectrum disorders workshop report. *Neurology, 81*(18), 1630–1636. doi:10.1212/WNL.0b013e3182a9f482.

Viscidi, E. W., Triche, E. W., Pescosolido, M. F., McLean, R. L., Joseph, R. M., Spence, S. J., et al. (2013). Clinical characteristics of children with autism spectrum disorder and co-occurring epilepsy. *PLoS One, 8*(7), e67797. doi:10.1371/journal.pone.0067797.

Volkmar, F. R., & Nelson, D. S. (1990). Seizure disorders in autism. *Journal of the American Academy of Child and Adolescent Psychiatry, 29*(1), 127–129.

Vorster, D. (1960). An investigation into the part played by organic factors in childhood schizophrenia. *The British Journal of Psychiatry, 106*(443), 494–522. doi:10.1192/bjp.106.443.494.

Weisbrot, D. M., Gadow, K. D., DeVincent, C. J., & Pomeroy, J. (2005). The presentation of anxiety in children with pervasive developmental disorders. *Journal of Child and Adolescent Psychopharmacology, 15*(3), 477–496.

Wetzel, R. J., Baker, J., Roney, M., & Martin, M. (1966). Outpatient treatment of autistic behavior. *Behaviour Research and Therapy, 4*(1–2), 169–177. doi:10.1016/0005-7967(66)90063-5.

White, P. T., DeMyer, W., & DeMyer, M. (1964). EEG abnormalities in early childhood schizophrenia: A double-blind study of psychiatrically disturbed and normal children during promazine sedation. *American Journal of Psychiatry, 120*(950–958).

White, S. W., Oswald, D., Ollendick, T., & Scahill, L. (2009). Anxiety in children and adolescents with autism spectrum disorders. *Clinical Psychology Review, 29*(3), 216–229.

Whittam, H., Simon, G. B., & Mittler, P. J. (1966). The early development of psychotic children and their sibs. *Developmental Medicine and Child Neurology, 8*(5), 552–560.

Wing, L. (1976). *Early Childhood Autism* (2nd ed.). Oxford: Pergamon Press.

Wing, L. (1981). Asperger's syndrome: A clinical account. *Psychological Medicine, 11*(1), 115–129. doi:10.1017/S0033291700053332.

Wing, L. (1991). The relationship between Asperger's syndrome and Kanner's autism. In U. Frith (Ed.), *Autism and Asperger syndrome* (pp. 93–121): Cambridge University Press.

Wood, J. J., & Gadow, K. D. (2010). Exploring the nature and function of anxiety in youth with autism spectrum disorders. *Clinical Psychology: Science and Practice, 17*(4), 281–292.

Zablotsky, B., Kalb, L. G., Freedman, B., Vasa, R. A., & Stuart, E. A. (2014). Health care experiences and perceived financial impact among families of children with an autism spectrum disorder. *Psychiatric Services, 65*(3), 395–398.

Chapter 2
Scope and Prevalence of the Problem

John F. Strang

Background Issues

Autism spectrum disorders (ASD) are often debilitating disorders, with only 9% of adults with ASD and average or above cognitive skills reaching full functional independence as adults (Farley et al. 2009). For more than 50% of individuals with co-occurring intellectual disability, outcomes are more bleak (LoVullo and Matson 2009). One of the primary complicating factors with ASD is the presence of co-occurring conditions (Matson and Goldin 2013). Depending on the study and characteristics of the groups studied, comorbid conditions are estimated to occur in about 70–80% of individuals with ASD (e.g., Leyfer et al. 2006; Mannion et al. 2013). In referred groups, the incidence of co-occurring conditions has been found to be even higher (Joshi et al. 2010).

Understanding the scope and the range of comorbidity in ASD is critical, as comorbid conditions often have a significant impact on the functioning of people with ASD (Kohane et al. 2012). Co-occurring conditions can exacerbate existing autism symptoms (Tureck et al. 2014) and make treatment less successful (Antshel et al. 2011). Co-occurring conditions can give rise to or make worse other comorbidities in an individual (Ming et al. 2008). Comorbidity makes ASD care more expensive, and families of individuals with ASD and comorbid conditions report a greater level of challenge in obtaining services for their children (Ahmedani and Hock 2011). Some studies have emphasized that apparent psychiatric and neurological comorbidities may obfuscate or delay a diagnosis of ASD, especially early on, and result in later identification of ASD as well as delayed ASD services (Gilmour et al. 2004; Mandell et al. 2007; Levy et al. 2010).

Separating out ASD symptoms versus additional diagnoses is particularly important for treatment planning, as different conditions may require different inter-

J. F. Strang (✉)
Center for Autism Spectrum Disorders, Children's National Medical Center,
Washington, D.C., USA
e-mail: jstrang@cnmc.org

Johnny L. Matson (ed.), *Comorbid Conditions Among Children with Autism Spectrum Disorders,* Autism and Child Psychopathology Series,
DOI 10.1007/978-3-319-19183-6_2

vention strategies. As important as diagnosing comorbidities is, however, the field can be challenging, with the diagnostic criteria for many co-occurring conditions overlapping with ASD symptom diagnostics (Matson and Nebel-Schwalm 2007; Mazefsky et al. 2012). Symptoms of ASD may also interfere with an individual's ability to report symptoms, and this may be particularly difficult in individuals with intellectual disability (Matson and Cervantes 2014). There have been efforts to develop new measures specifically designed for assessing comorbidity in ASD (e.g., Leyfer et al. 2006; Matson and Gonzalez 2007; Thorson and Matson 2012), as well as studies examining the performance of existing non-ASD specific measures in assessing comorbidity (Gjevik et al. 2014). Studies into comorbidities in ASD, in addition to informing clinical approaches and supports for individuals with ASD, may help to advance inquiries into the etiologies of ASD as well as specific etiological subgroups (Doshi-Velez et al. 2014).

In considering the literature to date on comorbidity in ASD, several biases have been discussed by investigators. Matson and Cervantes note the rapid increase in studies, but with a particular focus on studies of children and adolescents (Matson and Cervantes 2014). The authors also note the dearth of investigations into people with ASD and intellectual disability, with only a handful of studies available of adults with ASD and intellectual disability. This is problematic, as there is evidence of increased comorbidity among individuals with ASD and intellectual disability (LoVullo and Matson 2009). Few studies have investigated cross-cultural factors affecting diagnosis of comorbidities in ASD (e.g., Zachor et al. 2011).

Range and Rates of Comorbidities

Reported rates of comorbidities often vary significantly by study, related to factors of the study sample, such as population-based samples verses referred samples. Some disorders arise later in development, thus the age of study sample is critical in evaluating reported rates. Additionally, some disorders are particularly related to a subset of individuals with autism, such as those with intellectual disabilities.

Physical Conditions

Sleep

Sleep problems are among the most common comorbidities in children and adolescents with ASD, with approximately two-thirds of individuals experiencing at least one sleep problem in childhood (Richdale 2001; Richdale and Schreck 2009). This is in contrast to 25 % of children, in general, who experience sleep problems (Sheldon et al. 2005). Having intellectual disability and autism puts a child at particular risk for sleep problems, with up to 80 % experiencing sleep disturbance (Sheldon et al. 2005; Richdale and Schreck 2009). Sleep problems in adults with ASD are less well understood, though one study found lower rates of sleep problems among young adults than in children (Kohane et al. 2012). Sleep problems are related to many other areas of functioning, including autism severity (Schreck et al. 2004), anxiety (Rzepecka et al. 2011), and other physical conditions (Ming et al. 2008), as discussed below.

Epilepsy

Rates of comorbid epilepsy vary according to a report, from 7 % (Anne-Katrin et al. 2013) to 30 % (Tuchman and Rapin 2002), related to characteristics of the study sample. This is in contrast to rates of 2–3 % of the general population of children (Mannion and Leader 2013). A primary risk factor for epilepsy is co-occurring intellectual disability; Amiet and colleagues found that 21.4 % of the children with autism and intellectual disabilities had epilepsy, as compared to only 8 % of those with ASD and no intellectual disability (Amiet et al. 2008). Female sex is also related to higher rates of epilepsy in ASD, with findings that epilepsy occurred in 35 % of females and 18.5 % of males (Amiet et al. 2008). An epilepsy diagnosis often emerges later in childhood, which results in higher rates of epilepsy later in development (Bolton et al. 2011). In a study of 21-year olds with ASD, the average age of diagnosed epilepsy was 13 years, with most seizures beginning after the age of 10 years (Bolton et al. 2011).

Gastrointestinal Symptoms

There is a significant variability in reported rates of gastrointestinal symptoms (GI) (Mannion et al. 2013), with most common symptoms reported being abdominal pain, constipation, food refusal, diarrhea, and nausea (Mannion et al. 2013; Ibrahim et al. 2009). Reported rates of GI problems in children with ASD range from 9 to 84 % (Melmed et al. 2000; Horvath et al. 2000; Black et al. 2002; Kuddo and Nelson 2003), with some studies failing to find rates significantly higher than in the general population (Black et al. 2002). Apparently, there is no evidence for atypical motility in ASD (Buie et al. 2010). Although some emphasize that overly fixed/limited diets may lead to lack of fiber and fluids, the findings are mixed. One study failed to find a relationship between atypical diet and constipation (Gorrindo et al. 2012), while another reported a relationship between food intolerance and GI dysfunction (Ming et al. 2008). Nikolov and collaborators found that children with ASD and GI symptoms were no different from other ASD children in demographics, adaptive functioning, or ASD severity (Nikolov et al. 2009).

Other Physical/Medical Comorbidities

Many other physical/medical comorbidities have been reported, particularly among individuals with autism and intellectual disability (Hass 2010; Maski et al. 2011). Isaksen and colleagues performed comprehensive medical evaluations on 79 children diagnosed with ASD. Out of them, 10 % were found to have a specific medical syndrome in addition to ASD (Isaksen et al. 2013). Neurological findings, including brain nerve pathology, motor disturbances, nystagmus, cerebellar pathology, and sensory dysfunction were common, especially among the intellectual disability group (21.4 %). Dysmorphic findings were also common, occurring in 20.6 % of the patients.

Psychiatric Comorbidities

Attention Deficit/Hyperactivity Disorder

Recent studies of comorbid psychopathology in ASD have focused extensively on attention deficit/hyperactivity disorder (ADHD) over other psychopathologies, possibly due to apparent rates of comorbid ADHD in ASD of over 50 % (Matson and Goldin 2013). The literature reports a range of comorbidity rates for ADHD, from 30 to 80 % (Leyfer et al. 2006; Simonoff et al. 2008; Ames and White 2011). A study of younger children with ASD (4–6 years old) found 41 % met the criteria for comorbid ADHD (Carlsson et al. 2013). Individuals with ASD and lower cognitive skills may be more likely to have comorbid ADHD than those with greater cognitive skills (Lee and Ousley 2006). Rates of ADHD in adults with ASD have been understudied, but one group found that almost 37 % of the adults with ASD self-reported significant ADHD symptoms (Johnston et al. 2013). Prior to *The Diagnostic and Statistical Manual of Mental Disorders* 5th ed. (DSM–5; American Psychiatric Association 2013), ADHD symptoms were technically subsumed into the diagnosis of ASD, and a comorbid ADHD diagnosis was not permitted. Some studies have focused on the discernment of distinct symptoms of ADHD from ASD (e.g., Gadow et al. 2006). Others have emphasized the shared etiological factors of ASD and ADHD (van der Meer et al. 2012), with increased risk for both ASD and ADHD in families, with symptoms identified in the areas of executive function skills, motor speed, emotion recognition, and detail-focused processing (Corbett et al. 2009; Fine et al. 2008; Booth and Happé 2010).

Given shared etiological factors, some have considered that ADHD and ASD may be individual manifestations of a larger disorder. Analysis of symptom clusters has suggested that the two disorders are partly distinct, with three classes of symptoms identified: (1) ADHD symptoms only, (2) clinically significant ADHD and ASD symptoms, with ADHD as the most prominent symptom cluster, and (3) clinically significant ASD and ADHD symptoms, with ASD as the most prominent symptom cluster (van der Meer et al. 2012). Notably, in van der Meer et al.'s study, no class with just ASD symptoms was found; all the children who had ASD symptoms also presented with some level of ADHD symptoms, thus the two disorders are described as "partly distinct."

Anxiety Disorders

Anxiety disorders are reported to occur in 25–50 % of individuals with ASDs (Leyfer et al. 2006; Kuusikko et al. 2008; Sukhodolsky et al. 2008; Mattila et al. 2010). A meta-analysis of anxiety studies in children and adolescents with ASD found that almost 40 % of the young people with ASD met criteria for at least one anxiety disorder (Steensel et al. 2011). The most common was specific phobia (almost 30 %), followed by obsessive-compulsive disorder (OCD; 17.4 %) and social anxiety disorder (16.6 %). Studies are mixed in their findings of correlates to anxiety in ASD, with some finding anxiety symptoms pervasive across groups, regardless of age, IQ, or autism symptoms (e.g., Strang et al. 2012). Other studies have reported specific patterns of anxiety symptoms related to individual characteristics. For example, one study found a relationship between higher functioning ASDs and increased social worries, and lower functioning ASDs and increased avoidant and obsessive-compulsive ASD symptoms (White et al. 2009.) However, somewhat contrasting findings have also been reported, with lower IQ groups experiencing higher rates of anxiety in general and social anxiety, and higher IQ groups experiencing higher prevalence of OCD and separation anxiety. Greater age has been linked to increased incidence of anxiety disorders, though curiously, studies including younger children with ASD reported higher rates of OCD than studies with older children, which is the opposite pattern found in studies of OCD in general (Steensel et al. 2011). Atypical OCD age findings in ASD may reflect the diagnostic complexity of differentiating OCD from ASD core symptoms (see below, Symptom overlap).

Mood

Depression

Reported prevalence rates of depression in ASD vary widely, from 1.1 to 52 % (Levy et al. 2010; Hofvander et al. 2009). The comorbidity of ASD and depression has received significant attention, and findings have articulated a particularly complex and nuanced relationship between the disorders (Magnuson and Constantino 2011). Magnuson and Constantino summarize a case literature of presentations of depression in ASD, noting that clinicians often rely on self report of depression symptoms, which may be limited in ASD (Tager-Flusberg 1992). The authors identify several key diagnostic signs of depression in ASD, independent of self-report, based on previous studies: sadness, tearfulness, apathy, negative effect, anhedonia, changes in sleep/weight, decline in performance/skills, and preoccupation with death (Magnuson and Constantino 2011, citing Ghaziuddin et al. 2002; Stewart et al. 2006; Lainhart and Folstein 1994; Perry et al. 2001; Pollard and Predergast 2004; Janowksy and Davis 2005). In patients with ASD and intellectual disability, self-injurious behaviors are significantly related to depression (Janowsky and Davis 2005). Lower rates of depression are reported in studies of younger individuals (e.g., Levy et al. 2010), and several authors have noted greater depressive symptoms in individuals with less autism impairment, higher IQ, and greater insight into their condition (e.g., Vickerstaff et al. 2007; Sterling et al. 2008; Mazurek and Kanne 2010). However, several authors also report very high rates of mood disorders in people with autism and intellectual disability (Bradley et al. 2004; Bradley and Bolton 2006; Hill and Furniss 2006). These may be two different paths to depression, and the qualitative nature of the depression for high functioning and more insightful and intellectually disabled individuals may be very different. Rates of depression may increase into adulthood, with one study finding more than 50 % of the participants with ASD meeting criteria for depression (Hofvander et al. 2009). The quality of friendship has been related to experienced loneliness in ASD, which is related to increased depression (Whitehouse et al. 2009).

Bipolar Disorder

The comorbidity of bipolar disorder and autism is understudied and controversial (Matson and Nebel-Schwalm 2007). There is some evidence of an over-representation of bipolar disorder in referred adolescents and young adults with high functioning ASD (Munesue et al. 2008), as well as among adults (Stahlberg et al. 2004). Studies have indicated high rates of bipolar disorder among relatives of ASD probands (Bolton et al. 1998) as well as ASD among bipolar disorder probands (Joshi et al. 2013). Whereas some have suggested that bipolar disorder rates may be underestimated in ASD (Raja and Azzonoi 2008), others have noted that bipolar disorder may be over-diagnosed in ASD (Mazefsky et al. 2012).

Developmental Comorbidity—Intellectual Disability

Rates of co-occurring autism and intellectual disability vary by report. The Centers for Disease Control indicate 54 % of individuals with ASD in 2010 had concurrent intellectual disability (Centers for Disease Control and Prevention 2014). Former reports were often higher, with rates up to 70 % (La Malfa et al. 2004). The apparent drop in rates of ASD and intellectual disability over recent years has been attributed to the increasing number of individuals with higher cognitive abilities being diagnosed with ASD, and not to a decrease in the numbers of individuals with autism and intellectual disability (Keen and Ward 2004). Around 40% of individuals with intellectual disability are reported to have autism (Keen and Ward 2004).

The comorbidity of autism and intellectual disability results in striking impairments, far and above those experienced by individuals with intellectual disability alone (Brereton et al. 2006; Hill and Furniss 2006). Anxiety, mood disorders, problem behaviors, feeding issues, and stereotypies are greater in people with intellectual disability who also have autism (Hill and Furniss 2006; Bradley and Bolton 2006). Matson and Shoemaker's (2009) review of co-occurring autism and intellectual disability notes the dearth of studies on comorbidities in this area, as well as the over-focus on higher functioning individuals with autism in recent years, in spite of the greater numbers with intellectual disability and their higher levels of impairment (Matson and Shoemaker 2009).

Interrelatedness and Impact of Comorbidities

Comorbidities in ASD are often interrelated, and they can exacerbate ASD symptoms, reduce overall functioning, and result in poorer clinical outcomes over time. They are, therefore, a critical target for assessment and treatment. For example, children with comorbid ADHD and ASD had higher rates and intensity of other comorbidity than children with either ASD or ADHD (Gadow et al. 2009; Jang et al. 2013). The comorbidity of mood disorders in ASD may worsen the progression of ASD, with increased impairment of core skills (social and communication) and increased repetitive behaviors (Lainhardt 1999; Perry et al. 2001). Garcia-Willamisar and Rojahn found that comorbid psychopathology mediated the relationship between autistic traits and repetitive behaviors/restricted interests in adults with ASD and intellectual disability (Garcia-Villamisar and Rojahn 2013). The authors suggested that treating comorbid psychopathology and reducing stress could reduce the frequency and intensity of repetitive behaviors. It is important to consider the comorbidities caused by comorbidity. For example, epilepsy has its own comorbidity, including mood symptoms/suicidal ideation (Hecimovic et al. 2011).

Some investigators have found that medical comorbidities tend to cluster together, as psychiatric comorbidities (Ming et al. 2008). Others have found interrelatedness between medical and psychiatric symptoms (Rzepecka et al. 2011), particularly in the area of sleep and ASD. Sleep problems have been shown to be related to GI problems (Mannion et al. 2013); the greater a child's GI symptoms, the worse their sleep ratings. Sleep difficulties have also been linked to increased mood problems (Ming et al. 2008), as well as increased anxiety in children with ASD (Rzepecka et al. 2011). Sleep problems exacerbate ASD-related symptoms. Schreck et al. (2004) found less sleep was related to increased ASD severity ratings, increased stereotypic/repetitive behavior, and social skill weaknesses. Others have also reported a link between sleep problems in ASD and poorer social interactions (Malow et al. 2006), and too little sleep can reduce the ability to read social cues (van der Halm et al. 2010). Goldman et al. (2011) found that poor sleep in ASD was related to more behavior problems.

Comorbidities in ASD, and especially ADHD, may have significant impact on intervention. Antshel et al. (2011) examined the outcomes from social skill intervention for children with ASD, children with ASD + anxiety disorders, and children with ASD + ADHD and found that the intervention was effective for those with ASD or ASD + anxiety disorders, but not for those with ASD + ADHD. Results indicated that social skill intervention was particularly well suited for ASD + anxiety disorder; the authors note that social skill intervention is efficacious for both ASD and anxiety disorders, so the combination of both may lend itself to this type of treatment.

In a phone survey study, the presence of an ASD and a comorbid psychiatric condition related to significantly worse health outcomes as compared to having autism alone (Ahmedani et al. 2011); children with ASD and comorbid conditions were more likely to have poor overall health and "prevented in ability." Families of individuals with ASD and comorbidity were less satisfied with provider communications, and they were less likely to be successful in having insurance cover the necessary services for their child. Comorbidity in ASD also increases ASD-related expenditures. Children with autism have been found to have average medical expenditures 3–9 times higher than children without ASD (Amendah et al. 2011), though more recent studies have indicated even higher expenditure rates (Peacock et al. 2012). Peacock et al. looked at the impact of three co-occurring conditions with ASD on expenditures, according to a review of Medicaid records. Co-occurring autism and intellectual disability resulted in the greatest expense, 2.7 times more than for children with autism alone.

Symptom Overlap

Matson and Nebel-Schwalm (2007) highlight the heterogeneity in symptoms of ASD, which can make it difficult to differentiate ASD symptoms and commorbidities, and emphasize the importance of working to identify one comorbidity as primary in order to determine priority of intervention, long-term prognosis, and allocation of services. However, early in development this may be particularly challenging. Gillberg notes the complex overlap of symptom clusters, particularly in early childhood (Gillberg 2010). Carlsson et al. (2013) emphasize the importance of diagnosing over time in young children, as co-occurring disorders can make the diagnoses less clear at first. New instruments designed to assess comorbidity in ASD are being developed, such as the Autism Spectrum Disorder-Comorbidity for Children (ASD-CC; Matson and Gonzalez 2007).

Features of emotional dysregulation in ASD may result in inaccurate psychiatric diagnoses, or make diagnosing autism more difficult. Mazefsky et al. (2012) found that nearly 60 % of the prior psychiatric diagnoses given to a group of young people with ASD (age 10–17; IQ: 71–144) were not supported by a careful psychiatric interview that accounted for ASD-related impairment. Most notably, diagnoses of bipolar disorder or OCD were not supported in any of the individuals who had previously received these diagnoses. Almost one-third had a previous ADHD diagnosis that was not supported. Concordance for depression was higher, with 57% of the prior depressive disorder diagnoses maintained. Mazefsky et al. note that impediments to correct diagnosis such as diagnosing a psychiatric diagnosis instead of ASD, may delay the diagnosis of ASD, thereby preventing a child from receiving critical early intervention for ASD. The authors also cite Mandell's (2008) study, which found that later ASD diagnosis was related to higher chance of psychiatric hospitalization. In Mazefksy's study, out of eight children who had psychiatric hospitalizations only one was diagnosed with ASD prior to the hospitalization.

Similarly, Levy et al. (2010) in a population-based cohort, found a relationship between later diagnosis of ASD and the presence of co-occurring symptoms. Co-occurring non-ASD diagnoses were related to later age of ASD diagnosis. The authors note that "the symptomatology associated with non-ASD conditions might complicate recognition of ASDs and thus result in delayed identification" (Levy et al. 2010, p. 271). Pressures for billing may also complicate diagnostics; Leslie and Martin (2007) highlight that insurance reimbursements are often not made when a clinician bills under an autism diagnosis, which may lead clinicians to add, or put as primary, comorbid diagnoses.

OCD and social anxiety disorder each provide a rich example of the potential complexities of diagnosing comorbidities in ASD. OCD is typically diagnosed later in childhood and in adolescence, but studies in ASD have found a relationship between younger age and increased rates of OCD (Steensel et al. 2011), suggesting perhaps a different course for OCD in ASD, or more likely, diagnostic challenges. The core symptoms of ASD overlap with symptoms of OCD, and authors note the difficulty detangling symptoms of the two disorders (e.g., Matson and Cervantes 2014.) Van Steensel et al. (2011) have suggested that by assessing the nature of the special interests and routines, one can better differentiate ASD versus ASD+OCD, with each having a different character. Ruta and colleagues (Ruta et al. 2010) examined differences in symptoms between children with ASD and OCD, noting some areas that distinguished the groups, including higher frequencies of contamination and aggressive obsessions, as well as checking compulsions. Although diagnostic differentiation is a primary goal, there has been some suggestion that treatments appropriate for one disorder may transfer to the other, without a need for absolute diagnostic distinction (Rooney et al. 2011).

Difficulties in differentiating social anxiety from ASD core social symptoms are also notable. Van Steensal et al. (2011) suggest an important discriminating factor may be that the behavioral symptoms seen in both disorders such as social withdrawal, preferring to be alone, gaze avoidance, and not speaking in social situations may be more variable in children with social anxiety, whereas they would probably vary less in ASD without social anxiety. Summarizing several studies (Reaven and Hepburn 2003; Leyfer 2006; Matson and Nebel-Schwalm 2007), Rieske et al. (2012) note that features central to anxiety including unrealistic fears and sympathetic nervous system triggering, should be distinguished from impairment related to symptoms of ASD, such as a lack of engagement due to communication weaknesses or an over-focused interest.

Conclusions

Mazefsky et al. (2012) have outlined several possible understandings of high comorbidity in ASD:

1. Family history studies report high rates of emotional disorders in the relatives of children with ASD (e.g., Mazefsky, Folstein and Lainhardt 2008)), which suggests a genetic link between ASD and other disorders. Autism and ADHD run together in families (van der Meer et al. 2012), as do bipolar illness and ASD (Bolton et al. 1998; Joshi et al. 2013).
2. It may be the case that what is seen as a comorbidity is really a manifestation of ASD symptoms. Studies have shown that symptoms of apparent comorbidities can obfuscate an underlying ASD diagnosis (Mazefsky et al. 2012).
3. Varying progression of symptoms in an individual over time may appear as different disorders, but may be reflective of the same underlying pathology.
4. Having one disorder can increase the risk of a second. For example, more negative feedback from peers, awareness of social difficulties, etc., may contribute to the co-occurrence of ASD and social anxiety disorder (White et al., 2012)

Most comorbidity studies have focused on a single comorbidity or cluster of comorbidities. A new direction, now available with larger datasets, is analysis of symptom clusters. Doshi-Velez and colleagues 2014) examined electronic records, 4934 individuals of age 15 years and older. Although the study could only account for a small proportion of individuals included, the study identified three discernible symptom clusters:

1. A seizure group with high rates of intellectual disability (60 %) and lower rates of boys. The authors note the established diagnostic connections between the following: autism, seizures, intellectual disability, and increased rates of female gender.
2. A multisystemic disorders group with high rates (50 %) of intellectual disability. Disorders in this group included gastrointestinal, auditory disorders, and infections, and the authors noted previous studies suggesting an underlying biology for such interconnections.
3. A largely higher IQ group (only 28 % ID) with primarily psychiatric disorders, and especially anxiety.

Future directions in comorbidity and ASD research should further articulate symptom cluster groups, particularly in the overlap between ADHD and ASD, and the apparent emerging subgroups of individuals with components of each disorder. A particular need in the field is better tools to differentiate complex mood disorders from autism. Currently, problems diagnosing ASD in dysregulated children result in late diagnosis and poorer outcomes. As ASD treatment studies continue to develop, it will be helpful to study the impact of various comorbidities with ASD on treatment efficacy, and to tailor interventions accordingly. Finally, the interconnections between various comorbidities and ASD should be increasingly explored from a longitudinal perspective, as cross-sectional associational studies do not help us to understand the root causes of the associations.

References

Ahmedani, B. K., & Hock, R. M. (2011). Health care access and treatment for children with co-morbid autism and psychiatric conditions. *Social Psychiatry and Psychiatric Epidemiology, 47*(11), 1807–1804.

Amendah, D., Grosse, S. D., Peacock, G., & Mandell, D. S. (2011). The economic costs of autism: A review. In D.G. Amaral, G. Dawson, & D. H. Geschwind (Eds.), *Autism Spectrum Disorders* (2011: pp. 1343–1358). New York: Oxford University Press.

American Psychiatric Association. (2013). *Diagnostic and statistical manual of mental disorders* (5th ed.). Arlington, VA: American Psychiatric Publishing.

Ames, C. S., & White, S. J. (2011). Are ADHD traits dissociable from the autistic profile? Links between cognition and behavior. *Journal of Autism and Developmental Disabilities, 41,* 357–363.

Amiet, C., Gourfinkel-An, I., Bouzamondo, A., et al. (2008). Epilepsy in autism is associated with intellectual disability and gender: Evidence from a meta-analysis. *Biological Psychiatry, 64,* 577–582.

Anne-Katrin, K., Fernell, E., Gillberg, C., & Miniscalco, C. (2013). Autism in community pre-schoolers: Developmental profiles. *Research in Developmental Disabilities, 34,* 2900–2908.

Antshel, K. M., Placek, C., McMahon, M., et al. (2011). Comorbid ADHD and anxiety affect social skills group intervention treatment efficacy in children with autism spectrum disorders. *Journal of Developmental and Behavioral Pediatrics, 32,* 439–446.

Black, C., Kaye, J. A., & Jick, H. (2002). Relation of childhood gastrointestinal disorders to autism: Nested case-control study using data from the UK general practice research database. *British Medical Journal, 325*(7361), 419–421.

Bolton, P. F., Pickles, A., Murphy, M., & Rutter, M. (1998). Autism, affective and other psychiatric disorders: Patterns of familiar aggregation. *Psychological Medicine, 28*(2), 385–395.

Bolton, P. F., Carcani-Rathwell, I., Hutton, J., et al. (2011). Epilepsy in autism: Features and correlates. *British Journal of Psychiatry, 198*(4), 289–294.

Booth, R., & Happé, F. (2010). "Hunting with a knife and … fork": Examining central coherence in autism, attention deficit/hyperactivity disorder, and typical development with a linguistic task. *Journal of Experimental Child Psychology, 107,* 307–393.

Bradley, E., & Bolton, P. (2006). Episodic psychiatric disorders in teenagers with learning disabilities with and without autism. *The British Journal of Psychiatry, 189,* 361–366.

Bradley, E. A., Summers, J. A., Wood, H. L., & Bryson, S.E. (2004). Comparing rates of psychiatric and behavior disorders in adolescents and young adults with severe intellectual disability with and without autism. *Journal of Autism and Developmental Disorders, 34,* 151–161.

Brereton, A. V., Tonge, B. J., & Einfeld, S. L. (2006). Psychopathology in children and adolescents with autism compared to young people with intellectual disability. *Journal of Autism and Developmental Disorders, 36*(7), 863–870.

Buie, T., Fuchs, G. J. 3rd, Furuta, G. T., Kooros, K., Levy, J., Lewis, J. D., et al. (2010). Recommendations for evaluation and treatment of common gastrointestinal problems in children with ASDs. *Pediatrics, 125*(1), 19–29.

Carlsson, L. H., Norrelgen, F., Kjellmer, L., et al. (2013). Coexisting disorders and problems in preschool children with Autism Spectrum Disorders. *The Scientific World Journal, Vol, 2013,* 1–6.

Centers for Disease Control and Prevention. (2014). Prevalence of Autism Spectrum Disorder among children aged 8 years. *Morbidity and Mortality Weekly Report, 63(SS02)*, 1–21.

Corbett, B. A., Constantine, L. J., Hendren, R., et al. (2009). Examining executive functioning in children with autism spectrum disorder, attention deficit hyperactivity disorder and typical development. *Psychiatry Research, 166,* 210–222.

Doshi-Velez, F., Ge, Y., & Kohane, I. (2014). Comorbidity clusters in autism spectrum disorders: An electronic health record time-series analysis. *Pediatrics, 133(e4)*, 54–63.

Farley, M. A., McMahon, W. M., Fombonne, E., et al. (2009). Twenty-year outcome for individuals with Autism and average or near-average cognitive abilities. *Autism Research, 2,* 109–118.

Fine, J. G., Semrud-Clikeman, M., Butcher, B., & Walkowiak, J. (2008). Brief report: Attention effect on a measure of social perception. *Journal of Autism and Developmental Disorders, 38,* 1797–1802.

Gadow, K. D., DeVincent, C. J., & Pomeroy, J. (2006). ADHD symptom subtypes in children with pervasive developmental disorder. *Journal of Autism and Developmental Disorders, 36,* 271–283.

Gadow, K. D., DeVincent, C. J., & Schneider, J. (2009). Comparative study of children with ADHD only, autism spectrum disorder + ADHD, and chronic multiple tic disorder + ADHD. *Journal of Attention Disorders, 12,* 474–485.

García-Villamisar, D., & Rojahn, J. (2013). Comorbid psychopathology and stress mediate the relationship between autistic traits and repetitive behaviours in adults with autism. *Journal of Intellectual Disability Research.* doi:10.1111/jir.12083.

Ghaziuddin, M., Ghaziuddin N., & Greden J. (2002). Depression in persons with Autism: Implications for research and clinical care. *Journal of Autism and Developmental Disorders, 32,* 299–306.

Gillberg, C. (2010). The essence in child psychiatry: Early symptomatic syndromes eliciting neurodevelopmental clinical examinations. *Research in Developmental Disabilities, 31*(6), 1543–1551.

Gilmour, J., Hill, B., Place, M., Skuse, D. (2004). Social communication deficits in conduct disorders: A clinical and community survey. *Journal of Child Psychology and Psychiatry, 45,* 967–978.

Gjevik, E., Eldevik, S., Fjaeran-Granum, T., Sponheim, E. (2011). Kiddie-SADS reveals high rates of DSM- IV disorders in children and adolescents. *Journal of Autism and Developmental Disorders, 41,* 761–769.

Goldman, S. E., McGrew, S., Johnson, K. P., et al. (2011). Sleep is associated with problem behaviors in children and adolescents with Autism Spectrum Disorders. *Research in Autism Spectrum Disorders, 5,* 1223–1229.

Gorrindo, P., Williams, K. C., Lee, E. B., et al. (2012). Gastrointestinal dysfunction in autism: Parental report, clinical evaluation, and associated factors. *Autism Research, 5*(2), 101–108.

van der Halm, E., Gujar, N., Walker, M. P. (2010). Sleep deprivation impairs the accurate recognition of human emotions. *Sleep, 33,* 335–342.

Hass, R. H. (2010). Autism and mitochondrial disease. *Developmental Disabilities Research Reviews, 16,* 144–153.

Hecimovic, H., Salpekar, J., Kanner, A. M., Barry, J. J. (2011). Suicidality and epilepsy: a neuropsychobiological perspective. *Epilepsy & Behavior, 22*(1), 77–84.

Hill, J., & Furniss, F. (2006). Patterns of emotional and behavioural disturbance associated with autistic traits in young people with severe intellectual disabilities and challenging behaviours. *Research in Developmental Disabilities, 27,* 517–528.

Hofvander, B., Delorme, R., Chaste, P., et al. (2009). Psychiatric and psychosocial problems in adults with normal-intelligence autism spectrum disorders. *BMC psychiatry, 9,* 35.

Horvath, K., Medeiros, L., Rabsztyn, A., et al. (2000). High prevalence of gastrointestinal symptoms in children with autism spectrum disorder. *Journal of Pediatric Gastroenterology and Nutrition, 31*(Suppl. 2), 174.

Ibrahim, S. H., Voigt, R. G., Katusic, S. K., et al. (2009). Incidence of gastrointestinal symptoms in children with autism: A population based study. *Pediatrics, 124,* 680–868.

Isaksen, J., Bryn, V., Diseth, T. H., et al. (2013). Children with autism spectrum disorders—the importance of medical investigations. *European Journal of Paediatric Neurology, 17,* 68–76.
Jang, J., Matson, J. L., Williams, L. W., et al. (2013). Rates of comorbid symptoms in children with ASD, ADHD, and comorbid ASD and ADHD. *Research in Developmental Disabilities, 34,* 2369–2378.
Janowksy, D. S., & Davis, J. M. (2005). Diagnosis and treatment of depression in patients with mental retardation. *Current Psychiatry Reports, 7,* 421–428.
Johnston, K., Dittner, A., Bramham, J., et al. (2013). Attention deficit hyperactivity disorder symptoms in adults with autism spectrum disorders. *Autism Research, 6,* 225–236.
Joshi, G., Petty, C., Wozniak, J., et al. (2010). The heavy burden of psychiatric comorbidity in youth with autism spectrum disorders: A large comparative study of a psychiatrically referred population. *Journal of Autism and Developmental Disorders, 40,* 1361–1370.
Joshi, G., Biederman, J., Petty, C., et al. (2013). Examining the comorbidity of bipolar disorder and autism spectrum disorders: A large controlled analysis of phenotypic and familiar correlates in a referred population of youth with bipolar I disorder with and without autism spectrum disorders. *Journal of Clinical Psychiatry, 74*(6), 578–586.
Keen, D., & Ward, S. (2004). Autism spectrum disorder: a child population profile. *Autism: the International Journal of Research and Practice, 8,* 39–48.
Kohane, I. S., McMurry, A., Weber, G., et al. (2012). The co-morbidity burden of children and young adults with autism spectrum disorders. *PLoS One 7*: e3322410.1371/journal.pone.0033224.
Kuddo, T., & Nelson, K. B. (2003). How common are gastrointestinal disorders in children with autism? *Current Opinion in Pediatrics, 15,* 339–343.
Kuusikko, S., Pollock-Wurman, R., Jussila, K., et al. (2008). Social anxiety in high-functioning children and adolescents with Autism and Asperger syndrome. *Journal of Autism and Developmental Disorders, 38,* 1697–1709.
La Malfa, G., Lassi, S., Bertelli, M., et al. (2004). Autism and intellectual disability: A study of prevalence on a sample of the Italian population. *Journal of Intellectual Disability Research, 48*(3), 262–267.
Lainhardt, J. E. (1999). Psychiatric problems in individuals with autism, their parents, and siblings. *International Review of Psychiatry, 11*(4), 278–298.
Lainhart, J. E., & Folstein, S. E. (1994). Affective disorders in people with autism: A review of published cases. *Journal of Autism and Developmental Disorders, 24,* 587–601.
Lee, D. O., & Ousley, O. Y. (2006). Attention-deficit hyperactivity disorder symptoms in a clinic sample of children and adolescents with pervasive developmental disorders. *Journal of Child and Adolescent Psychopharmacology, 16,* 737–746.
Leslie, D. L., & Martin, A. (2007). Health care expenditures associated with autism spectrum disorders. *Archives of Pediatrics and Adolescent Medicine, 161,* 350–355.
Levy, S. E., Giarelli, E., Lee, L., et al. (2010). Autism Spectrum Disorder and co-occurring developmental, psychiatric, and medical conditions among children in multiple populations of the United States. *Journal of Developmental and Behavioral Pediatrics, 31,* 267–275.
Leyfer, O. T., Folstein, S. E., Bacalman, S., et al. (2006). Comorbid psychiatric disorders in children with autism: Interview development and rates of disorders. *Journal of Autism and Developmental Disorders, 36,* 849–861.
LoVullo, S. V., & Matson, J. L. (2009). Comorbid psychopathology in adults with Autism Spectrum Disorders and intellectual disabilities. *Research in Developmental Disabilities, 30,* 1288–1296.
Magnuson, K. M., & Constantino, J. N. (2011). Characterization of depression in children with autism spectrum disorders. *Journal of Developmental and Behavioral Pediatrics, 32,* 332–340.
Malow, B. A., Marzec, M. L., McGrew, S. G., et al. (2006). Characterizing sleep in children with autism spectrum disorders: A multidimensional approach. *Sleep, 29,* 1563–1571.
Mandell, D. S. (2008). Psychiatric hospitalization among children with autism spectrum disorders. *Journal of Autism and Developmental Disorders, 37,* 1795–1802.
Mandell, D. S., Ittenbach, R. F., Levy, S. E., Pinto-Martin, J. A. (2007). Disparities in diagnoses received prior to a diagnosis of autism spectrum disorder. *Journal of Autism and Developmental Disorders, 37,* 1795–1802.

Mannion, A., & Leader, G. (2013). Comorbidity in autism spectrum disorder: A literature review. *Research in Autism Spectrum Disorders, 7,* 1595–1616.

Mannion, A., Leader, G., Healy, O. (2013). An investigation of comorbid psychological disorders, sleep problems, gastrointestinal symptoms and epilepsy in children and adolescents with Autism Spectrum Disorder. *Research in Autism Spectrum Disorders, 7,* 35–42.

Maski, K. P., Jeste, S. S., Spence, S. J. (2011). Common neurological co-morbidities in autism spectrum disorders. *Current Opinion in Pediatrics, 23,* 609–615.

Matson, J. L., & Cervantes, P. E. (2014). Commonly studied comorbid psychopathologies among persons with autism spectrum disorder. *Research in Developmental Disabilities, 35,* 952–962.

Matson, J. L., & Goldin, R. L. (2013). Comorbidity and autism: trends, topics and future directions. *Research in Autism Spectrum Disorders, 7,* 1228–1233.

Matson, J. L., & Gonzalez, M. (2007). Autism spectrum disorder—comorbid for children. Baton Rouge: Disability Consultants, LLC.

Matson, J. L., & Nebel-Schwalm, M. S. (2007). Comorbid psychopathology with autism spectrum disorder in children: An overview. *Research in Developmental Disabilities, 28*(4), 341–351.

Matson, J. L., & Shoemaker, M. (2009). Intellectual disability and its relationship to Autism spectrum disorders. *Research in Developmental Disabilities, 30,* 1107–1114.

Mattila, M. L., Hurtig, T., Haapsamo, H., et al. (2010). Comorbid psychiatric disorders associated with Asperger syndrome/high-functioning autism: A community- and clinic-based study. *Journal of Autism and Developmental Disorders, 40,* 1080–1093.

Mazefsky, C. A., Folstein, S. E., & Lainhart, J. E. (2008). Brief report: Overrepresentation of mood and anxiety disorders in adults with autism and their first degree relatives: What does it mean? *Autism Research, 1,* 193–197.

Mazefsky, C. A., Oswald, D. P., Day, T. N., et al. (2012). ASD, a psychiatric disorder, or both? Psychiatric diagnoses in adolescents with high-functioning ASD. *Journal of Clinical Child & Adolescent Psychology, 41*(4), 516–523.

Mazurek, M. O., & Kanne, S. M. (2010). Friendship and internalizing symptoms among children and adolescents with ASD. *Journal of Autism and Developmental Disorders, 40,* 1512–1520.

van der Meer, J. M. J., Oerlemans, A. M., van Steijn, D. J., et al. (2012). Are autism spectrum disorder and attention-deficit/hyperactivity disorder different manifestations of one overarching disorder? Cognitive and symptom evidence from a clinical and population-based sample. *Journal of the American Academy of Child & Adolescent Psychiatry, 55*(11), 1160–1172.

Melmed, R. D., Schneider, C. K., Fabes, R. A., et al. (2000). Metabolic markers and gastrointestinal symptoms in children with autism and related disorders. *Journal of Pediatric Gastroenterology and Nutrition, 31*(Suppl. 2), 31.

Ming, X., Brimacombe, M., Chaaban, J., et al. (2008). Autism spectrum disorders: Concurrent clinical disorders. *Journal of Child Neurology, 23,* 6–13.

Munesue, T., Ono. Y., Mutoh, K., et al. (2008). High prevalence of bipolar disorder comorbidity in adolescents and young adults with high-functioning autism spectrum disorder: A preliminary study of 44 outpatients. *Journal of Affective Disorders, 111*(2–3), 170–175.

Nikolov, R. N., Bearss, K. E., Lettinga, J., et al. (2009). Gastrointestinal symptoms in a sample of children with pervasive developmental disorders. *Journal of Autism and Developmental Disorders, 30,* 405–413.

Peacock, G., Amendah, D., Ouyang, L., & Grosse, S. (2012). Autism spectrum disorders and health care expenditures: The effects of co-occurring conditions. *Journal of Developmental Behavioral Pediatrics, 33,* 2–8.

Perry, D. W., Marston, G. M., Hinder, S. A., et al. (2001). The phenomenology of depressive illness in people with a learning disability and autism. *Autism: The International Journal of Research and Practice, 5,* 265–275.

Pollard, A. J., & Predergast, M. (2004). Depressive pseudodementia in a child with autism. *Developmental Medicine and Child Neurology, 46,* 485–489.

Raja, M., & Azzoni, A. (2008). Comorbidity of Asperger's syndrome and bipolar disorder. *Clinical Practice and Epidemiology in Mental Health, 4,* 26.

Reaven, J., & Hepburn, S. (2003). Cognitive-behavioral treatment of obsessive-compulsive disorder in a child with Asperger's syndrome: a case report. *Autism: the International Journal of Research and Practice, 7,* 145–164.
Richdale, A. (2001). Sleep disorders in autism and Asperger's syndrome. In G. Stores, L. Wiggs (Eds.), *Sleep disturbances in disorders of development: its significance and management* (pp. 181–191). London: MacKeith.
Richdale, A. L., & Schreck, K. A. (2009). Sleep problems in autism spectrum disorders: prevalence, nature, & possible biopsychosocial aetiologies. *Sleep Medicine Reviews, 13,* 403–411.
Rieske, R. D., Matson, J. L., May, A. C., & Kozlowski, A. M. (2012). Anxiety in children with high functioning autism spectrum disorders: Significant differences and the moderating effects of social impairments. *Journal of Physical and Developmental Disabilities, 24,* 167–180.
Rooney, M., Alfano, C. A., Walsh, K. S., & Parr, A. F. (2011). Differential diagnosis and treatment of obsessive-compulsive, inattentive, and sleep symptoms in a 7-year-old with PDD-NOS. *Clinical Case Studies*, published online 21 February 2011. doi:10.1177/1534650111398123.
Ruta, L., Mugno, D., D'Arrigo, V. G., et al. (2010). Obsessive-compulsive traits in children and adolescents with Asperger syndrome. *European Child & Adolescent Psychiatry, 19*(1), 17–24.
Rzepecka, H., McKenzie, K., McClure, I., & Murphy, S. (2011). Sleep, anxiety and challenging behavior in children with intellectual disability and/or autism spectrum disorder. *Research in Developmental Disabilities,* 32, 2758–2766.
Schreck, K. A., Mulick, J. A., & Smith, A. F. (2004). Sleep problems as possible predictors of intensified symptoms of autism. *Research in Developmental Disabilities, 25,* 57–66.
Sheldon, S. H., Ferber, R., & Kryger, M. H. (Eds.). (2005). *Principles and practice of pediatric sleep medicine.* Philadelphia: Elseview Saunders.
Simonoff, E., Pickles, A., Charman, T., et al. (2008). Psychiatric disorders in children with autism spectrum disorders: Prevalence, comorbidity and associated factors in a population-driven sample. *Journal of the American Academy of Child and Adolescent Psychiatry, 47*(8), 921–929.
Stahlberg, O., Soderstrom, H., Rastam, M., & Gillberg, C. (2004). Bipolar disorder, schizophrenia, and other psychotic disorders in adults with childhood onset AD/HD and/or autism spectrum disorders. *Journal of Neural Transmissions, 111*(7), 891–902.
van Steensel, F. J. A., Bögels, S. M., & Perrin, S. (2011). Anxiety disorders in children and adolescents with autistic spectrum disorders: A meta-analysis. *Clinical Child and Family Psychological Review, 14,* 302–317.
Sterling, L., Dawson, G., Estes, A., & Greenson, J. (2008). Characteristics associated with presence of depressive symptoms in adults with autism spectrum disorder. *Journal of Autism and Developmental Disorders, 38,* 1011–1018.
Stewart, M. E., Barnard, L., Pearson, J., et al. (2006). Presentation of depression in autism and Asperger syndrome: A review. *Autism: The International Journal of Research and Practice, 10,* 103–116.
Strang, J. F., Kenworthy, L., Daniolos, P., et al. (2012). Depression and anxiety symptoms in children and adolescents with autism spectrum disorders without intellectual disability. *Research in Autism Spectrum Disorders, 6*(1), 406–412.
Sukhodolsky, D. G., Scahill, L., Gadow, K.D., et al. (2008). Parent-rated anxiety symptoms in children with pervasive developmental disorders: Frequency and association with core autism symptoms and cognitive functioning. *Journal of Abnormal Child Psychology, 36,* 117–128.
Tager-Flusberg, H. (1992). Autistic children's talk about psychological states: Deficits in the early acquisition of a theory of mind. *Child Development, 63,* 161–172.
Thorson, R. T., & Matson, J. L. (2012). Cutoff scores for the Autism Spectrum Disorder—comorbid for children (ASD-CC). *Research in Autism Spectrum Disorders, 6*(1), 556–559.
Tuchman, R. F., & Rapin, I. (2002). Epilepsy in autism. *The Lancet Neurology, 1,* 352–357.
Tureck, K., Matson, J. L., Cervantes, P., Konst, M. J. (2014). An examination of the relationship between autism spectrum disorder, intellectual functioning, and comorbid symptoms in children. *Research in Developmental Disabilities, 35*(7), 1766–1772.

Vickerstaff, S., Heriot, S., Wong, M., et al. (2007). Intellectual ability, self-perceived social competence, and depressive symptomatology in children with high-functioning autistic spectrum disorders. *Journal of Autism and Developmental Disorders, 37,* 1647–1664.

White, S. W., Oswald, D., Ollendick, T., & Scahill, L. (2009). Anxiety in children and adolescents with autism spectrum disorders. *Journal of Developmental and Physical Disabilities, 22,* 367–380.

White, S. W., Bray, C. B., & Ollendick, T. H. (2012). Examining shared and unique aspects of social anxiety disorders and autism spectrum disorders using factor analysis. *Journal of Autism and Developmental Disorders, 42*(5), 874–884.

Whitehouse, A. J., Durkin, K., Jaquet, E., & Ziatas, K. (2009). Friendship, loneliness and depression in adolescents with Asperger's syndrome. *Journal of Adolescence, 32,* 309–322.

Zachor, D., Yang, J.-W., Itzchak, E. B., et al. (2011). Cross-cultural differences in comorbid symptoms of children with autism spectrum disorders: An international examination between Israel, South Korea, the United Kingdom and the United States of America. *Developmental Neuro.*

Part II
Assessment

Chapter 3
Methods and Procedures for Measuring Comorbid Disorders: Psychological

Amanda M. Pearl and Susan D. Mayes

Autism spectrum disorder (ASD) is a complex neurodevelopmental disorder that persists throughout a person's lifetime. Individuals with ASD have challenges with social interaction/communication and evidence overly restrictive and repetitive patterns of behavior (DSM-5, American Psychiatric Association 2013). Prevalence statistics from the Centers for Disease Control and Prevention (CDC) estimate that 1 in 68 children have ASD (CDC; 2014). The lifetime per capita cost of caring for and treating a person with an ASD is estimated to be $ 1.4 million for those without co-occurring intellectual disability (ID) (Ganz 2007). When factoring in indirect costs (loss of productivity for the individual with ASD and his/her caregivers), the expense may rise to $ 3.2 million lifetime cost per individual with ASD (Mandell 2012). In 2012, Mandell estimated that autism costs society $ 126 billion per year in the USA, more than triple since 2006. Mortality rates for individuals with ASD are approximately 2–6 times higher than for individuals without ASD (Gillberg et al. 2010; Mouridsen 2008).

ASD affects quality of life beyond the societal impact. Individuals with ASD report significantly lower social and physical quality of life, and ASD was found to contribute more to family stress than other chronic conditions affecting children and adolescents such as cystic fibrosis (Bouma and Schweitzer 1990; Jennes-Coussens et al. 2006). Approximately 50 % of adults with ASD report that they have no same-age friendships and many have challenges finding and maintaining employment despite high levels of education (Gerhardt and Lainer 2011; Orsmond et al. 2004; Seltzer et al. 2003). Approximately 20 % of individuals with ASD have reported living independently or semi-independently, and 25 % reported having at least one friend (Howlin and Moss 2012). Only 14 % report a long-term intimate relationship (Gerhardt and Lainer 2011).

Despite improvements in earlier diagnosis and entry into services, social outcomes for individuals with ASD remain poor and there is emerging evidence that

A. M. Pearl (✉) · S. D. Mayes
Department of Psychiatry, Penn State College of Medicine, Hershey, PA, USA
e-mail: apearl@hmc.psu.edu

Johnny L. Matson (ed.), *Comorbid Conditions Among Children with Autism Spectrum Disorders,* Autism and Child Psychopathology Series,
DOI 10.1007/978-3-319-19183-6_3

young adults with ASD and *without* a diagnosis of ID may fare worse than those with a comorbid diagnosis of ID (Taylor and Seltzer 2011). It is likely that comorbid psychological difficulties, such as anxiety, depression, and/or disruptive behavior in childhood and adolescence, are contributing to these poor outcomes in adulthood. Therefore, it is imperative that clinicians use accurate and reliable assessment batteries when assessing for potential comorbidities in children with ASD.

Previous research has found that the majority of children with ASD meet criteria for a clinical diagnosis of at least one comorbid disorder, often disruptive behavior disorders (e.g., attention-deficit/hyperactivity disorder (ADHD), oppositional defiant disorder (ODD)), anxiety, or affective disorders (Green et al. 2000; Mattila et al. 2010). Using a modified structured interview for psychiatric disorders to assess for comorbidities in ASD, Leyfer et al. (2006) found that the median number of diagnoses for children with ASD was three. Additionally, Leyfer et al. (2006) found that while approximately 75 % met criteria for one additional diagnosis besides ASD, 52 % of these children had two additional diagnoses, and 38 % of these children had three or more disorders in addition to ASD. More recently, the Bureau of Autism Services, Pennsylvania Department of Public Welfare (2012) completed a statewide needs assessment to better understand how individuals and families were impacted by ASD. More than 3500 families and individuals responded, making it one of the most comprehensive surveys of individuals with ASD and their caregivers to date (Bureau of Autism Services, Pennsylvania Department of Public Welfare 2012). In this survey, 85 % of individuals with ASD reported having a co-occurring disorder requiring additional services.

Psychiatric comorbidities in children diagnosed with ASD are notoriously difficult to identify. In general, in comparison to adolescents and adults, children present with unique challenges are associated with the assessment of psychiatric diagnoses. Children with ASD by definition present with significant difficulties with social communication, which may make more traditional methods of assessment (e.g., clinical interview) at best difficult and at worst impossible. Additionally, children with ASD may present with deficits in theory of mind, central coherence, and executive functioning, which may hinder the assessment process (Leyfer et al. 2006).

Typically, a clinician's goal in diagnostic assessment is to determine if the presenting symptoms are clinically significant warranting a diagnosis. Second, the clinician must determine if the symptoms are not better accounted for by another diagnosis. This second goal of assessment is particularly tricky for clinicians when assessing for comorbidities in children with ASD. That is, the clinician must determine if the presenting problems are best explained by the ASD diagnosis or by a comorbid disorder above and beyond the diagnosis of ASD (DSM-5, American Psychiatric Association 2013).

There are several well-established, validated, and standardized measures to assess psychiatric symptoms in typically developing children. However, although the measures the authors summarize here have been used to assess psychopathology in children with ASD, the majority of these instruments have not yet been standardized specifically for children with ASD. To the authors' knowledge, the few assessment tools specifically designed to assess for comorbid psychiatric symptoms in children with ASD are still in their infancy (Leyfer et al. 2006; McBrien 2003).

Some of the core symptoms of ASD may overlap with or be difficult to differentiate from other comorbid psychiatric disorders. For example, it may be difficult to distinguish repetitive behaviors from compulsive behaviors within obsessive compulsive disorder (OCD), stereotypies from tic disorders, deficits in social communication from social anxiety or ADHD, and stereotyped speech, restricted interests, and/or repetitive thinking from psychotic symptoms (Zandt et al. 2007). Beyond the primary reason of assessment of getting the "right" answer, the much more salient concern for accuracy in assessment is to pave the road for accessing services, inform treatment priorities, and facilitate an accurate case conceptualization for intervention. For instance, in the examples cited above, if repetitive behaviors are diagnosed as part of the presentation of ASD or if they are diagnosed as a comorbid diagnosis of OCD in addition to the ASD diagnosis, the course of treatment should vary significantly. Although behavioral techniques may be used in both circumstances, the specific techniques will differ.

General Psychopathology

Often the first choice of assessment for a clinician is to administer a broadband assessment for general psychopathology. Broadband assessments should not be used in isolation to diagnose, but can often be a first step of screening for symptoms of psychopathology within the structure of the diagnostic and statistical manual of mental disorders (DSM) (Gadow et al. 2006). Several self- and other-report broadband questionnaires such as the Achenbach System of Empirically Based Assessment (ASEBA; Achenbach and Rescorla 2001) and the behavior assessment system for children, Second Edition (BASC-2; Reynolds 2004) have been extensively researched and applied clinically in typically developing children with a wide range of clinically significant presenting issues. Recently, some studies have found empirical support for the use of these questionnaires when assessing children with ASD using the ASEBA (Achenbach et al.1991; Decker et al. 2002; Duarte et al. 2003; Holtmann et al. 2005; Mazefsky et al. 2011) and the BASC-2 (Bellini 2004; Mahan and Matson 2011; Vickerstaff et al. 2007; Bellini 2004). One of biggest benefits of the use of these questionnaires is the ability to assess for general psychopathology from the perspective of different reports in multiple environments, including the home and school.

In addition to broadband questionnaires for psychopathology, several well-established structured and semi-structured interviews exist to screen for symptoms of clinical disorders in children. The Kiddie-SADS Present and Lifetime Version (K-SADS-PL; Kaufman et al. 1997), the diagnostic interview schedule for children (DISC-IV; Shaffer et al. 2000), and the child and adolescent psychiatric assessment (CAPA; Angold et al. 1995) have been used in empirical assessments to examine rates of comorbidities in children with ASD (Dekker et al. 2002; Gjevik et al. 2011; Masi et al. 1999; Shaffer et al. 2000; Simonoff et al. 2008).

However, only one structured assessment was revised and examined specifically within an ASD population. The K-SADS-PL was revised and renamed as autism comorbidity interview (ACI)-present/lifetime (ACI-PL; Leyfer et al. 2006) to assess for comorbid disorders specifically in children with ASD per primary caregiver report. Using the ACI-PL, Leyfer et al. (2006) found that 72 % of the children with ASD in their study met criteria for a comorbid diagnosis. Some of the specific revisions made to the K-SADS-PL in creating the ACI-PL included a section to establish the child's emotions and behaviors at baseline, descriptions of how each disorder may manifest in a child with ASD, as well as revisions to specific screening questions related to the presentation of specific symptoms (e.g., depression, anxiety, and ADHD) in children with ASD (Leyfer et al. 2006). Although, the ACI-PL is promising and has shown good reliability and validity in a community sample of children with ASD, at this time, there is no "gold standard" assessment for diagnosing comorbid psychopathology in children with ASD.

Autism diagnostic instruments with established validity and reliability that assess the core symptoms of ASD, as well as common comorbid problems (e.g., behavior problems, emotional dysregulation, sleep disturbance, feeding problems, fears, ADHD symptoms, and language problems) may be helpful in differentiating ASD from other disorders, as well as in identifying comorbid problems in a child with ASD. Such instruments include rating scales like the childhood autism rating scale (Schopler et al. 1986; Schopler et al. 2010) and parent diagnostic interview measures such as the Checklist for Autism Spectrum Disorder (Mayes 2012).

Finally, there are several instruments which have been specifically created for use with individuals with developmental disorders, but not specifically for children with ASD. These questionnaires include the Aberrant Behavior Checklist (ABC; Aman et al. 1985), the Developmental Behavior Checklist (Einfeld and Tonge 1995), the Behavior Problems Inventory (Rojahn et al. 2001), and the Anxiety, Depression, and Mood Scale (Esbensen et al. 2003). Although these measures were not specifically validated and standardized for use with children with ASD, there are several well-documented empirical examinations of the use of these instruments in children with developmental disabilities which may have included children with ASD (Clarke et al. 2003; McCracken et al. 2002; Rojahn et al. 2003).

Disruptive Behavior Disorders

Disruptive behavior disorders, which include ADHD, ODD, and conduct disorder (CD), are often the primary reason, children are referred to outpatient psychiatric clinics either by caregivers in the home or school personnel (National Research Council (NRC) 2001). This is often the case for children with ASD as well (Gadow et al. 2008; Gadow et al. 2004; Lecavalier 2006; Tonge and Einfeld 2003). The specific reason for referral for children with ASD can range from verbal or physical aggression to general noncompliance, inattention, and/or other symptoms consistent with a disruptive behavior diagnosis (de Bruin et al. 2007; Gadow et al. 2004; Gillberg 2002; Klin and Volkmar 2000). However, symptoms of disruptive behavior disorders are not part of the core feature of ASD but are to be examined to determine if a comorbid diagnosis is appropriate. Specific caution must be used in assessing for disruptive behavior disorders in children with ASD, as the presentation may differ from disruptive behavior in typically developing children.

Attention-Deficit/Hyperactivity Disorder ADHD is defined by developmentally inappropriate symptoms of inattention, impulsiveness, and/or hyperactivity that are present in multiple areas of daily life (e.g., home, school; DSM-5, American Psychiatric Association 2013). Both ASD and ADHD are neurodevelopmental disorders which affect circuits in the brain which are related to use of executive functions (e.g., working memory, planning, flexibility; Hill 2004; Willcutt et al. 2005). Prior to the most recent update to the DSM, ADHD could not be diagnosed if ASD had been given as a primary diagnosis (DSM-IV, American Psychiatric Association 2010). However, ASD and ADHD can now be dually diagnosed under the DSM-5 (American Psychiatric Association 2013). Researchers have found that approximately 25–50% of children with ASD have a comorbid diagnosis of ADHD (Gadow et al. 2004; Gjevik et al. 2011; Goldstein and Schwebach 2004; Simonoff et al. 2008; Yoshida and Uchiyama 2004). In a study of approximately 1000 referred children with ASD or ADHD, differences in maternal ratings of attention deficit, impulsivity, and hyperactivity and performance on neuropsychological tests measuring attention did not differ between the two groups (Mayes et al. 2012a). Given these rates of comorbidity, there is a clear need for accurate assessment tools to identify the presence of ADHD in ASD (Gjevik et al. 2011).

Children with ASD are frequently misdiagnosed as having ADHD (Keen and Ward 2004; Perry 1998). Differentiating between ASD, particularly individuals with less impairing ASD, and ADHD can be difficult due to similarity in symptom presentation (Barkley 1990; Clark et al. 1999). Researchers have found that in comparison to typically developing peers, children with ASD score higher on parent-report of ADHD symptoms on the Child Behavior Checklist (CBCL; ASEBA parent report) and BASC-2's attention problems subscale, hyperactivity subscale, and externalizing composite (Mahan and Matson 2011; Mazefsky et al. 2011). However, several studies have found that the core symptoms of ADHD in individuals with ASD do not present differently from individuals who have been diagnosed with ADHD only (Gadow et al. 2006; Goldstein and Schewbach 2004; Hattori et al. 2006; Luteijn et al. 2000). Additionally, the developmental trend for ADHD symptoms found in typically developing children, that is hyperactivity/impulsivity declining with age while inattention remains stable, has been found to hold in individuals with ASD (DuPaul et al. 1998; Lee and Ousley 2006; Sinzig et al. 2009; Ousley 2006).

Some children with ADHD may present with social difficulties which may be somewhat difficult to differentiate from ASD. Individuals with ADHD only have been found to present with more ASD symptoms than typically developing children (Buitelaar et al. 1999; Hattori et al. 2006; Luteijn et al. 2000; Mulligan et al. 2009; Santosh et al. 2006). These difficulties include social problems (e.g., poor social interactions, decreased social reciprocity), theory of mind deficits, and language impairments (Buitelaar et al. 1999; Clark et al. 1999; Reiersen et al. 2007; Santosh et al. 2006). Additionally, research has found that individuals with ADHD may present with stereotypies, as well as restricted and repetitive interests (Clark et al. 1999; Hattori et al. 2006).

Children with ASD often present with more significant social interaction impairments as compared to individuals with ADHD (Hattori et al. 2006; Luteijn et al. 2000). More specifically, in comparison to individuals with ADHD, individuals with ASD present with impairment in nonverbal communication used to regulate social interaction (e.g., eye contact, gestures) and may present with insistence on sameness, hyper- or hyporeactivity to sensory input, and/or restricted interests that are abnormal in focus (Anckarsater et al. 2006; Mulligan et al. 2009). Finally, in comparison to individuals with ASD, overall individuals with ADHD have been found to be more motivated to engage in social interaction (Geurts et al. 2008).

Teasing out a diagnosis of ADHD in a child with ASD is a topic of significant discussion in the current literature (Frazier et al. 2001; Gadow et al. 2006; Holtmann et al. 2005). The core question is "are the presenting symptoms of ADHD a reflection of a true comorbid diagnosis or are they evidence of the ASD diagnosis?" Even given the similarity between ADHD and ASD, there are several significant differences to be assessed that can aid in determining if a comorbid diagnosis of ADHD is warranted. Standard clinical assessment of ADHD often includes the completion of ADHD-specific questionnaires which are completed by parents, teachers, and/or other adults with knowledge of the child's behavior in various environments, as well as standardized assessments of executive functioning within a psychological test battery.

An autism diagnostic instrument that has good discriminative validity for ASD and ADHD is the Checklist for Autism Spectrum Disorder. In a study of 847 children with ASD and 158 children with ADHD, all children with ASD had a score in the autism range (mean 22), and all children with ADHD scored below the autism cutoff with a mean score of 4 (Mayes et al. 2012a). Few studies have utilized questionnaires only to attempt differential diagnosis between ASD and ADHD. Geurts et al. (2004) used the Children's Communication Checklist (Bishop 1998), while Luteijn et al. (2000) used the children behavior checklist (Achenbach 1992). Additionally, several studies examining the efficacy of treatments for ADHD (e.g., stimulants) used questionnaires measuring ADHD symptoms as outcomes suggesting possible use in children with ASD. Findings by the Research Units on Pediatric Psychopharmacology Autism Network (2005), as well as Handen et al. (2000) indicated that following pharmacological treatment for ADHD symptoms, teacher ratings on the hyperactivity subscale of the ABC (Aman et al. 1985), were sensitive to change. Handen et al. (2000) also utilized the Conners Teacher Scale Hyperactivity Index (Goyette et al. 1978) and the IOWA Conners Teacher Rating Scale (Loney and Milich 1982) aggression and hyperactivity subscales to effectively measure change in ADHD symptoms in children with ASD.

As always with the use of questionnaires to aid in diagnosis, certain items on ADHD assessments must be examined more closely than others in light of ASD. For example, "often does not seem to listen when spoken to directly," "often talks excessively," and "often interrupts or intrudes on others" may reflect deficits in social communication/interaction as opposed to inattention and/or hyperactivity/impulsivity. Specifically, reports or observations suggesting a child has deficits in the ability to listen and attend when spoke to can be indicative of a deficit in nonverbal communicative behavior *or* a symptom of inattention. Likewise, a child who talks excessively or often interrupts or intrudes on others could be better accounted for by a deficit in social–emotional reciprocity or by difficulties with hyperactivity/im pulsivity.

In addition to questionnaires, clinicians often rely on standardized psychological testing to identify deficits associated with ADHD and/or ASD, particularly assessment of executive functioning. Empirical examinations of the pattern of executive functioning deficits in children with ASD as compared to children with ADHD have identified some notable patterns in the children's cognitive profiles; unfortunately, no clear patterns of executive functioning deficits have been delineated to differentiate between ASD and ADHD. Children with ASD have been found to demonstrate deficits in flexibility (Geurts et al. 2004; Ozonoff and Jensen 1999; Sinzig et al. 2008; Jensen 1999), while there have been mixed findings on deficits in inhibition (Happé et al. 2006; Johnson et al. 2007; Nydén et al. 1999) and planning (Happé 1999; Sinzig et al. 2008). Both children with ASD and ADHD have been found to demonstrate deficits in working memory (Geurts et al. 2004; Goldberg et al. 2005; Happé 1999; Sinzig et al. 2008). More recently, Sinzig et al. (2008) found that children with ASD and ADHD were significantly more impaired on tasks measuring inhibition and flexibility. However, most of these findings have not been replicated and are likely specific to certain presentations of ASD and/or ADHD (i.e., severity of symptoms/impairment, age, intelligence).

Conduct Problems Children with ASD frequently present with symptoms of conduct problems (e.g., ODD or CD) which often is reported in terms of challenging behaviors ranging from noncompliance and tantrums to self-injury, aggression, and/or property destruction (Horner et al. 2002; Matson and Minshawi 2007). Studies report a range of 27–42% of children to have a comorbid diagnosis of ODD (de Bruin et al. 2007; Mayes et al. 2012b; Simonoff et al. 2008). When examining the presentation of ODD symptoms in children with ASD, Gadow et al. (2008) found that the clinical characteristics of ODD in children with ASD had very similar presentations in children without ASD.

On the other hand, in regards to CD, rates of comorbid CD in children with ASD have been found to be quite low ranging from 3 to 10% (de Bruin et al. 2007; Gjevik et al. 2011; Leyfer et al. 2006; Simonoff et al. 2008). It has been posited that these lower rates of CD can be attributed to children with ASD having difficulties with social communication and cognition which are directly related to behaviors displayed in children with CD (Horner et al. 2002). However, lower levels of empathy have been found to be an area of deficiency in both children with ASD and CD (Baron-Cohen and Wheelwright 2004; Decety and Moriguchi 2007; Woodworth and Waschbusch 2008). Smith's empathy imbalance theory (2006) suggests that ASD and CD can be differentiated by levels of emotional versus cognitive empathy. Specifically, children with ASD have deficits in cognitive empathy (e.g., the ability to take the perspective of others in terms of his/her emotional distress) while children with CD display deficits in emotional empathy (e.g., an individual's emotional reaction to another's emotional state). Unfortunately, there is scant empirical evidence to support this theory, although it appears promising (Jones et al. 2010).

Several empirical studies have identified higher rates of aggressive behavior as reported by others in children with ASD as compared to typically developing children (Matson et al. 2009; Matson and Nebel-Schwalm 2007; Nicholas et al. 2008). Additionally, Gjevik et al. (2011) found children with less severe ASD symptoms had higher rates of conduct problems as compared to children with higher levels of impairment. Currently, to the authors' knowledge, there are no specific questionnaires that assess conduct problems symptoms specifically in children with ASD. The Nisonger Child Behavior Rating Form (Aman et al. 1996; Tassé et al. 1996) has been used to measure conduct problems and irritability in children who are diagnosed with a developmental disability by both parents and teachers (Lecavalier et al. 2006).

Anxiety Disorders

The most common comorbid disorders for children with ASD are anxiety disorders. Estimates often range from 40 to 60 % in individuals with ASD (Gjevik et al. 2011; Leyfer et al 2006; Simonoff et al. 2008; White et al. 2009). Simonoff et al. (2008) found the most common anxiety disorders diagnosed in children with ASD which include social anxiety disorder (29 %), generalized anxiety disorder (13 %), panic disorder (10 %), and OCD (8 %). Anxiety is a frequent barrier to successful peer engagement for individuals with ASD (White et al. 2009). Many times, as children with ASD age into adolescence, they experience setbacks as a result of increasing social processing demands and newly emerging areas of concern such as anxiety.

Some studies have found higher rates of clinically significant anxiety in individuals with less severe symptoms of ASD, often times called "high functioning" (Ghaziuddin et al. 1998; Gillott et al. 2001; Kim et al. 2000). In fact, in a study of over 1000 referred children, the frequency of maternal reported anxiety did not differ significantly between children with ASD and normal intelligence and children with an anxiety disorder and no ASD, whereas children with ASD and below normal intelligence had significantly lower levels of anxiety (Mayes et al. 2011). It has been proposed that higher functioning individuals with ASD may have more insight or awareness of their disability, as by definition they are not as impaired in symptoms related to ASD such as theory of mind and perspective-taking (Kim et al. 2000; Klin et al. 2005; Kim et al. 2000). Recent work has indicated that adolescents with ASD who successfully participate in extracurricular activities with peers have more successful adult transitions, where successful adult transition is defined as community engagement (employment, postsecondary education or training, or community-based services post high school).

Traditionally, the best reporters of anxiety are the individuals themselves as symptoms of anxiety can go unnoticed by others (e.g., internal emotional distress, somatic symptoms), while caregivers and/or teachers are better reporters of behavioral symptoms of anxiety (e.g., escape). However, traditional means of anxiety assessment, particularly via self-report, in children with ASD must be interpreted with caution. Few of most commonly used measures of anxiety in typically developing children have been standardized or validated for use with children with ASD.

Social Anxiety Disorder Research has found rates of social anxiety in individuals with ASD to vary from 7 to 29 % (Gjevik et al. 2011; Leyfer et al. 2006; Muris et al. 1998; Simonoff et al. 2008). According to the DSM-5, social anxiety disorder (social phobia) is defined as fear or anxiety about social situations where the individual is exposed to possible scrutiny of others and is fearful of this perceived judgment. A salient question would be to determine if the social avoidance is to be accounted for by ASD or if it is a symptom of anxiety. Therefore, to meet criteria for social anxiety disorder, the individual must indicate anxiety related to evaluation by others. While some individuals with ASD will report being stressed or anxious in crowds, it may be better accounted for by a hyperactivity to sensory input (e.g., loud noises) as opposed to anxiety related to being viewed as incompetent by people in the crowd. However, some individuals with ASD will report significant anxiety in situations where they require interaction with or performance in front of peers or individuals in authority where a diagnosis of social anxiety disorder is appropriate.

Obsessive Compulsive Disorder Rates between 8 and 37 % for comorbid diagnoses of OCD have been found in individuals with ASD (Gjevik et al. 2011; Leyfer et al. 2006; Muris et al 1998; Simonoff et al. 2008). The majority of studies have found the rates to fall in the lower end of this range, while higher rates have been found by modifying the criteria to include the ability of others to report the presence of compulsions. OCD is defined as the presence of obsessions (i.e., recurrent and persistent thoughts, urges, or images that are unwanted and cause distress) and/or compulsions (i.e., repetitive behaviors or mental acts that are performed in response to the anxiety caused by an obsession). As mentioned previously, individuals with ASD may present with stereotyped or repetitive motor movements, use of objects, or speech that are attributed to being a core symptom of ASD. Some individuals with OCD present with good to fair insight where they recognize that these beliefs are likely not true, which will help to confirm a comorbid OCD diagnosis. However, some individuals with OCD may have poor or absent insight. When an individual presents with obsessions which lead to anxiety and behaviors/acts that engage in to reduce this anxiety, a diagnosis of comorbid OCD is likely warranted.

Repetitive motor behaviors in individuals with ASD often serve an automatic function, in that they provide the individual with reinforcing sensory input (Lovaas et al. 1987). However, some repetitive behavior in individuals with ASD may not be inherently pleasurable, and may be driven by need to maintain sameness or by anxiety. Some researchers argue that these behaviors may serve the role of reducing sensory hyperarousal or anxiety (Leekam et al. 2011). When individuals with ASD experience anxiety, they may display increased repetitive behaviors, although the same individuals may display these behaviors in response to excitement. It is not fully understood at this time the relation between the etiology of anxiety in OCD and the need for sameness in individuals with ASD (Leekman et al. 2011).

Specific Phobias Rates of specific phobias have been found to range from approximately 8–31 % in children with ASD (Gjevik et al. 2011; Simonoff et al. 2008). Gjevik et al. (2011) found that the most commonly reported specific phobia was a fear of loud noises. In a sample of 1033 children with ASD, 41 % of mothers reported that their child had unusual fears (Mayes et al. 2013a). More than half who had unusual fears had fears of mechanical things, heights, and/or weather. Many additional children had common childhood fears (e.g., dogs, bugs, and the dark). Amazingly, many of the fears reported in this sample were described in children with autism more than 70 years ago by Kanner (1943), including fear of vacuum cleaners, elevators, mechanical toys, swings, and the wind.

Anxiety-Specific Measures The Revised Children's Anxiety and Depression Scale (RCADS; Chorpita et al. 2005) has been found to be promising as a measure to assess for anxiety in children with ASD, particularly as a screener to evaluate the necessity for a full evaluation (Sterling et al. 2014).

Depression

Researchers have found relatively lower rates of general depressive disorders (1–10 %) in individuals with ASD (Gjevik et al. 2011; Simonoff et al. 2008). However, studies that have found rates in the lower end of this range, found up to 11 % of individuals with ASD who reported symptoms of depression that fell below clinical threshold (Simonoff et al. 2008). Similar rates have been found in previous studies for DSM-IV-TR diagnosis of autistic disorder (Ghaziuddin 1992), although much higher rates (30 %) were found in individuals diagnosed with Asperger's disorder (Ghaziuddin et al. 1998). The most common diagnosis found by Gjevik et al. 2011 using the Kiddie-SADS was depressive disorder not otherwise specified. The specified most common symptoms included anhedonia, irritability, anger, and apathy. Rates of bipolar disorder in ASD have been found to range from less than 2–20 % (de Bruin et al. 2007; Gjevik et al. 2011; Leyfer et al. 2006; Wozniak et al. 1997). However, the majority of research has found rates to be less than 5 %.

Children with ASD were found to have higher rates of depressive symptoms as rated by parents on the BASC-2 than same-age, typically developing children (Kim et al 2000; Mahan and Matson 2011). Among 350 children with ASD, mothers of 54 % of children with normal intelligence and 42 % with below normal intelligence reported depressed mood in their children (Mayes et al. 2011). Individuals who have more severe presentations of ASD may present with depression differently than those with less severe ASD (Matson and Nebel-Schwalm 2007).

Approximately 30 years ago, several researchers stated that depression is likely a common comorbidity missed in individuals with ASD, along with a comorbid diagnosis of (ID; formerly Mental Retardation; Kazdin et al. 1983; Matson et al. 1984). Individuals with less severe or mild ID likely present with similar symptom presentations as individuals with average intelligence, while individuals with moderate to severe ID may present with different symptom patterns. In the latter population, a clinician may need to focus more on observable behaviors associated with depression observed by others, including vegetative symptoms, along with family history (Ghaziuddin et al. 2002; Matson et al. 1999).

Suicidality In a sample of 791 children with ASD, mothers reported that 14% of the children had suicide ideation or attempts sometimes to very often, which was 28 times greater than the percentage for typical children, but less than 43% for depressed children (Mayes et al. 2013b). However, a clinician must closely assess the nature of the behavior which may or may not be indicative of suicidality. For example, given the high rate of self-injurious behavior in children with ASD, a clinician must carefully assess whether or not there is intention of death behind the observed behaviors. In the presence of comorbid depression with ASD, clinicians should regularly assess for suicidal ideation.

Miscellaneous Disorders

Tic Disorders Rates of comorbid tic disorders in individuals with ASD ranged from 11 to 22% (Canitano and Vivanti 2007; Gjevik et al. 2011; Simonoff et al. 2008).

Psychosis Few studies have empirically examined the presence of psychosis in children and adolescents with ASD. Examinations of the presence of comorbidities in large samples of ASD using semi-structured or structured diagnostic interviews have found very low rates of comorbid psychosis (Gjevik et al. 2011; Simonoff et al. 2008).

Eating Disorders Although feeding and eating problems are often found in children and adolescents with ASD (e.g., 69% have limited food preferences, Mayes and Calhoun 2011), systematic examinations of the presence of traditional eating disorders (e.g., anorexia nervosa, Bulimia Nervosa) have found very low rates of comorbidities (Schreck et al. 2004). Gjevik et al. (2011) found children with ASD to have significant difficulties with eating, but few report fear of gaining weight or binge eating followed by compensatory behaviors to prevent weight gain. However, some studies have found individuals with anorexia nervosa report symptoms of ASD (Wentz et al. 2005).

Related Psychological Problems

Sleep Disturbance Mothers of 63% of children with autism (vs. 5% in typical children) report a sleep disturbance in their children, including 60% who have trouble falling asleep, 50% who wake during the night, and 45% who wake early in the morning (Mayes 2012; Mayes and Calhoun 2009).

Learning Disabilities and Dysgraphia A study of referred children with ASD and normal intelligence found that 64 % had a learning disability in written expression (vs. 13 % in reading and 22 % in math), and that almost all had a weakness in handwriting compared with other ability scores (Mayes and Calhoun 2007). This was highly significant for 50 % of the children with ASD whose score on the developmental test of visual-motor integration (requiring them to copy geometric forms with a pencil, Beery 2010), was more than 15 points below their intelligence quotient (IQ). Because the majority of children with ASD and normal intelligence have writing problems, it is essential that a comprehensive assessment battery include not only a measure of intelligence but also measures of written expression (e.g., Wechsler Individual Achievement Test-III, Wechsler 2009) and graphomotor skills (e.g., Developmental Test of Visual-Motor Integration, Beery 2010).

Sources of Information for Assessment

Traditionally, primary caregivers of children with ASD are the principal sources of information gathered by a clinician during a clinical assessment. These individuals, often mothers and/or fathers, as well as extended family members including siblings, are usually privy to an individual's behavior in multiple contexts over an extended period of time. Gathering this information can give a clinician salient information about the pervasiveness of symptoms across contexts, as well as the ebb and flow of symptoms over time. Traditionally, the best reporters of disruptive behavior disorders are caregivers and/or school personnel who have regular contact with the child, as symptoms of these comorbid disorders are often manifested behaviorally.

Conclusion

In general, the rules of gold standard clinical assessments hold, and are perhaps even more salient, for assessing comorbidities in children with ASD. That is, a clinician will likely need information from multiple reporters who know the child's typical behavior in multiple environments over an extended period of time. Finally, the clinician will likely need to capitalize on multiple assessment techniques including self- and other-report (i.e., questionnaires), semi- and/or structured interviews, as well as observation of either past (i.e., via home movies, etc.) or present behavior.

Accurate diagnosis of comorbidities in children with ASD will have several benefits. In regards to efficiency and effectiveness of treatment, targeted interventions for comorbidities will result in greater improvement in functioning as opposed to general, nonspecific treatment (Leyfer et al. 2006). It is imperative that comorbid diagnoses are accurately identified and incorporated in the case conceptualization for clinical treatment of children with ASD. Additionally, comorbid mental health diagnoses for children with ASD may result in the ability to access additional services.

The unmet need for mental health services substantially increases as individuals age due to both increasing need for and lack of services. Lack of access to well-qualified professionals with experience addressing the needs of individuals with ASD was often highlighted as a barrier to obtaining needed services in the Pennsylvania Department of Public Welfare Bureau of Autism Services (2012) statewide survey. As a result of these unmet needs, individuals with ASD are more likely to experience an unwanted outcome such as police contact (16.3 % of adults) or inpatient psychiatric hospitalization (7.6 % of adolescents), as they age. Therefore, although there are the beginnings of an empirical base for assessing comorbidities in ASD, there is significantly more work that needs to be done in order to increase sensitivity and specificity in this area of assessment.

References

Achenbach, T. M. (1992). *Child Behavior Checklist*. Burlington, VT: Department of Psychiatry, University of Vermont.

Achenbach, T. M., & Rescorla, L. (2001). *ASEBA school-age forms and profiles*. Burlington, VT: ASEBA.

Achenbach, T. M., Howell, C. T., Quay, H. C., Conners, C. K., & Bates, J. E. (1991). National survey of problems and competencies among four- to sixteen-year-olds: Parents' reports for normative and clinical samples. *Monographs of the Society for Research in Child Development*, 56(3), i—130.

Aman, M. G., Singh, N. N., Stewart, A. W., & Field, C. J. (1985). The Aberrant Behavior Checklist: A behavior rating scale for the assessment of treatment effects. *American Journal of Mental Deficiencies, 89*(5), 485–491.

Aman, M. G., Tassé, M. J., Rojahn, J., & Hammer, D. (1996). The Nisonger CBRF: A child behavior rating form for children with developmental disabilities. *Research in Developmental Disabilities, 17*(1), 41–57.

American Psychiatric Association. (2010). *Diagnostic and statistical manual of mental disorders* (4th ed.TR). Arlington, VA: American Psychiatric Publishing.

American Psychiatric Association. (2013). *Diagnostic and statistical manual of mental disorders* (5th ed.). Arlington: American Psychiatric Publishing.

Anckarsater, H., Stahlberg, O., Larson, T., Hakansson, C., Jutblad, S. B., Niklasson, L., et al. (2006). The impact of ADHD and autism spectrum disorders on temperament, character, and personality development. *American Journal of Psychiatry, 163*(7), 1239–1244.

Angold, A., Prendergast, M., Cox, A., Harrington, R. C., Simonoff, R., & Rutter, M. (1995). The child and adolescent psychiatric assessment (CAPA). *Psychological Medicine, 25,* 739–753.

Barkley, R. A. (1990). *Attention deficit hyperactivity disorder: A handbook for diagnosis and treatment*. New York: Guilford Press.

Baron-Cohen, S., & Wheelwright, S. (2004). The empathy quotient: An investigation of adults with Asperger Syndrome or high functioning autism, and normal sex differences. *Journal of Autism and Developmental Disorders, 34*(2), 163–175.

Beery, K. E., & Beery, N. A. (2010). *Developmental test of visual-motor integration* (6th edn.). San Antonio: Pearson.

Bellini, S. (2004). Social skills deficits and anxiety in high-functioning adolescents with autism spectrum disorders. *Focus on Autism and Other Developmental Disabilities, 19*(2), 78–86.

Bishop, D. V. (1998). Development of the Children's Communication Checklist (CCC): A method for assessing qualitative aspects of communicative impairment in children. *Journal of Child Psychology and Psychiatry, 39*(6), 879–891.

Bouma, R., & Schweitzer, R. (1990). The impact of chronic childhood illness on family stress: A comparison between autism and cystic fibrosis. *Journal of Clinical Psychology, 46*(6), 722–730.

Buitelaar, J. K., Van Der Wees, M., Swaab-Barneveld, H., & Van Der Gaag, R. J. (1999). Theory of mind and emotion-recognition functioning in autistic spectrum disorders and in psychiatric control and normal children. *Development and Psychopathology, 11*(1), 39–58.

Bureau of Autism Services, Pennsylvania Department of Public Welfare. (2012). Pennsylvania autism needs assessment: A survey of individuals and families living with autism: Statewide summary. http://www.paautism.org/asert/Needs%20Assess_Stateswide%20Summary%20May%20202012.pdf. Accessed 26 june 2015

Canitano, R., & Vivanti, G. (2007). Tics and tourette syndrome in autism spectrum disorders. *Autism: The International Journal of Research and Practice, 11*(1), 19–28.

Centers for Disease Control and Prevention. (2014). Prevalence of autism spectrum disorder among children aged 8 years—autism and developmental disabilities monitoring network, 11 sites, United States, 2010. *MMWR Surveillance Summaries, 63*(SS02), 1–21.

Chorpita, B. F., Moffitt, C. E., & Gray, J. (2005). Psychometric properties of the revised child anxiety and depression scale in a clinical sample. *Behavior Research and Therapy, 43*(3), 309–322.

Clark, T., Feehan, C., Tinline, C., & Vostanis, P. (1999). Autistic symptoms in children with attention-deficit/hyperactivity disorder. *European Child & Adolescent Psychiatry, 8*(1), 50–55.

Clarke, A. R., Tonge, B. J., Einfeld, S. L., & Mackinnon, A. (2003). Assessment of change with the developmental behavior checklist. *Journal of Intellectual Disability Research, 47*(3), 210–212.

de Bruin, E. I., Ferdinand, R. F., Meester, S., de Nijs, P. F., & Verheij, F. (2007). High rates of psychiatric co-morbidity in PDD—NOS. *Journal of Autism and Developmental Disorders, 37*(5), 877–886.

Decety, J., & Moriguchi, Y. (2007). The empathic brain and its dysfunction in psychiatric populations: Implications for intervention across different clinical conditions. *BioPsychoSocial Medicine, 1*(1), 22.

Dekker, M. C., Koot, H. M., Van der Ende, J. V. D., & Verhulst, F. C. (2002). Emotional and behavioral problems in children and adolescents with and without intellectual disability. *Journal of Child Psychology and Psychiatry, 43*(8), 1087–1098.

Duarte, C. S., Bordin, I. A., DeOliveira, A., & Bird, H. (2003). The CBCL and the identification of children with autism and related conditions in Brazil: Pilot findings. *Journal of Autism and Developmental Disorders, 33*(6), 703–707.

DuPaul, G. J., Power, T. J., Anastopoulos, A. D., & Reid, R. (1998). *ADHD Rating Scale-IV: Checklists, norms, and clinical interpretation.* New York: Guilford Press.

Einfeld, S. L., & Tonge, B. J. (1995). The developmental behavior checklist: The development and validation of an instrument to assess behavioral and emotional disturbance in children and adolescents with mental retardation. *Journal of Autism and Developmental Disorders, 25*(2), 81–104.

Esbensen, A. J., Rojahn, J., Aman, M. G., & Ruedrich, S. (2003). Reliability and validity of an assessment instrument for anxiety, depression, and mood among individuals with mental retardation. *Journal of Autism and Developmental Disorders, 33*(6), 617–629.

Frazier, J. A., Biederman, J., Bellordre, C. A., Garfield, S. B., Geller, D. A., Coffey, B. J., et al. (2001). Should the diagnosis of attention-deficit/hyperactivity disorder be considered in children with pervasive developmental disorder? *Journal of Attention Disorders, 4*(4), 203–211.

Gadow, K. D., DeVincent, C. J., Pomeroy, J., & Azizian, A. (2004). Comparison of DSM-IV symptoms in elementary school-age children with PDD versus clinic and community samples. *Autism: The International Journal of Research and Practice, 9*(4), 392–415.

Gadow, K. D., DeVincent, C. J., & Pomeroy, J. (2006). ADHD symptom subtypes in children with pervasive developmental disorder. *Journal of Autism and Developmental Disorders, 36*(2), 271–283.

Gadow, K. D., DeVincent, C. J., & Drabick, D. A. (2008). Oppositional defiant disorder as a clinical phenotype in children with autism spectrum disorder. *Journal of Autism and Developmental Disorders, 28*(7), 1302–1310.

Ganz, M. L. (2007). The lifetime distribution of the incremental societal costs of autism. *Archives of Pediatric and Adolescent Medicine,* 161(4), 343–349.

Gerhardt, P. F., & Lainer, I. (2011). Addressing the needs of adolescents and adults with autism: A crisis on the horizon. *Journal of Contemporary Psychotherapy, 41,* 37–45.

Geurts, H. M., Verté, S., Oosterlaan, J., Roeyers, H., & Sergeant, J. A. (2004). How specific are executive functioning deficits in attention deficit hyperactivity disorder and autism? *Journal of Child Psychology and Psychiatry, 45*(4), 836–854.

Geurts, H. M., Grasman, R. P., Verté, S., Oosterlaan, J., Roeyers, H., van Kammen, S. M., et al. (2008). Intra-individual variability in ADHD, autism spectrum disorders and Tourette's syndrome. *Neuropsychologia, 46*(13), 3030–3041.

Ghaziuddin, M., Tsai, L. Y., & Ghaziuddin, N. (1992). Brief report: A comparison of the diagnostic criteria for Asperger syndrome. *Journal of Autism and Developmental Disorders, 22*(4), 543–649.

Ghaziuddin, M., Weidmer-Mikhail, E., & Ghaziuddin, N. (1998). Comorbidity of Asperger syndrome: A preliminary report. *Journal of Intellectual Disability Research, 4,* 279–283.

Ghaziuddin, M., Ghaziuddin, N., & Greden, J. (2002). Depression in persons with autism: Implications for research and clinical care. *Journal of Autism and Developmental Disorders, 32,* 299–306.

Gillberg, C. (2002). *A guide to asperger syndrome*. Cambridge: Cambridge.

Gillberg, C., Billstedt, E., Sundh, V., & Gillberg, I. C. (2010). Mortality in autism: A prospective longitudinal community-based study. *Journal of Autism and Developmental Disorders, 40*(3), 352–357.

Gillott, A., Furniss, F., & Walter, A. (2001). Anxiety in high-functioning children with autism. *Autism: The International Journal of Research and Practice, 5*(3), 277–286.

Gjevik, E., Eldevik, S., Fjæran-Granum , T., & Sponheim, E. (2011). Kiddie-SADS reveals high rates of DSM-IV disorders in children and adolescents with autism spectrum disorders. *Journal of Autism and Developmental Disorders, 41*(6), 761–769.

Goldberg, H. M., Mostowsky, S. H., Cutting, L. E., Mahone, E. M., Astor, B. C., Denckla, M. B., et al. (2005). Subtle executive impairment in children with autism and children with ADHD. *Journal of Autism and Developmental Disorders, 35,* 279–293.

Goldstein, S., & Schwebach, A. J. (2004). The comorbidity of pervasive developmental disorder and attention deficit hyperactivity disorder: Results of a retrospective chart review. *Journal of Autism and Developmental Disorders, 34*(3), 329–339.

Goyette, C. H., Conners, C. K., & Ulrich, R. F. (1978). Normative data on revised Conners parent and teacher rating scales. *Journal of Abnormal Child Psychology, 6*(2), 221–236.

Green, J., Gilchrist, A., Burton, D., & Cox, A. (2000). Social and psychiatric functioning in adolescents with asperger syndrome compared with conduct disorder. *Journal of Autism and Developmental Disorders, 30*(4), 279–293.

Handen, B. L., Johnson, C. R., & Lubetsky, M. (2000). Efficacy of methylphenidate among children with autism and symptoms of attention-deficit hyperactivity disorder. *Journal of Autism and Developmental Disorders, 30*(3), 245–255.

Happé, F. (1999). Autism: Cognitive deficit or cognitive style? *Trends in Cognitive Sciences, 3*(6), 216–222.

Happé, F., Booth, R., Charlton, R., & Hughes, C. (2006). Executive function deficits in autism spectrum disorders and attention-deficit/hyperactivity disorder: Examining profiles across domains and ages. *Brain and Cognition, 61*(1), 25–39.

Hattori, J., Ogino, T., Abiru, K., Nakano, K., Oka, M., & Ohtsuka, Y. (2006). Are pervasive developmental disorders and attention-deficit/hyperactivity disorder distinct disorders? *Brain and Development, 28*(6), 371–374.

Hill, E. L. (2004). Executive dysfunction in autism. *Trends in Cognitive Sciences, 8*(1), 26–32.

Holtmann, M., Bolte, S., & Poutska, F. (2005). Attention-deficit/hyperactivity disorder symptoms in pervasive developmental disorders: Association with autistic behavior domains and coexisting psychopathology. *Psychopathology, 40,* 172–177.

Horner, R. H., Carr, E. G., Strain, P. S., Todd, A. W., & Reed, H. K. (2002). Problem behavior interventions for young children with autism: A research synthesis. *Journal of Autism and Developmental Disorders, 32*(5), 423–446.

Howlin, P., & Moss, P. (2012). Adults with autism spectrum disorders. *The Canadian Journal of Psychiatry/La Revue Canadienne De Psychiatrie, 57*(5), 275–283.

Jennes-Coussens, M., Magill-Evans, J., & Koning, C. (2006). The quality of life of young men with Asperger Syndrome: A brief report. *Autism: The International Journal of Research and Practice, 10*(4), 403–414.

Johnson, K. A., Robertson, I. H., Kelly, S. P., Silk, T. J., Barry, E., Dáibhis, A., Watchorn, A., et al. (2007). Dissociation in performance of children with ADHD and high-functioning autism on a task of sustained attention. *Neuropsychologia, 45*(10), 2234–2245.

Jones, A. P., Happé, F. G., Gilbert, F., Burnett, S., & Viding, E. (2010). Feeling, caring, knowing: Different types of empathy deficit in boys with psychopathic tendencies and autism spectrum disorder. *Journal of Child Psychology and Psychiatry, 51*(11), 1188–1197.

Kanner, L. (1943). Autistic disturbances of affective contact. *Nervous Child, 2,* 217–250.

Kaufman, J., Birmaher, E., Brent, D., Rao, U., Flynn, C., Moreci, P., et al. (1997). Schedule for affective disorders and schizophrenia for school-age children-present and lifetime version (K-SADS-PL): Initial reliability and validity data. *Journal of the American Academy for Child and Adolescent Psychiatry, 36*(7), 980–988.

Kazdin, A. E., Matson, J. L., & Senatore, V. (1983). Assessment of depression in mentally retarded adults. *American Journal of Psychiatry, 140*(8), 1040–1043.

Keen, D., & Ward, S. (2004). Autism spectrum disorder: A child population profile. *Autism: The International Journal of Research and Practice, 8*(1), 39–48.

Kim, J. A., Szatmari, P., Bryson, S. E., Steiner, D. L., & Wilson, F. J. (2000). The prevalence of anxiety and mood problems among children with autism and asperger syndrome. *Autism: The International Journal of Research and Practice, 4*(2), 117–132.

Klin, A., & Volkman, F. R. (2000). Treatment and intervention guidelines for individuals with asperger syndrome. In A. Klin, F. R. Volkmar, & S. S. Sparrow (Eds.), *Asperger syndrome*. New York: Guilford Press.

Klin, A., McPartland, J., & Volkmar, F. R. (2005). Asperger syndrome. *Handbook of Autism and Pervasive Developmental Disorders, 1,* 88–125.

Lecavalier, L. (2006). Behavioral and emotional problems in young people with pervasive developmental disorders: Relative prevalence, effects of subject characteristics, and empirical classification. *Journal of Autism and Developmental Disorders, 26*(8), 1101–1114.

Lecavalier, L., Leone, S., & Wiltz, J. (2006). The impact of behavior problems on caregiver stress in young people with autism spectrum disorders. *Journal of Intellectual Disability Research, 50*(3), 172–183.

Lee, D. O., & Ousley, O. Y. (2006). Attention-deficit hyperactivity disorder symptoms in a clinic sample of children and adolescents with pervasive developmental disorders. *Journal of Child and Adolescent Psychopharmacology, 16*(6), 737–746.

Leekam, S. R., Prior, M. R., & Uljarevic, M. (2011). Restricted and repetitive behaviors in autism spectrum disorders: A review of research in the last decade. *Psychological Bulletin, 137*(4), 562.

Leyfer, O. T., Folstein, S. E., Bacalman, S., Davis, N. O., Dinh, E., Morgan, J., et al. (2006). Comorbid psychiatric disorders in children with autism: Interview development and rates of disorders. *Journal of Autism and Developmental Disorders, 36*(7), 849–861.

Loney, J., & Milich, R. (1982). Hyperactivity, inattention, and aggression in clinical practice. In M. Wolraich & D. K. Routh (Eds.), *Advances in developmental and behavioral pediatrics*. Greenwich: JAI Press.

Lovaas, I., Newsom, C., & Hickman, C. (1987). Self-stimulatory behavior and perceptual reinforcement. *Journal of Applied Behavior Analysis, 20*(1), 45–68.

Luteijn, E. F., Serra, M., Jackson, S., Steenhuis, M. P., Althaus, M., Volkman, F., et al. (2000). How unspecified are disorders of children with a pervasive developmental disorder not otherwise specified? A study of social problems in children with PDD-NOS and ADHD. *European Child and Adolescent Psychiatry, 9*(3), 168–179.

Mahan, S., & Matson, J. L. (2011). Children and adolescents with autism spectrum disorders compared to typically developing controls on the behavioral assessment system for children, second edition (BASC-2). *Research in Autism Spectrum Disorders, 5*(1), 119–125.

Mandell, D. (2012). Autism costs nation $ 126 billion annually. *Education Daily,* 45(64), 4.

Masi, G., Mucci, M., Favilla, L., Romano, R., & Poli, P. (1999). Symptomatology and comorbidity of generalized anxiety disorder in children and adolescents. *Comprehensive Psychiatry, 40*(3), 210–215.

Matson, J. L., & Minshawi, N. F. (2007a). Functional assessment of challenging behavior: Toward a strategy for applied settings. *Research in Developmental Disabilities, 28*(4), 353–361.

Matson, J. L., & Nebel-Schwalm, M. S. (2007b). Comorbid psychopathology with autism spectrum disorder in children: An overview. *Research in Developmental Disabilities, 28*(4), 341–352.

Matson, J. L., Kazdin, A. E., & Senatore, V. (1984). Psychometric properties of the psychopathology instrument for mentally retarded adults. *Applied Research in Mental Retardation, 5*(1), 81–89.

Matson, J. L., Rush, K. S., Smiroldo, B. B., Hamilton, M., Anderson, S. J., Baglio, C. S., et al. (1999). Characteristics of depression as assessed by the diagnostic assessment for the severely handicapped II (DASH-II). *Research in Developmental Disabilities, 20,* 305–313.

Matson, J. L., Boisjoli, J., Rojahn, J., & Hess, J. (2009). A factor analysis of challenging behaviors assessed with the baby and infant screen for children with autism traits. *Research in Autism Spectrum Disorders, 3*(3), 714–722.

Mattila, M., Hurtig, T., Haapsamo, H., Jussila, K., Kuusikko-Gauffin, S., Keilinen, M., et al. (2010). Comorbid psychiatric disorders associated with asperger syndrome/high-functioning autism: A community and clinic-based study. *Journal of Autism and Developmental Disorders, 40*(9), 1080–1093.

Mayes, S. D. (2012). *Checklist for autism spectrum disorder*. Wood Dale: Stoelting.

Mayes, S.D., & Calhoun, S.L. (2007). Learning, attention, writing, and processing speed in typical children and children with ADHD, autism, anxiety, depression, and oppositional-defiant disorder. *Child Neuropsychology, 13,* 469–493.

Mayes, S. D., & Calhoun, S. L. (2009). Variables related to sleep problems in children with autism. *Research in Autism Spectrum Disorders, 3,* 931–941.

Mayes, S. D., & Calhoun, S. L. (2011). Impact of IQ, age, SES, gender, and race on autistic symptoms. *Research in Autism Spectrum Disorders, 5,* 749–757.

Mayes, S. D., Calhoun, S. L., Murray, M. J., Ahuja, M., & Smith, L. A. (2011). Anxiety, depression, and irritability in children with autism relative to children with other neuropsychiatric disorders and typical development. *Research in Autism Spectrum Disorders, 5,* 474–485.

Mayes, S. D., Calhoun, S. L., Mayes, R. D., & Molitoris, S. (2012a). Autism and ADHD: Overlapping and discriminating symptoms. *Research in Autism Spectrum Disorders, 6,* 277–285.

Mayes, S. D., Calhoun, S. L., Aggarwal, R., Baker, C., Mathapati, S., Anderson, R., et al. (2012b). Explosive, oppositional, and aggressive behavior in children with autism compared to other clinical disorders and typical development. *Research in Autism Spectrum Disorders, 6,* 1–10.

Mayes, S. D., Calhoun, S. L., Aggarwal, R., Baker, C., Mathapati, S., Molitoris, S., et al. (2013a). Unusual fears in children with autism. *Research in Autism Spectrum Disorders, 7,* 151–158.

Mayes, S. D., Gorman, A. A., Hillwig-Garcia, J., & Syed, E. (2013b). Suicide ideation and attempts in children with autism. *Research in Autism Spectrum Disorders, 7,* 109–119.

Mazefsky, C. A., Anderson, R., Conner, C. M., & Minshew, N. (2011). Child Behavior Checklist scores for school-aged children with autism: Preliminary evidence of patterns suggesting the need for referral. *Journal of Psychopathology and Behavioral Assessment, 33*(1), 31–37.

McBrien, J. A. (2003). Assessment and diagnosis of depression in people with intellectual disability. *Journal of Intellectual Disability Research, 47*(1), 1–13.

McCracken, J. T., McGough, J., Shah, B., Cronin, P., Hong, D., Aman, M. G., et al. (2002). Risperidone in children with autism and serious behavior problems. *New England Journal of Medicine, 347,* 314–321.

Mouridsen, S. E., Bronnum-Hansen, H., Rich, B., & Isager, T. (2008). Mortality and causes of death in autism spectrum disorders: An update. *Autism: The International Journal of Research and Practice, 12*(4), 403–414.

Mulligan, A., Anney, R. J., O'Regan, M., Chen, W., Butler, L., Fitzgerald, M., Buitelaar, J. K., et al. (2009). Autism symptoms in attention-deficit/hyperactivity disorder: A familiar trait which correlates with conduct, oppositional defiant, language and motor disorders. *Journal of Autism and Developmental Disorders, 39*(2), 197–209.

Muris, P., Steerneman, P., Merckelbach, H., Holdrinet, I., & Meesters, C. (1998). Comorbid anxiety symptoms in children with pervasive developmental disorders. *Journal of Anxiety Disorders, 12*(4), 387–393.

National Research Council. (2001). *Educating children with autism*. Washington, DC: National Academy Press.

Nicholas, J. S., Charles, J. M., Carpenter, L. A., King, L. B., Jenner, W., & Spratt, E. G. (2008). Prevalence and characteristics of children with autism-spectrum disorders. *Annals of Epidemiology, 18*(2), 130–136.

Nydén, A., Gillberg, C., Hjelmquist, E., & Heiman, M. (1999). Executive function/attention deficits in boys with Asperger's Syndrome, attention disorder and reading/writing disorder. *Autism: The International Journal of Research and Practice, 3*(3), 213–228.

Orsmond, G. I., Krauss, M. W., & Seltzer, M. M. (2004). Peer relationships and social and recreational activities among adolescents and adults with autism. *Journal of Autism and Developmental Disorders, 34*(3), 245–256.

Ozonoff, S., & Jensen, J. (1999). Brief report: Specific executive function profiles in three neurodevelopmental disorders. *Journal of Autism and Developmental Disorders, 29*(2), 171–177.

Perry, R. (1998). Misdiagnosed ADD/ADHD: Rediagnosed PDD. *Journal of the American Academy of Child and Adolescent Psychiatry, 37*(1), 113–114.

Reiersen, A. M., Constantino, J. N., Volk, H. E., & Todd, R. D. (2007). Autistic traits in a population-based ADHD twin sample. *Journal of Child Psychology and Psychiatry, 48*(5), 464–472.

Research Units on Pediatric Psychopharmacology Autism Network. (2005). Risperidone treatment of autistic disorder: Longer-term benefits and blinded discontinuation after 6 months. *American Journal of Psychiatry, 162,* 1361–1369.

Reynolds, C. R. (2004). *Behavior assessment system for children*. New York: Wiley.

Rojahn, J., Matson, J. L., Lott, D., Esbensen, A. J., & Smalls, Y. (2001). The behavior problems inventory: An instrument for the assessment of self-injury, stereotyped behavior, and aggression/destruction in individuals with developmental disabilities. *Journal of Autism and Developmental Disorders, 31*(6), 577–588.

Rojahn, J., Aman, M. G., Matson, J. L., & Mayville, E. (2003). The aberrant behavior checklist and the behavior problems inventory: Convergent and divergent validity. *Research in Developmental Disabilities, 24*(5), 391–404.

Santosh, P. J., Baird, G., Pityaratstian, N., Tavare, E., & Gringas, P. (2006). Impact of comorbid autism spectrum disorders on stimulant response in children with attention deficit hyperactivity disorder: A retrospective and prospective effectiveness study. *Child: Care, Health, and. Development, 32*(5), 575–583.

Schopler, E., Reichler, R. J., & Renner, B. R. (1986). *The childhood autism rating scale* (*CARS*). Los Angeles: Western Psychological Services.

Schopler, E., Van Bourgondien, M. E., Wellman, G. J., & Love, S. R. (2010). *The childhood autism rating scale, second edition* (*CARS2*). Los Angeles: WesternPsychological Services.

Schreck, K. A., Williams, K., & Smith, A. F. (2004). A comparison of eating behaviors between children with and without autism. *Journal of Autism and Developmental Disorders, 34*(4), 433–438.

Seltzer, M. M., Krauss, M. W., Shattuck, P. T., Orsmond, G., Swe, A., & Lord, C. (2003). The symptoms of autism spectrum disorders in adolescence and adulthood. *Journal of Autism and Developmental Disorders, 33*(6), 565–581.

Shaffer, D., Fisher, P., Lucas, C. P., Dulcan, M. K., & Schwab-Stone, M. E. (2000). NIMH Diagnostic interview schedule for children version IV (NIMH DISC-IV): Description, differences from previous versions, and reliability of some common diagnoses. *Journal of the American Academy of Child and Adolescent Psychiatry, 39*(1), 28–38.

Simonoff, E., Pickles, A., Charman, T., Chandler, S., Loucas, T., & Baird, G. (2008). Psychiatric disorders in children with autism spectrum disorders: Prevalence, comorbidity, and associated factors in a population-derived sample. *Journal of the American Academy of Child and Adolescent Psychiatry, 47*(8), 921–929.

Sinzig, J., Morsch, D., Bruning, N., Schmidt, M. H., & Lehmkuhl, G. (2008). Inhibition, flexibility, working memory and planning in autism spectrum disorders with and without comorbid ADHD symptoms. *Child and Adolescent Psychiatry and Mental Health, 2*(1), 4.

Sinzig, J., Walter, D., & Doepfner, M. (2009). Attention deficit/hyperactivity disorder in children and adolescents with autism spectrum disorder: Symptom or syndrome? *Journal of Attention Disorders, 13*(2), 117–126.

Smith, A. (2006). Cognitive empathy and emotional empathy in human behavior and evolution. *Psychological Record, 56*(1), 3.

Sterling, L., Renno, P., Storch, E. A., Ehrenreich-May, J., Lewin, A. B., Arnold, E., et al. (2014). Validity of the revised children's anxiety and depression scale for youth with autism spectrum disorders. *Autism: The International Journal of Research and Practice*. doi:10.1177/1362361313510066.

Tassé, M. J., Aman, M. G., Hammer, D., & Rojahn, J. (1996). The nisonger child behavior rating form: Age and gender effects and norms. *Research in Developmental Disabilities, 17*(1), 59–75.

Taylor, J. L., & Seltzer, M. M. (2011). Employment and postsecondary educational activities for young adults with autism spectrum disorders during the transition to adulthood. *Journal of Autism and Developmental Disorders, 41*(5), 566–574.

Tonge, B. J., & Einfeld, S. L. (2003). Psychopathology and intellectual disability: The Australian child to adult longitudinal study. *International Review of Research in Mental Retardation, 26,* 61–91.

Vickerstaff, S., Heriot, S., Wong, M., Lopes, A., & Dossetor, D. (2007). Intellectual ability, self-perceived social competence, and depressive symptomatology with children with high-functioning autistic spectrum disorders. *Journal of Autism and Developmental Disorders, 37,* 1647–1664.

Wechsler, D. (2009). *Wechsler individual achievement test* (3rd ed.). San Antonio: Pearson.

Wentz, E., Lacey, J.H., Waller, G., Råstam, M., Turk, J., & Gillberg, C. (2005). Childhood onset neuropsychiatric disorders in adult eating disorder patients. *European Child and Adolescent Psychiatry, 14*(8), 431–437.

White, S. W., Oswald, D., Ollendick, T., & Scahill, L. (2009). Anxiety in children and adolescents with autism spectrum disorders. *Clinical Psychology Review, 29*(3), 216–229.

Willcutt, E. G., Doyle, A. E., Nigg, J. T., Faraone, S. V., & Pennington, B. F. (2005). Validity of the executive function theory of attention-deficit/hyperactivity disorder: A meta-analytic review. *Biological Psychiatry, 57*(11), 1336–1346.

Woodworth, M., & Waschbusch, D. (2008). Emotional processing in children with conduct problems and callous/unemotional traits. *Child: Care, Health, and Development, 32*(2), 234–244.

Wozniak, J., Biederman, J., Faranoe, S. V., Frazier, J., Kim, J., Millstein, R., et al. (1997). Mania in children with pervasive developmental disorder revisited. *Journal of the American Academy of Child and Adolescent Psychiatry, 36*(11), 1552–1559.

Yoshida, Y., & Uchiyama, T. (2004). The clinical necessity for assessing attention deficit/hyperactivity disorder (AD/HD) symptoms in children with high-functioning pervasive developmental disorder (PDD). *European Child and Adolescent Psychiatry, 13*(5), 307–314.

Zandt, F., Prior, M., & Kyrios, M. (2007). Repetitive behavior in children with high functioning autism and obsessive compulsive disorder. *Journal of Autism and Developmental Disabilities, 37*(2), 251–259.

Chapter 4
Methods and Procedures for Measuring Comorbid Disorders: Medical

Paige Cervantes and Jina Jang

Autism spectrum disorder (ASD) is characterized by social communication impairments and the presence of restricted, repetitive behaviors (RRBs; Fodstad et al. 2009; Matson et al. 2009). Additionally, individuals with ASD often experience a range of comorbid symptoms. For example, rates of co-occurring psychopathology in individuals with ASD have been estimated as high as 70 % (Simonoff et al. 2008). Several medical conditions, such as gastrointestinal (GI) conditions, cerebral palsy (CP), and intellectual disabilities (ID), have been suggested to occur at high rates with ASD as well. However, prevalence estimates of these medical conditions in the ASD population have varied widely within the research (Bauman 2010).

Variance in research findings may be due to the complexity of medical assessment for individuals with ASD. Contributing to this complexity are pervasive communication and socialization impairments, challenging behaviors, high distractibility, motivational deficits, and sensory impairments in the recognition or localization of pain (Bauman 2010; Coury et al. 2012; Koegel et al. 1997; Mannion and Leader 2014; Ozonoff et al. 2005). Additionally, individuals with ASD may not present with the same symptom profile that medical professionals use to identify conditions in individuals with typical development (Bauman 2010). For example, a sudden exacerbation of ASD symptomology (e.g., RRBs) and/or challenging behaviors (e.g., aggression) may signal an underlying medical condition (Bauman 2010).

Though medical evaluation may be challenging, it is imperative that service providers and medical professionals ensure appropriate assessment and diagnostic procedures when working with clients with ASD. Recognition of medical comorbidities would inform treatment planning and medical management and thus, results in improved health status, more effective educational and intervention programs, and a better quality of life (Bauman 2010; Mannion and Leader 2014).

P. Cervantes (✉) · J. Jang
Department of Psychology, Louisiana State University, Baton Rouge, LA, USA
e-mail: pcerva2@tigers.lsu.edu

Johnny L. Matson (ed.), *Comorbid Conditions Among Children with Autism Spectrum Disorders,* Autism and Child Psychopathology Series,
DOI 10.1007/978-3-319-19183-6_4

Increased accurate identification of medical conditions in individuals with ASD may also help to inform researchers about the biological and genetic nature of ASD. Researchers anticipate that medical conditions relating to specific organ systems may help to identify unique phenotypic and genetic subgroups of ASD. Although this topic warrants a great deal of additional research, identifying subtypes of ASD would result in a better understanding of the etiological and biological factors involved in ASD (Bauman 2010; Gorrindo et al. 2012).

The rate of medical comorbidities in individuals with ASD has been the subject of debate; however, it is presumed that individuals with ASD experience many of the same medical conditions at the same or higher rates than individuals with typical development (Bauman 2010). Individuals with ASD often present several complications to the assessment process. Therefore, clinicians and physicians working with individuals with ASD should be aware of assessment challenges as well as several considerations for mediating those challenges (Bauman 2010). This chapter will work to provide an overview of methods and procedures used to measure medical problems in individuals with ASD. Further, several considerations for the evaluation of GI problems, CP, and ID are discussed.

Gastrointestinal (GI) Problems in ASD

The pervasiveness of GI problems within the ASD population is largely debated. The research methodology in available GI studies is often flawed (Erickson et al. 2005; Myers and Johnson 2007). Sound conclusions are difficult to deduce due to differences in populations being studied and in how data are collected (e.g., medical records review, clinical evaluation by physicians, and parent-report questionnaires), variations in operational definitions for GI problems, and frequent lack of comparison groups (Erickson et al. 2005; Gorrindo et al. 2012; Mannion and Leader 2014). As such, prevalence estimates range extensively from 9 to 91 % of the ASD population experiencing GI dysfunction (Coury et al. 2012; Kral et al. 2013; Mannion and Leader 2014; Myers and Johnson 2007).

Due to conflicting research findings and aforementioned flawed methodology, it is unclear whether GI problems are more common in individuals with ASD (Coury et al. 2012). However, it can be assumed that GI symptoms and conditions are at least as prevalent as in the general population with a possibility of higher rates of GI problems within the ASD population (Coury et al. 2012; Myers and Johnson 2007; Valicenti-McDermott et al. 2006). GI problems, such as chronic constipation, diarrhea, and abdominal pain, are a major source of pain and discomfort. Individuals with ASD are often deficient in or lack the communication skills necessary to express their symptoms or feelings of pain to caregivers or healthcare providers (Coury et al. 2012). This communication obstacle could complicate the assessment process, and lead to prolonging or worsening GI symptoms, increase in challenging behaviors, and a decrease in quality of life (Mannion and Leader 2014).

Common GI Symptoms and Conditions

GI symptoms and conditions found commonly within the general population are also prevalent among the ASD population (Buie et al. 2010). Researchers have focused on both organic GI conditions as well as functional GI disorders in individuals with ASD. Organic GI disorders have an identifiable anatomic, metabolic, or pathologic cause, while functional GI disorders do not have an identifiable cause (Gorrindo et al. 2012). Similar to the trend seen in the general population, Gorrindo and colleagues (2012) found that the majority of children with ASD and GI problems had functional rather than organic GI disorders.

The most common GI symptoms in individuals with ASD include chronic constipation, chronic diarrhea, abdominal pain with or without diarrhea, chronic reflux/vomiting, and encopresis with constipation (Gorrindo et al. 2012; Molloy and Manning-Courtney 2003). The most prevalent GI disorder diagnoses include functional constipation and reflux (Gorrindo et al. 2012). Other GI conditions that have been observed in people with ASD are gastroesophageal reflux diseaese (GERD), abdominal bloating, enzyme deficiencies (e.g., disaccharidase), and inflammation of the GI tract (Gorrindo et al. 2012).

More intrusive clinical evaluation (e.g., endoscopy, histopathology) studies suggest greater prevalence of various organic GI disorders in individuals with ASD compared to the general population. However, due to methodology issues, no conclusions can be drawn (Myers and Johnson 2007). Specifically, researchers have suggested that individuals with ASD have a different bacterial makeup of the gut flora (Kral et al. 2013). The gut flora is a group of bacteria that resides in the digestive tract and carries out important tasks such as aiding in digestion and synthesizing vitamins (Guarner and Malagelada 2003). An affected gut flora in ASD is hypothesized to cause increased GI problems (Kral et al. 2013). A group of researchers have also suggested that individuals with ASD have increased intestinal permeability, or a "leaky gut." The "leaky gut hypothesis" asserts that dietary peptides leak out of the intestines due to increased permeability, causing disruption of neurological functioning and brain development. The ingestion of gluten is said to worsen these effects (de Magistris et al. 2010; Kral et al. 2013). However, the research is inconclusive and the existence of ASD-specific GI conditions has not been established (Buie et al. 2010; Kral et al. 2013).

Causes of GI Problems in ASD

Individuals with ASD often display high rates of food selectivity and food refusal. The resulting restricted diet may lack important nutrients and thus, contribute to GI problems (Coury et al. 2012; Mannion and Leader 2014). Children with ASD may also be on medications that cause changes in gut function. Among these GI-related side effects are increased constipation, diarrhea, vomiting, and weight fluctuation (Gorrindo et al. 2012; Kral et al. 2013; Mannion and Leader 2014).

Although these behavioral and environmental causes have been indicated, biological and genetic contributions to GI problems cannot be ruled out. Researchers have found evidence for genetic differences between groups of individuals with ASD with and without GI conditions (Gorrindo et al. 2012). Taken together, results of the available literature suggest that a subgroup of individual with ASD may exist who are at greater risk for GI problems due to the interaction of environmental and genetic components (Gorrindo et al. 2012).

Effect of GI Problems on ASD Symptom Presentation

GI conditions frequently present in an atypical manner (i.e., non-GI symptoms; Buie et al. 2010). The onset or worsening of challenging behaviors may indicate pain or discomfort in individuals with ASD. Because of this, parents and service providers should be aware of changes in challenging behaviors such as sobbing, screaming, increased irritability and agitation, noncompliance, property destruction, aggression, and self-injurious behavior (e.g., biting self, head banging; Buie et al. 2010; Maenner et al. 2012). In terms of ASD-specific symptomology, GI problems have been associated with greater sensitivity to sensory input and higher rates of RRBs (Buie et al. 2010; Mannion and Leader 2014).

Additionally, individuals with ASD and GI conditions were found to have greater sleep problems including more disturbed sleep and nighttime awakenings (Kral et al. 2012; Mannion and Leader 2014). Researchers indicated an association between chronic GI problems (e.g., chronic constipation, bloating, nausea, and abdominal pain) and higher anxiety scores (Mannion and Leader 2014). Further, increased anxiety may exacerbate GI problems.

Researchers have suggested greater GI problems are associated with autistic regression, as well as larger language and social deficits (Gorrindo et al. 2012; Valicenti-McDermott et al. 2008); however, results have been inconclusive with several studies indicating no such relationships (Chandler et al. 2013; Mannion and Leader 2014; Molloy and Manning-Courtney 2003). Further, no relationship between autism severity and degree of GI problems has been found (Chander et al. 2013).

Because pain caused by GI problems may exacerbate ASD symptomology and associated challenging behaviors, GI conditions may lead to increased difficulty in learning environments, decreased effectiveness of intervention, and reduced quality of life (Mannion and Leader 2014). Additionally, medical and psychological evaluation is often complicated when GI problems in individuals with ASD present behaviorally (Buie et al. 2010).

Assessment of GI Problems

Identifying GI symptoms in individuals with ASD can be a difficult task (Buie et al. 2010; Mannion and Leader 2014; Myers and Johnson 2007). Given that the ASD population is characterized by deficits in social communication, individuals with ASD may not be able to communicate symptoms effectively. Further, behavior change is commonly the only indicator of GI discomfort in individuals with ASD (Buie et al. 2010; Mannion and Leader 2014). Therefore, there are several indirect cues of pain and discomfort caregivers and service providers should be aware of. In addition to the aforementioned challenging behaviors that may indicate GI problems (e.g., sleep problems, aggression, and irritability), caregivers of individuals with ASD should be conscious of vocal behaviors such as moaning, echolalia that includes reference to pain, and pain-related verbalizations, as well as motor behaviors such as grimacing, wincing, and unusual posturing (Buie et al. 2010).

Currently, the research concerning the pervasiveness of GI problems in the ASD population does not support routine, universal GI assessment (Myers and Johnson 2007). The evaluation of potential GI or other medical conditions is also often neglected in individuals with ASD (Buie et al. 2010; Mannion and Leader 2014). However, individuals with ASD presenting with GI symptoms or common behavioral manifestations of GI problems require further evaluation. At this time, there are no empirically supported assessment procedures of GI problems specifically for the ASD population (Buie et al. 2010). Therefore, because GI conditions that are common in the general population are also common in individuals with ASD, clinical practice guidelines available for the general population should be utilized (Buie et al. 2010; Mannion and Leader 2014).

Screening

The evaluation and management of GI conditions in individuals with ASDs should begin with the primary care provider (e.g., pediatrician, general physician; Buie et al. 2010) and may require further consultation with specialists. Routine screens for indicators of GI problems should be carried out at every checkup. Height, weight, and body mass index as well as any significant changes in growth rate should be recorded. Signs of limited growth could serve as an indicator of poor nutrition and/or abnormal or inadequate performance of the GI system (Buie et al. 2010). Other variables that should be explored include abdominal pain or distention, frequency of constipation and diarrhea, presence of pica, and possible rectal fissures or infections (Buie et al. 2010; Kral et al. 2013). Significant aberrations detected in these observations are grounds for consultation with or referral to specialist teams (e.g., nutritionists, gastroenterologists, and allergists).

A detailed medical, dietary, and behavioral history is necessary to obtain in the evaluation of possible GI conditions. Frequency, intensity, and duration of GI symptoms should be explored. As previously stated, many medications commonly prescribed to individuals with ASD may cause side effects related to GI functioning (e.g., abdominal pain, constipation, indigestion, nausea, vomiting, and diarrhea; Gorrindo et al. 2012; Kral et al. 2013; Mannion and Leader 2014). Therefore, medication monitoring and management is of paramount importance and consultation with a psychiatrist may be essential. In cases of severe food selectivity, nutritional deficiencies may be evident in individuals with ASD and contribute to GI problems (Coury et al. 2012; Mannion and Leader 2014). Thus, acquiring a dietary history is important to ensure appropriate steps in care be taken. Working with a nutritionist or dietician may be necessary (Buie et al. 2010). Food selectivity and GI problems may also be caused by food allergies. The rate of food allergies in the general population has been estimated at 6–8 % of children and 4 % of adolescents and adults; and, the prevalence is assumed to be similar in the ASD population. Structured interview regarding client history may help identify potential allergies; follow-up assessment with an allergist is encouraged if symptoms appear allergy-related (Buie et al. 2010).

Measures

There are also several caregiver-report measures that may aid in the evaluation of GI conditions. Gorrindo and colleagues (2012) found that parents of individuals with ASD were reliable reporters on GI questionnaires of the presence, although not the nature, of GI problems. This finding supports the approach of administering GI parent-report measures may be a good starting place in the assessment process. Two such measures include the *Gastrointestinal Symptoms Inventory* (Autism Treatment Network 2005) and the *Questionnaire on Pediatric Gastrointestinal Symptoms-Rome III Version (QPGS-RIII*; van Tilburg et al. 2013; Walkeret al. 2000).

Gastrointestinal Symptoms Inventory

The *Gastrointestinal Symptoms Inventory* consists of 77 items in total and assesses for the presence and duration of GI problems specifically in individuals with ASD. The measure was developed by the Autism Treatment Network, a group of hospitals and physicians working to develop a comprehensive medical care model for the ASD population. The items of the *Gastrointestinal Symptoms Inventory* were created according to the steps of clinical GI symptom assessment and symptoms of commonly identified GI disorders. The broad GI symptoms targeted by the measure include abdominal pain, nausea, bloating, diarrhea, and other GI symptom. Further, specific areas measured include abdominal pain, abnormal bowel movements, reflux, and food insensitivity. The *Gastrointestinal Symptoms Inventory* has not been validated (Mannion and Leader 2014).

Questionnaire on Pediatric Gastrointestinal Symptoms-Rome III Version (QPGS-RIII)

The *QPGS-RIII* is a parent-report measure that assesses for GI symptoms and functional GI disorders. The measure is made up of 71 items assessing for symptoms consistent with functional GI disorders (Gorrindo et al. 2012; Mannion and Leader

2014; van Tilburg et al. 2013). The *QPGS-RIII* is not designed specifically for children with ASD. While previous versions of the *QPGS* have been found to hold sound psychometrics, research concerning the psychometric properties of the *QPGS-RIII* is limited (van Tilburg et al. 2013). However, van Tilburg and colleagues (2013) found adequate reliability estimates for the measure.

Behavioral Strategies

Because GI problems often manifest behaviorally in individuals with ASD, collaboration between medical and behavioral professionals would be beneficial in the assessment and management processes. If an onset or worsening of challenging behaviors occurs, a functional assessment should be conducted to identify the maintaining variables (Buie et al. 2010). The four most commonly cited functions of a behavior include automatic reinforcement, attention, access to tangibles, and escape from demands. Behavioral function can be assessed indirectly through interview, descriptively through direct behavior observations, or experimentally through functional analysis (Tarbox et al. 2009).

Additionally, concurrent behavioral treatment employed during the medical assessment process may aid in the evaluation and management of GI conditions. Functional communication training may be used to target identifying and communicating the nature of GI symptoms in individuals with ASD. Coping skills for GI pain can also be targeted with behavioral intervention, such as teaching a client to appropriately ask for a break when symptoms arise (Buie et al. 2010).

Intrusive Procedures

The assessment procedures for GI problems can differ according to the presentation of symptoms (i.e., frequency, severity, and duration) and of associated symptoms (e.g., challenging behaviors, weight fluctuation) as well as the possibility of an organic cause to GI dysfunction (Buie et al. 2010; Gorrindo et al. 2012). Consultation with specialist teams is warranted for individuals whose symptoms persist or worsen despite receiving standard treatment from their primary physician. As previously stated, specialists involved could include allergists, nutritionists, dieticians, gastroenterologists, and behavior therapists (Buie et al. 2010).

After less intrusive evaluation strategies have been used and when GI symptoms are theorized to be organic, more intrusive measures, like laboratory tests, endoscopies, and histopathological examinations, may be necessary. Laboratory tests that may be utilized include a comprehensive metabolic panel, sedimentation rate, a complete blood count with differential, and screening panels for potential food allergies and Celiac disease. Endoscopies can be used to internally examine the esophagus, stomach, and duodenum (esophagogastroduodenoscopy), the small intestine (enteroscopy), and the large intestine and colon (sigmoidoscopy, colonoscopy; Gorrindo et al. 2012). Histopathologies involve evaluating tissue biopsies from the GI tract for possible disease (Gorrindo et al. 2012). These procedures would be carried out by an experienced specialist, such as a gastroenterologist.

Future Directions

Currently, the research literature concerning GI problems in ASD is inconclusive and a greater understanding is necessary to help improve care. Further research targeting prevalence rates using sound methodology is imperative. Studies examining risk factors as well as possible subpopulations of ASD who experience GI problems would benefit the field. Greater research on differences in the presentation of GI disorders in individuals with ASD would enhance assessment procedures (Coury et al. 2012). Clinically, the ruling out of medical causes to challenging behavior is necessary when conducting functional assessments and implementing interventions (Buie et al. 2010). Although the field requires a great deal of additional research on this topic, dispersing knowledge of GI problems to parents and service providers is imperative for effective intervention and preserving the quality of life of individuals with ASD.

Cerebral Palsy in ASD

Cerebral Palsy (CP)

CP refers to a group of disorders characterized by nonprogressive, motor impairments that occur in the early stages of development due to lesions or anomalies of the brain (Bax 1964; Meyns et al. 2011; Pakula et al. 2009; Rosen and Dickinson 1992; Rosenbaum et al. 2007). CP affects about 1.5–4 per 1000 children (Arneson et al. 2009; Bhasin et al. 2006; Kirby et al. 2011; Yeargin-Allsopp et al. 2008), making it one of the most common motor disorders in childhood. The brain injury that causes CP may be prenatal, natal, or postnatal, though most of CP cases are due to prenatal injuries (MacLennan 1999). Prenatal causes and risk factors include disturbance of brain cell migration, poor myelination of developing nerve cell fibers, intrauterine infections, chromosome abnormalities, placental insufficiency, multiple births, maternal infections and fever, etc. (Nelson and Grether 1999; Sankar and Mundkur 2005). Perinatal causes include hypoxia, periventricular leukomalacia (PVL), intracranial hemorrhage, fetal stroke, hyperbilirubinemia, hypoglycemia, and birth asphyxia; postnatal causes include inappropriate connections between brain cells due to trauma, infectious meningitis, toxic, and encephalitis (Dodge 2008; Sankar and Mundkur 2005).

Early Signs and Symptoms of CP

A general delay in motor milestones may be a sign of CP. More specifically, some early signs of CP of those less than 6 months of age include: stiffness, floppiness, and not overextending his or her neck and back. For those who are more than 6 months of age, not rolling over, not being able to bring his or her hands together, having trouble bringing the hands to mouth, and reaching out with one hand while keeping the other fisted may be some signs of CP. For those who are older than 1 year of age, difficulties in crawling and standing may be a sign of CP (Centers for Disease Control and Prevention [CDC] 2014).

Classifications of CP

Since there are various types and severity levels of CP, a myriad of classifications exist today. CP can be classified based on motor functions: spastic, dyskinetic, ataxic, and mixed (Dodge 2008; Rethlefsen et al. 2010). Spastic CP is the most common type of CP, affecting about 70–80 % of CP cases (CDC 2014). Spastic CP implies increased muscle tone, meaning that their muscles are stiff; individuals with spastic CP often have awkward and jerky movements. Spastic CP is often described by affected body parts (i.e., diplegia, hemisparesis, quadriplegia). Among the CP population, 33 % are reported to have hemiplegic CP, 44 % diplegic, and 6 % quadriplegic (Hagberg et al. 2001).

Non-spastic CP implies decreased muscle tone and is mainly characterized by involuntary movements and make up about 20 % of CP cases. Non-spastic CP is divided into two groups: ataxic and dyskinetic. Ataxic CP affects balance and coordination. Individuals with ataxic CP have wide and irregular walking gait and impaired fine motor skills. Individuals with dyskinetic CP are affected by involuntary movements, especially in the hands, arms, and legs. Individuals with more than one type of CP are referred to as having mixed CP (CDC 2014).

Prevalence Rates of Comorbid CP and ASD

In addition to motor, sensory, cognitive, and verbal impairments, comorbid conditions such as epilepsy and ASD are common in individuals with CP (Kirby et al. 2011; Sankar and Mundkur 2005; Singhi et al. 2003; Smits et al. 2011). Although, prevalence rates of CP and co-occurring developmental disabilities vary widely due to different assessment instruments and sample characteristics, comorbid rates of CP and ASD may be higher than previously believed.

Goodman and Graham (1996) examined the prevalence rate of associated psychiatric problems in 149 children with hemiplegia and reported 3 % of the participants as having autistic disorder. Nordin and Gillberg (1996) assessed the prevalence of pervasive developmental disorders (PDD) in children with neurological and neurodevelopmental disorders and found that 10.5 % of their CP sample (n=38) had an ASD. More recently, Kilincaslan and Mukaddes (2009) evaluated 126 children and adolescents with CP and reported that 15 % of the participants had a diagnosis of PDD. In a study assessing associated medical disorders in children with ASD, Kielinen and colleagues (2004) found that 4.8 % of their sample children with ASD had a diagnosis of CP. Also, Kirby et al. (2011) conducted a population-based surveillance of 8-year-old children and found that 8 % of their sample children with CP had a comorbid ASD. Christensen et al. (2013) reported findings of the autism and developmental disabilities monitoring (AADM) Network, a population-based surveillance monitoring CP and ASD across the USA. The authors found that co-occurring ASD rate was 6.9 % among their sample of children with CP.

Cause of ASD and CP

Although causes of ASD and CP overlap are not well known, overlap in behavioral and motor findings may suggest common risk factors and shared etiologies (Christensen et al. 2013). Specific genetic variants affecting both motor and social communication may contribute to potential shared etiologies of these two disorders (Zwaigenbaum 2014). Future research is needed to investigate various factors (i.e., genetically influence developmental versus injury-related processes) underlying the overlap of ASD and CP (Zwaigenbaum 2014).

Comorbid CP and ASD Symptoms

Children with a dual diagnosis of CP and ASD are reported to have a high rate of cognitive impairment. In addition to cognitive delays, affected children are more likely to have a higher prevalence of other medical conditions including asthma and constipation (Smile et al. 2013). Children with comorbid CP and ASD were also reported to have higher rates of aggression compared to the children with CP only (Smile et al. 2013). Children with comorbid CP and ASD were reported to exhibit more impairment in RRBs than those with CP only. Greater impairments in RRBs include limited number of interests, curiosity with surroundings, and expecting others to know their thoughts, experiences, and opinions without communicating them (Hattier et al. 2012).

Previous researchers stated that in addition to physical and neurological problems in CP, social and communication problems may also be present (Kilincaslan and Mukaddes 2009; Pennington 2008). More specifically, children with CP may have impaired speech, language, and communication development as the intelligibility of speech, communicative gestures, facial expressions, and understanding of language may be delayed (Pennington 2008). These delays in communication may lead to social isolation in children with CP. Hattier et al. (2012) examined impairments in communication in children with comorbid CP and ASD and found that children with a dual diagnosis exhibited greater communication impairments compared to those with CP only.

Assessment of CP

The diagnosis of CP usually begins with observations by the child's primary physician or parents when the child is not reaching age appropriate motor milestones. The assessment and diagnosis of CP may take some time, as there is no one definitive test to confirm or rule out CP. CP is usually diagnosed at the ages of 1 or 2 years unless the symptoms are severe. If the symptoms are milder, a diagnosis may take several more years (CDC 2014). A comprehensive medical and developmental history, functional assessment, neuroimaging, and a thorough physical examination are necessary for the assessment and diagnosis of CP.

Medical and Developmental Evaluations

The child's motor skills will be evaluated during regular visits. The child's development, growth, muscle tone, reflexes, motor control, posture, and a medical history will be examined by the primary care doctor or by a specialist such as developmental pediatricians, child neurologists, and pediatric physiatrists (CDC 2014; National Institute of Neurological Disorders and Stroke [NIH] 2014). Because CP is not a progressive disorder, if the child is continuously losing motor skills, CP can be ruled out. Then the problems will more likely be due to genetic or muscle disease, metabolism disorder, or tumors (NIH 2014).

Functional Assessment

In this chapter, three commonly used functional assessment tools for CP, the *Gross Motor Function Classification System (GMFCS)*, the *Gross Motor Function Measure (GMFM)*, and the *Pediatric Evaluation of Disability Inventory (PEDI)*, will be discussed.

Gross Motor Function Classification System (GMFCS)

In order to increase consistency in CP research, researchers have developed a universally accepted classification system, *GMFCS*, which is another way to classify CP (Palisano et al. 2008, Rethelefsen et al. 2010). The *GMFCS* uses age-specific gross motor activity (0–2; 2–4; 4–6; 6–12; and 12–18 age groups) to classify children with CP into five different levels, level I being the mildest to V being most severe. More specifically, level I is described as walking without limitations, level II as walking with limitations such as walking long distances and balancing, and level III as walking with adaptive equipment assistance (hand-held mobility assistance indoors, wheeled mobility outdoors). In level IV, self-mobility is limited and supported by powered mobility assistance; affected children are usually supported when sitting. Affected children in level V have severe head and trunk control limitations, as extensive use of assistance is required.

Gross Motor Function Measure (GMFM)

The *GMFM* is a reliable and valid measure developed especially for children with CP (Russell et al. 1993). The *GMFM,* a standardized observational instrument, consists of 88 items that measure change in gross motor function over time for children of 5 months to 16 years of age. It is subdivided into five dimensions: lying and rolling; sitting; crawling and kneeling; standing; and walking, running, and jumping. Detailed guidelines for administration and scoring are included in the manual. Inter-observer and intra-observer reliability and validity of the measure were reported to be high (Russell et al. 1993).

Pediatric Evaluation of Disability Inventory (PEDI)

The *PEDI* is a standardized assessment instrument developed to measure functional ability of chronically ill and disabled children of 6 months to 7 years of age (Haley et al. 1992). The *PEDI* consists of three scales: typical functional skill level, physical assistance typically required of the caregiver, and modifications or adaptive equipment used such as braces and wheelchairs. Each scale is further divided into three domains: self-care, mobility, and social function. The judgment of the clinicians or educators who know the child and his or her function very well or the child's primary caretaker's interviews may be used to administer the inventory. Numerous studies reported that the *PEDI* is a reliable and valid assessment (Feldman et al. 1990; Haley et al. 1991; Nichols and Case-Smith 1996; Wright and Boschen 1993). The advantage of the *PEDI* includes its intrinsic relevance to daily functioning (e.g., dressing, eating, drinking, bathing, toileting, etc.) of the children and the inclusion of contextual influences (Ketelaar and Vermeer 1998).

Neuroimaging

In addition to the developmental evaluations, noninvasive neuroimaging tests are commonly used in CP diagnosis to acquire pictures of the brain. While, the neuroimaging cannot predict the effect of an injury, it still is a dependable tool in diagnosing CP. Three types of neuroimaging include cranial ultrasound, magnetic resonance imaging (MRI), and Computed tomography (CT) scans.

Cranial Ultrasound

Cranial ultrasound uses high-frequency sound waves and its results can reveal abnormalities of the brain. It does not produce high quality results as an MRI or a CT scan, but is the least intrusive technique to capture the brain image. The cranial ultrasound is commonly used on an infant from birth to age 18 months before the cranial bones are fully formed (NIH 2014).

Magnetic Resonance Imaging (MRI)

Magnetic resonance imaging (MRI), which uses a magnetic field and radio waves to create the picture of the brain, is most preferred neuroimaging as it produces the clearest results, showing the location and type of damage. It requires the child to remain still during the exam, which lasts approximately 30 min. Sedation is often used during MRIs in order to minimize movements. Also, loud noises during the exam may be uncomfortable for young children. Magnetic resonance imagings (MRIs) capture accurate images of the brain and the spinal cord structure and their abnormalities (NIH 2014).

Computed Tomography (CT)

Computed tomography (CT) scans produce cross-sectional views of the brain; CT scans are known to have better results than cranial ultrasounds, but are not as accurate as MRIs. Since CT scans use high levels of ionizing radiation, the use of CT scans on young, developing brain should be used with extra caution.

Laboratory Tests

Laboratory tests such as blood work, urinalysis, and genetic testing are commonly used rule out other conditions that are not CP. Blood tests including chemistry panels, plasma screens, chromosome analysis, and creatine phosphokinase (CPK) isoenzymes tests are used to detect other hereditary conditions. Similarly, urine tests are utilized to rule out various conditions examining the levels of chemical contents, amino acids, organic acids, and other molecules.

Future Directions

Although a dual diagnosis of ASD and CP has been reported, research examining the relationship between these two disorders is limited. Existing research reported that the prevalence rate of comorbid CP and ASD is higher than previously believed.

Difficulties with communication, socialization, and other ASD-related symptoms in children with CP may be overlooked, as all functional impairments may mistakenly be thought of as a part of CP. When the potential ASD diagnoses are overlooked, it may delay early diagnosis and intervention, which is critical to ASD treatment. Therefore, it is of utmost importance that clinicians and professionals develop a better understanding of the presence, topography, and overlapping symptoms of ASD and CP and actively improve the assessment of ASD in the presence of CP.

Intellectual Disability (ID) in ASD

Intellectual Disability (ID) is characterized by long-term impairment in cognitive functioning and deficits in adaptive skills. Marked communication and social difficulties as well as motor problems and behavioral excesses (e.g., stereotypies, aggression, self-injurious behavior) are often associated with ID (Kozlowski et al. 2011; Matson and Cervantes 2013). Level of ID can range from mild to profound based on degree of intellectual and adaptive impairment related to conceptual, social, and practical domains (American Psychiatric Association [APA] 2013). Researchers have found that individuals with greater intellectual deficits are more likely to have ASD (Matson and Shoemaker 2009; Vig and Jedrysek 1999). Further, ID is among the most common comorbid disorders in individuals with ASD. It has been estimated that as many as 50–70 % of individuals with ASD have ID (Artigas-Pallares et al. 2007; Matson and Shoemaker 2009).

Because the overlap between ASD and ID is substantial, cognitive and adaptive testing should be a routine component of every ASD evaluation (Tomanik et al. 2007). The recognition of ID in individuals with ASD has important implications. First, the presence of ID is associated with poorer prognosis in people with ASD. ID has also been found to affect severity of ASD symptomology and challenging behaviors as well as levels of comorbid psychopathology (Matson and Shoemaker 2009; Matson et al. 1997). Proper evaluation and diagnosis of co-occurring ASD and ID would help inform treatment and educational planning and lead to better care. However, the assessment of ID in individuals with ASD can be complex. Confounding variables, such as deficits in attention and motivation, the presence of challenging behaviors during testing, and differences in the measures used to assess cognitive and adaptive abilities, can result in misrepresentation of abilities and flawed diagnostic conclusions (Koegel et al. 1997; Ozonoff et al. 2005). Therefore, it is imperative that clinicians become familiar with the unique assessment needs of individuals with ASD when evaluating for ID.

Common Symptoms

The presence of ID in individuals with ASD has been found to correlate with ease of skill acquisition as well as level of adaptive functioning. Further, level of intellectual functioning, along with autism symptom severity, functions as an important outcome predictor for individuals diagnosed with ASD (Ozonoff et al. 2005).

Adaptive functioning refers to behaviors necessary for success in living independently. Adaptive skills include daily living skills (e.g., dressing and feeding oneself, personal hygiene), social skills (e.g., interpersonal relationships, coping skills), motor skills (e.g., fine motor skills, running, jumping), and communication skills (e.g., ability to express wants and needs, following instructions; Kenworthy et al. 2010). Individuals with ASD not only display deficits in communication and socialization, but also often experience impairment across all domains of adaptive functioning (Kenworthy et al. 2010). Kanne and colleagues (2011) found that when controlling for autism severity and age, intellectual level significantly predicted level of adaptive functioning in individuals with ASD. Further, as intellectual level (i.e., IQ) decreased, adaptive abilities decreased as well (Kanne et al. 2011). Similarly, Green and Carter (2014) found that children with ASD and low IQ demonstrated slow development of daily living skills, such as grooming, dressing, awareness of safety rules, and carrying out chores.

Individuals with ASD and ID experience substantial cognitive deficits as well; however, unique to the ASD population, there is often a disproportion in cognitive skills (Coolican et al. 2008; Johnson and Myers 2007; Matson and Shoemaker 2009; Ozonoff et al. 2005). Uneven subtest score patterns on standardized intelligence tests have been found in individuals with ASD. Verbal IQ scores are often significantly lower than performance IQ scores (Ozonoff et al. 2005). Relatedly, researchers have found strengths in visual-motor abilities within the ASD population (Coolican et al. 2008; Matson and Shoemaker 2009). However, this pattern of intellectual functioning has not been found throughout the autism spectrum (Ozonoff et al. 2005).

Effect of ID on ASD Symptom Presentation

Comorbid ID is associated with increased ASD symptom severity in individuals with ASD (Matson and Shoemaker 2009). Individuals with ASD and ID have been found to have more deficits in verbal and nonverbal communication than individuals with ASD alone (Matson and Shoemaker 2009). People with ASD and greater ID have also been found to engage in greater rates of RRBs (Bishop, Richler and Lord 2006; Matson and Shoemaker 2009). Further, researchers have suggested that intellectual functioning affects not only rate, but also typography of RRBs (Gabriels et al. 2005). Individuals with ASD and typical intellectual functioning engage in greater rates of repetitive speech as well as have more unusual attachment to objects and restricted interests. Individuals with ASD and low intellectual ability demonstrate more sensory and motor stereotypies and self-injurious behaviors (SIB; Gabriels et al. 2005; Goldman et al. 2009). Severity of challenging behaviors rises with greater ID in individuals with ASD (Matson and Shoemaker 2009). Further, the challenging behaviors of individuals with comorbid ASD and ID often persist across the lifespan (Murphy et al. 2005).

A high rate of comorbid psychopathology has been found in ASD on its own, with estimates as great as 70 % of children with ASD meeting criteria for at least one comorbid disorder (Simonoff et al. 2008). However, the co-occurrence of ASD and ID has been associated with an even greater increase in rates of comorbid psychopathology (LoVullo and Matson 2009). The most common co-occurring disorders found in individuals presenting with both ASD and ID include depression, bipolar disorder, schizophrenia, and anxiety (Matson and Shoemaker 2009).

Causes of ID and ASD Overlap

Because ASD and ID hold significant overlap, it is believed the two disorders may share genetic or neurodevelopmental etiologies. Researchers have theorized that common deletions and/or duplications of various chromosomes underlie this overlap. However, the existence of shared biological etiology is not yet well established (Matson and Shoemaker 2009).

Assessment of ID

The *Diagnostic and Statistical Manual of Mental Disorders, Fifth Edition* (*DSM-5*; APA 2013) defines ID according to three criteria: (1) deficits in intellectual functioning (e.g., problem solving, reasoning, planning, abstract thinking, judgment, academic learning, learning from experience) confirmed by clinical assessment as well as individualized, standardized intelligence testing; (2) deficits in adaptive functioning that prevent individuals from meeting developmental or sociocultural milestones for personal autonomy and social responsibility, and limit functioning in one or more everyday life activities (e.g., communication, socialization, independent living) across multiple environments (e.g., home, school, work, community); and (3) onset of deficits occurs during the developmental period. Severity specifiers, ranging from mild to profound ID, are assigned based on degree of deficit in conceptual (e.g., language, academic skills, knowledge of time, money), social (e.g., interpersonal skills, social judgment and decision-making) and practical (e.g., eating, dressing, toileting, occupational skills) domains (APA 2013; Schalock and Luckasson 2004).

Therefore, to assess for ID, it is necessary for clinicians to administer standardized measures of both intellectual and adaptive functioning as well as obtain a documented age of onset. Further, several considerations for selecting instruments and interpreting results must be factored into diagnostic decisions making clinical interview and clinician acumen integral components of the evaluation process as well (Schalock and Luckasson 2004). For example, client age, culture, language and communication, and community environment may relate to opportunities, motivation, and performance of skills (Schalock and Luckasson 2004).

Assessment of Intellectual Functioning

The American Association on Intellectual and Developmental Disabilities (AAIDD) defines intelligence as a general mental ability that includes skills related to reasoning, abstract thinking, planning, and problem solving (Schalock and Luckasson 2004). Assessment of intellectual functioning with a measure of IQ is a basic component of an ID evaluation and aids in the identification of cognitive strengths and weaknesses as well as suggested prognosis (Ozonoff et al. 2005; Schalock and Luckasson 2004).

However, measures of IQ may be unstable in younger populations, may change over the course of development and/or treatment, and may differ depending on the instrument administered (Ozonoff et al. 2005). When selecting an IQ test to administer, clinicians must ensure the test is appropriate for the individual (e.g., age, culture, language, challenging behaviors), is sensitive to measure a wide range of abilities, and measures verbal and nonverbal abilities independently (Filipek et al. 1999; Ozonoff et al. 2005). Further, because individuals with ASD may present disproportionate abilities, results should not be interpreted in isolation or used on their own to formulate diagnostic decisions (Matson and Shoemaker 2009).

Measures of Intellectual Functioning

Stanford-Binet Intelligence Scales, Fifth Edition (SB5)

The *Stanford-Binet Intelligence Scales, Fifth Edition (SB5;* Roid 2003) is a norm-referenced measure of cognitive functioning intended for use with individuals aged 2 to 85 years. The *SB5* results in a full scale intelligence quotient (FSIQ), nonverbal and verbal IQ domain scores, and five index scores (i.e., fluid reasoning, knowledge, quantitative reasoning, visual-spatial processing, working memory). The *SB5* consists two routing subtests (i.e., object series/matrices and vocabulary) and eight subtests. The routing subtests are administered first to identify on which items to start for subsequent subtests. Four subtests and the object series/matrices routing subtest are used to calculate nonverbal IQ and four subtests and the Vocabulary routing subtest are used to calculate verbal IQ. Based on assessment needs and client characteristics, the clinician can administer solely the verbal or nonverbal IQ domain (Roid 2003). Administered in full, the *SB5* takes approximately 1 h. The normative sample for the *SB5* included 108 children with ASD and worked to improve the assessment of younger individuals, lower-functioning individuals, and individuals with comorbid ID (Ozonoff et al. 2005).

Additionally, there is an abbreviated battery IQ (ABIQ) available based on the two routing subtests. The ABIQ has been found to strongly correlate with FSIQ in a majority of cases (Coolican et al. 2008). Due to short administration time (15–20 min), the abbreviated battery may be beneficial for use with individuals with ASD.

Wechsler Intelligence Scales for Children, Fourth Edition (WISC-IV)

The *Wechsler Intelligence Scales for Children, Fourth Edition* (*WISC-IV;* Wechsler 2003*)* is a standardized, individually administered test of intelligence for children aged 6 to 16 years old. The *WISC-IV* consists of four indexes (verbal comprehension index [VCI], perceptual reasoning index [PRI], working memory index [WMI], and processing speed index [PSI]) and results in a FSIQ as well as four index scores. The *WISC-IV* is made up of 15 subtests, 10 of which are core subtests and five subtests are supplemental. Supplemental tests are provided to correct for potential error made in administering a core subtest. Administration of the *WISC-IV* takes about 50–70 min (Ozonoff et al. 2005; Wechsler 2003). Because the verbal requirements of the *WISC-IV* may underestimate intellectual abilities, the instrument would be most appropriate for use on children with spoken language (Ozonoff et al. 2005; Shah and Holmes 1985). The *WISC-IV* is currently one of the most popular measures of IQ (Ozonoff et al. 2005).

Also available are the *Wechsler Preschool and Primary Scale of Intelligence, Fourth Edition (WPPSI-IV;* Wechsler 2012), an IQ measure intended for use with young children aged 2 years, 6 months to 7 years, 7 months old and the *Wechsler Adult Intelligence Scale, Fourth Edition (WAIS-IV;* Wechsler 2008) for use with adults aged 16 years and older.

Leiter International Performance Scale, Third Edition (Leiter-3)

The *Leiter International Performance Scale, Third Edition (Leiter-3; Roid et al.* 2013) assesses nonverbal cognitive abilities and is intended for use with individuals 3 to 75 years old. The administration of the *Leiter-3* is primarily nonverbal. Test items require only gestures and manipulating test stimuli for response. No receptive or expressive language skills are needed for the *Leiter-3* (Ozonoff et al. 2005). The *Leiter-3* includes cognitive and attention and memory scales. The *Leiter-3* yields an overall nonverbal IQ composite, nonverbal memory and processing speed scores, as well as standard scores for each of ten subtests (Kranzler and Floyd 2013; Roid et al. 2013).

The *Leiter* was designed for use with difficult-to-test populations and has traditionally been used with individuals who are young, nonverbal, and/or have moderate to severe ID (Ozonoff et al. 2005). Due to its nonverbal nature, the measure has particular utility with individuals with ASD. However, this instrument should be used with caution as researchers have found that the *Leiter* may overestimate intellectual abilities (Shah and Holmes 1985).

Considerations for Assessing IQ in Individuals with ASD

Intellectual assessment of individuals with ASD is often challenging due to pervasive socialization and communication deficits, difficulty staying on-task and focused, challenging behaviors, and decreased motivation (Koegel et al. 1997;

Ozonoff et al. 2005). These variables may lead to misinterpretation of standardized test results and underestimations of ability. Underestimations of ability may hold serious consequences for individuals with ASD such as inappropriate educational decisions and flawed treatment planning. Further, treatment gains measured by IQ score may represent a decrease in challenging behaviors or increased familiarity with the examiner rather than a true increase in intellectual functioning (Koegel et al. 1997). These problems are exacerbated when a clinician who is inexperienced in the nature of ASD or unfamiliar with the client is conducting the assessment (Koegel et al. 1997).

Koegel and colleagues (1997) suggest that few individuals with ASD should be unable to complete an intellectual assessment. Important considerations for appropriate testing include clinician experience and the selection of appropriate tests. Clinicians should have experience with the ASD population as well as knowledge of the challenging behaviors and idiosyncrasies of the specific client before conducting the assessment. Because several measures may not be appropriate or validated for use on younger, lower functioning, or nonverbal individuals with ASD, the clinician must take time in selecting appropriate tests based on individualized needs (Koegel et al. 1997).

Client motivation requires clinician consideration in administering measures and interpreting scores as well (Koegel et al. 1997). Because standardized measures of intellectual functioning do not provide contingencies for responding, motivation for emitting correct responses may be low in individuals with ASD. Therefore, clinicians should work to improve motivation during testing without departing from administration guidelines. This can be done by providing reinforcement for on-task responding and requiring the client to attend to test materials to earn a reward (Koegel et al. 1997).

Recommendations for testing include providing breaks for preferred activities contingent upon on-task behavior, presenting test material in different locations (e.g., on the floor, at the table), administering the test with a caregiver in the room, and instructing the client to repeat directions before providing a response (Koegel et al. 1997). When conducting an assessment for an individual with ASD, more breaks during testing or testing over several sessions may be warranted (Koegel et al. 1997; Ozonoff et al. 2005).

Assessment of Adaptive Functioning

Adaptive skills relate to those learned conceptual, social, and practical behaviors that allow individuals to be successful in day-to-day functioning (Schalock and Luckasson 2004). In the evaluation of ID, adaptive functioning impairment should be identified using standardized, norm-referenced assessments of adaptive skills (Schalock and Luckasson 2004). Standardized measures of adaptive behavior provide age-referenced results regarding an individual's ability in several areas (e.g., communication, socialization, motor skills, cognitive skills; Kenworthy et al. 2010;

Schalock and Luckasson 2004). Because adaptive functioning should be evaluated relative to expected developmental milestones, these instruments are beneficial.

Measures of Adaptive Functioning

Vineland Adaptive Behavior Scales, Second Edition (Vineland-II)

The *Vineland Adaptive Behavior Scales, Second Edition (Vineland-II;* Sparrow et al. 2005) is a widely utilized measure of adaptive skills intended for use with individuals from birth to 90 years of age. The *Vineland-II* consists of interviews (i.e., Survey Interview Form, Expanded Interview Form) and rating scales (i.e., Parent/Caregiver Rating Form, Teacher Rating Form) completed by parents or caregivers and teachers. Informants are asked to rate the client on the presence of ability in specific adaptive behaviors on a Likert scale. The Survey Interview Form and the rating forms use a 3-point Likert scale (i.e., never, sometimes or partially, or usually); and, the Expanded Interview Form utilizes a 5-point Likert scale (i.e., never, rarely, sometimes, often, almost always).

The instrument assesses an individual's adaptive skill performance within four domains: communication, daily living skills, socialization, and motor skills. Communication subdomains include receptive and expressive language. Subdomains for daily living skills include personal, domestic, and community skills. Socialization subdomains are interpersonal relationships, play and leisure time, and coping skills. The motor skills domain includes fine and gross motor skill subdomains. The *Vineland-II* yields an adaptive behavior composite score, as well as standard scores for each domain and subdomain (Sparrow et al. 2005).

Battelle Developmental Inventory, Second Edition (BDI-2)

The *Battelle Developmental Inventory, Second Edition* (*BDI-2*; Newborg 2005) is a measure used to evaluate the development of children from birth to 7 years old. Administration of the *BDI-2* includes structured play-based activities, observation, and caregiver and/or teacher interviews. The *BDI-2* assesses five domains: adaptive, personal-social, communication, motor, and cognitive. Adaptive subdomains include self-care and personal responsibility. Personal-social subdomains are adult interaction, peer interaction, and self-concept and social role. The communication domain includes receptive and expressive communication subdomains, and the motor domain includes gross and fine motor subdomains. The cognitive domain consists of attention and memory, reasoning and academic skills, and perception and concepts subdomains.

Items are administered based upon the child's age and scored on a 3-point Likert scale. A score of 0 indicates the child has no ability in the skill, a score of 1 indicates emerging ability, and a score of 2 indicates ability. Item responses formulate a total developmental quotient (DQ) as well as a DQ for each domain (Newborg 2005).

Considerations for Assessing Adaptive Functioning in Individuals with ASD

Standardized measures of adaptive functioning often assess for acquisition deficits (not knowing how to engage in a skill) and performance deficits (not knowing when to use a skill) but lack sensitivity to delineate motivational deficits in performing adaptive skills (Schalock and Luckasson 2004). Additionally, many of the behaviors comprising adaptive skills cannot be observed in the clinic during formal assessment sessions. Therefore, comprehensive interview of caregivers and the employment of clinical judgment are necessary to avoid misrepresentations of ability (Schalock and Luckasson 2004).

Many individuals with ASD engage in a variety of challenging behaviors (e.g., tantrums, RRBs). These behaviors may intrude on the acquisition or performance of adaptive skills. However, challenging behaviors are not frequently included as a necessary component of standardized adaptive functioning measures (Schalock and Luckasson 2004). Therefore, clinicians must consider the role of these behaviors in adaptive skill deficits when evaluating for ID.

Future Directions

It is important to recognize that these standardized instruments should work to provide an evidence base from which to employ clinical judgment when diagnosing ID in individuals with ASD. Clinical judgment should be systematic and take into consideration the previously mentioned factors of potential influence (e.g., culture, language, opportunity, motivation, challenging behaviors; Schalock and Luckasson 2004).

Because ASD is such a heterogeneous condition, uniform procedures for ID evaluation would be difficult to offer. Intellectual and adaptive assessment of people with ASD needs to be individualized. However, because the ASD-ID overlap is substantial and ID serves as a significant risk factor for poorer prognosis, it is imperative to increase clinician awareness of important considerations within ID assessment as well as provide guidelines for evaluation procedures.

Conclusion

ASD itself is a complex disorder, and assessing and diagnosing ASD is not a brief process. To further complicate matters, children with ASD often are affected by a variety of medical problems such as GI problems, CP, and ID at high rates. It is important to recognize symptoms of medical conditions in ASD, as medical comorbidities associated with ASD may exacerbate symptoms.

As discussed, individuals with comorbid ASD and GI conditions were reported to exhibit more sleep difficulties (Kral et al. 2013; Mannion and Leader 2014), and increased anxiety may worsen GI conditions (Mannion and Leader 2014). Further, pain caused by GI conditions may exacerbate ASD symptomology. Similarly, individuals with comorbid ASD and CP were reported to exhibit more cognitive impairment, RRBs, aggression, communication difficulties, and other medical conditions such as asthma and constipation. Moreover, the presence of ID in ASD is associated with poorer prognosis, severe ASD symptomology, challenging behaviors, and comorbid psychopathology.

Because some medical conditions and associated problems may present symptoms that are similar to ASD, it is imperative to distinguish ASD from other conditions. Early autism identification and intervention is critical as it increases the likelihood of a positive outcome and provides opportunities to reach maximum potential. When the identification and treatment of ASD is delayed, it may limit the development of social relationships and interfere with effective education and quality of life.

In order to accurately assess and differentiate ASD from other comorbid condition, clinicians must be able to distinguish between core symptoms of ASD, symptoms solely attributed to other comorbid conditions and psychopathology, and overlapping symptoms of ASD and associated conditions. It is important to involve a multidisciplinary team of doctors including a psychologist, pediatrician, and speech therapist, especially when medical conditions are suspected in ASD. Further, ASD assessments must be conducted by a qualified clinician with extensive experience and training, using a comprehensive assessment battery including structured interviews, behavioral observation, reliable and valid assessment tools, and developmental/medical history. Medical problems that have been identified to covary with ASD and current methods and procedures used to measure these problems were discussed in the current chapter. More research in this area, especially in the assessment of co-occurring conditions in ASD, is needed to enhance the potential to all affected individuals.

References

American Psychiatric Association (2013). *Diagnostic and Statistical Manual of Mental Disorders, (5th ed.)*. Washington, DC: Author.

Arneson, C. L., Durkin, M. S., Benedict, R. E., Kirby, R. S., Yeargin-Allsopp, M., Van Naarden Braun, K., et al. (2009). Prevalence of cerebral palsy: Autism and developmental disabilities monitoring network, three sites, United States, 2004. *Disability Health Journal, 2,* 45–48.

Artigas-Pallarés, J., Rigau-Ratera, E., & García-Nonell, C. (2007). The relation between borderline intellectual capacity and neurodevelopmental disorders. *Revista de Neurologia, 44,* 739–744.

Autism Treatment Network. (2005). *GI symptom inventory questionnaire, version 3.0*. New York: Autism Speaks.

Bauman, M. L. (2010). Medical comorbidities in autism: Challenges to diagnosis and treatment. *Neurotherapeutics, 7,* 320–327.

Bax, M. (1964). Terminology and classification of cerebral palsy. *Developmental Medicine & Child Neurology, 6,* 295–307.

Bhasin, T. K., Brocksen, S., Avchen, R. N., & Van Naarden Braun, K. (2006). Prevalence of four developmental disabilities among children aged 8 years-Metropolitan Atlanta Developmental Disabilities Surveillance Program, 1996 and 2000. *MMWR. Surveillance Summaries, 55,* 1–9.

Bishop, S. L., Richler, J., & Lord, C. (2006). Association between restricted and repetitive behaviors and nonverbal IQ in children with autism spectrum disorders. *Child Neuropsychology, 12,* 247–267.

Buie, T., Campbell, D. B., Fuchs, G. J., Furuta, G. T., Levy, J., VandeWater, J., et al. (2010). Evaluation, diagnosis, and treatment of gastrointestinal disorders in individuals with ASDs: A consensus report. *Pediatrics, 125,* S1–S18.

Centers for Disease Control and Prevention. (2014). Screening and diagnosis of cerebral palsy. http://www.cdc.gov/features/cerebralpalsy/. Accessed 26 April 2014.

Chandler, S., Carcani-Rathwell, I., Charman, T., Pickles, A., Loucas, T., Meldrum, D., et al. (2013). Parent-reported gastro-intestinal symptoms in children with autism spectrum disorders. *Journal of Autism and Developmental Disorders, 43,* 2737–2747.

Christensen, D., Van Naarden Braun, K., Doernberg, N. S., Maenner, M. J., Arneson, C. L., Durkin, M. S., et al. (2013). Prevalence of cerebral palsy, co-occurring autism spectrum disorders, and motor functioning—autism and developmental disabilities monitoring network, USA, 2008.

Coolican, J., Bryson, S., & Zwaigenbaum, L. (2008). Brief report: Data on the Stanford–Binet Intelligence Scales (5th ed.) in children with autism spectrum disorder. *Journal of Autism and Developmental Disorders, 38,* 190–197.

Coury, D. L., Ashwood, P., Fasano, A., Fuchs, G., Geraghty, M., Kaul, A., et al. (2012). Gastrointestinal conditions in children with autism spectrum disorder: Developing a research agenda. *Pediatrics, 130,* S160–S168.

de Magistris, L., Familiari, V., Pascotto, A., Sapone, A., Frolli, A., Iardino, P., et al. (2010). Alterations of the intestinal barrier in patients with autism spectrum disorders and in their first-degree relatives. *Journal of Pediatric Gastroenterology and Nutrition, 51,* 418–424.

Dodge, N. N. (2008). Cerebral palsy: Medical aspects. *Pediatric Clinics of North America, 55,* 1189–1207.

Erickson, C. A., Stigler, K. A., Corkins, M. R., Posey, D. J., Fitzgerald, J. F., & McDougle, C. J. (2005). Gastrointestinal factors in autistic disorder: A critical review. *Journal of Autism and Developmental Disorders, 35,* 713–727.

Feldman, A. B., Haley, S. M., & Coryell, J. (1990). Concurrent and construct validity of the pediatric evaluation of disability inventory. *Physical Therapy, 70,* 602–610.

Filipek, P. A., Accardo, P. J., Baranek, G. T., Cook, E. H. Jr., Dawson, G., Gordon, B., et al. (1999). The screening and diagnosis of autistic spectrtim disorders. *Journal of Autism and Developmental Disorders, 29,* 439–484.

Fodstad, J. C., Matson, J. L., Hess, J., & Neal, D. (2009). Social and communication behaviours in infants and toddlers with autism and pervasive developmental disorders-not otherwise specified. *Developmental Neurorehabilitation, 12,* 152–157.

Gabriels, R. L., Cuccaro, M. L., Hill, D. E., Ivers, B. J., & Goldson, E. (2005). Repetitive behaviors in autism: Relationships with associated clinical features. *Research in Developmental Disabilities, 26,* 169–181.

Goldman, S., Wang, C., Salgado, M. W., Greene, P. E., Kim, M., & Rapin, I. (2009). Motor stereotypies in children with autism and other developmental disorders. *Developmental Medicine and Child Neurology, 51,* 30–38.

Goodman, R., & Graham, P. (1996). Psychiatric problems in children with hemiplegia: Cross sectional epidemiological survey. *British Medical Journal, 312,* 1065–1069.

Gorrindo, P., Williams, K. C., Lee, E. B., Walker, L. S., McGrew, S. G., & Levitt, P. (2012). Gastrointestinal dysfunction in autism: Parental report, clinical evaluation, and associated factors. *Autism Research, 5,* 101–108.

Green, S. A., & Carter, A. S. (2014). Predictors and course of daily living skills development in toddlers with autism spectrum disorders. *Journal of Autism and Developmental Disorders, 44,* 256–263.

Guarner, F., & Malagelada, J. R. (2003). Gut flora in health and disease. *Lancet, 361,* 512–519.

Hagberg, B., Hagberg, G., Beckung, E., & Uvebrant, P. (2001). Changing panorama of cerebral palsy in Sweden. VIII. Prevalence and origin in the birth year period 1991–94. *Acta Paediatrica, 90,* 271–277.

Haley, S. M., Coster, W. J., & Faas, R. M. (1991). A content validity study of the pediatric evaluation of disability inventory. *Pediatric Physical Therapy, 3,* 177–184.

Haley, S. M., Coster, W. J., Ludlow, L., Haltiwanger, J., & Andrellos, P. (1992). *Pediatric Evaluation of Disability Inventory (PEDI): Development, standardization, and administration manual.* Boston: New England Medical Center Hospitals.

Hattier, M. A., Matson, J. L., May, A. C., & Whiting, S. E. (2012). Repetitive/restricted behaviours and interests in children with cerebral palsy and autism spectrum disorder. *Developmental Neurorehabiliation, 15,* 178–184.

Hattier, M. A., Matson, J. L., & Kozlowski, A. M. (2012). Communication skills in children with cerebral palsy and autism spectrum disorders. *Journal of Developmental and Physical Disabilities, 24,* 85–93.

Johnson, C. P., & Myers, S. M. (2007). Identification and evaluation of children with autism spectrum disorders. *Pediatrics, 120,* 1183–1215.

Kanne, S. M., Gerber, A. J., Quirmbach, L. M., Sparrow, S. S., Cicchetti, D. V., & Saulnier, C. A. (2011). The role of adaptive behavior in autism spectrum disorders: Implications for functional outcome. *Journal of Autism and Developmental Disorders, 41,* 1007–1018.

Kenworthy, L., Case, L., Harms, M. B., Martin, A., & Wallace, G. L. (2010). Adaptive behavior ratings correlate with symptomatology and IQ among individuals with high-functioning autism spectrum disorders. *Journal of Autism and Developmental Disorders, 40,* 416–423.

Ketelaar, M., & Vermeer, A. (1998). Functional motor abilities of children with cerebral palsy: A systematic literature review of assessment measures. *Clinical Rehabilitation, 12,* 369–380.

Kielinen, M., Rantala, H., Timonen, E., Linna, S. L., & Moilsanen, I. (2004). Associated medical disorders and disabilities in children with autistic disorder: A population-based study. *Autism, 8,* 49–60.

Kilincaslan, A., & Mukaddes, N. M. (2009). Pervasive developmental disorders in individuals with cerebral palsy. *Developmental Medicine and Child Neurology, 51,* 289–294.

Kirby, R. S., Wingate, M. S., Van Naarden Braun, K., Doernberg, N. S., Arneson, C. L., Benedict, R. E., et al. (2011). Prevalence and functioning of children with cerebral palsy in four areas of the United States in 2006: A report from the autism and developmental disabilities monitoring network. *Research in Developmental Disabilities, 32,* 462–469.

Koegel, L. K., Koegel, R. L., & Smith, A. (1997). Variables related to differences in standardized test outcomes for children with autism. *Journal of Autism and Developmental Disorders, 27,* 233–243.

Kozlowski, A. M., Matson, J. L., Sipes, M., Hattier, M. A., & Bamburg, J. W. (2011). The relationship between psychopathology symptom clusters and the presence of comorbid psychopathology in individuals with severe and profound intellectual disability. *Research in Developmental Disabilities, 32,* 1610–1614.

Kral, T. V., Eriksen, W. T., Souders, M. C., & Pinto-Martin, J. A. (2013). Eating behaviors, diet quality, and gastrointestinal symptoms in children with autism spectrum disorders: A brief review. *Journal of Pediatric Nursing, 28,* 548–556.

Kranzler, J. H., & Floyd, R. G. (2013). *Assessing intelligence in children and adolescents: A practical guide.* New York: Guilford Press.

LoVullo, S. V., & Matson, J. L. (2009). Comorbid psychopathology in adults with autism spectrum disorders and intellectual disabilities. *Research in Developmental Disabilities, 30,* 1288–1296.

MacLennan, A. (1999). A template for defining a causal relation between acute intrapartum events and cerebral palsy: International consensus statement. *British Medical Journal, 319,* 1054–1059.

Maenner, M. J., Arneson, C. L., Levy, S. E., Kirby, R. S., Nicholas, J. S., & Durkin, M. S. (2012). Brief report: Association between behavioral features and gastrointestinal problems among children with autism spectrum disorder. *Journal of Autism and Developmental Disorders, 42,* 1520–1525.

Mannion, A., & Leader, G. (2014). Gastrointestinal symptoms in autism spectrum disorder: A literature review. *Review Journal of Autism and Developmental Disorders, 1*(1), 1–7.

Matson, J. L., & Cervantes, P. E. (2013). Comorbidity among persons with intellectual disabilities. *Research in Autism Spectrum Disorders, 7,* 1318–1322.

Matson, J. L., & Shoemaker, M. (2009). Intellectual disability and its relationship to autism spectrum disorders. *Research in Developmental Disabilities, 30,* 1107–1114.

Matson, J. L., Smiroldo, B. B., Hamilton, M., & Baglio, C. (1997). Do anxiety disorders exist in persons with severe and profound mental retardation? *Research in Developmental Disabilities, 18,* 39–44.

Matson, J. L., Dempsey, T., & Fodstad, J. C. (2009). Stereotypies and repetitive behaviors in infants with autism and pervasive developmental disorder. *Developmental Neurorehabilitation, 12,* 122–127.

Meyns, P., van Gestel, L., Massaad, F., Desloovere, K., Malenaers, G., & Duysens, J. (2011). Arm swing during alking at different speeds in children with cerebral palsy and typically developing children. *Research in Developmental Disabilities, 32,* 1957–1964.

Molloy, C. A., & Manning-Courtney, P. (2003). Prevalence of chronic gastrointestinal symptoms in children with autism and autistic spectrum disorders. *Autism, 7,* 165–171.

Murphy, G. H., Beadle-Brown, J., Wing, L., Gould, J., Shah, A., & Nan, H. (2005). Chronicity of challenging behaviours in people with severe intellectual disabilities and/or autism: A total population sample. *Journal of Autism and Developmental Disorders, 35,* 405–418.

Myers, S. M., & Johnson, C. P. (2007). Management of children with autism spectrum disorders. *Pediatrics, 120,* 1162–1182.

National Institute of Neurological Disorders and Stroke. (2014). Cerebral palsy: Hope through research. http://www.ninds.nih.gov/disorders/cerebral_palsy/detail_cerebral_palsy.htm#263843104. Accessed 1 May 2014.

Nelson, K. B., & Grether, J. K. (1999). Causes of cerebral palsy. *Current Options in Pediatric, 11,* 487–491.

Newborg, J. (2005). *Battelle developmental inventory* (2nd edn.). Itasca: Riverside.

Nichols, D. S., & Case-Smith, J. (1996). Reliability and validity of the pediatric evaluation of disability inventory. *Pediatric Physical Therapy, 8,* 15–24.

Nordin, V., & Gillberg, C. (1996). Autism spectrum disorders in children with physical or mental disability or both. I: Clinical and epidemiological aspects. *Developmental Medicine & Child Neurology, 38,* 297–313.

Ozonoff, S., Goodlin-Jones, B. L., & Solomon, M. (2005). Evidence-based assessment of autism spectrum disorders in children and adolescents. *Journal of Clinical Child and Adolescent Psychology, 34,* 523–540.

Pakula, A. T., Van Naarden Braun, K., & Yeargin-Allsopp, M. (2009). Cerebral palsy: Classification and epidemiology. *Physical Medicine and Rehabilitation Clinics of North America, 20,* 425–452.

Palisano, R., Rosenbaum, P., Walter, S., Russell, D., Wood, E., & Galuppi, B. (2008). Development and reliability of a system to classify gross motor function in children with cerebral palsy. *Developmental Medicine & Child Neurology, 39,* 214–223.

Pennington, L. (2008). Cerebral palsy and communication. *Pediatrics and Child Health, 18,* 405–409.

Rethlefsen, S. A., Ryan, D. D., & Kay, R. N. (2010). Classification systems in cerebral palsy. *Orthopedic Clinics of North America, 41,* 457–467.

Roid, G. (2003). *Stanford-Binet intelligence scales fifth edition (SB5).* Itasca: Riverside Publishing.

Roid, G. H., Miller, L. J., Pomplun, M., & Koch, C. (2013). *Leiter international performance scale, third edition (Leiter 3).* Wood Dale: Stoelting.

Rosen, M. G., & Dickinson, J. C. (1992). The incidence of cerebral palsy. *American Journal of Obstetrics & Gynecology, 167,* 417–423.

Rosenbaum, P., Paneth, N., Leviton, A., Goldsten, M., Bax, M., Damiano, D., et al. (2007). A report: The definition and classification of cerebral palsy April 2006. *Developmental Medicine & Child Neurology, 49,* 8–14.

Russell, D. J., Rosenbaum, P. L., Gowland, C., Hardy, S., Lane, M., Plews, N., et al. (1993). *Manual for the gross motor function measure.* Hamilton: McMaster University.

Sankar, C., & Mundkur, N. (2005). Cerebral palsy-definition, classification, etiology, and early diagnosis. *Indian Journal of Pediatric, 72,* 865–868.

Schalock, R. L., & Luckasson, R. (2004). American association on mental retardation's efinition, classification, and system of supports and its relation to international trends and issues in the field of intellectual disabilities. *Journal of Policy and Practice in Intellectual Disabilities, 1,* 136–146.

Shah, A., & Holmes, N. (1985). The use of the Leiter International Performance Scale with autistic children. *Journal of Autism and Developmental Disorders, 15,* 195–203.

Simonoff, E., Pickles, A., Charman, T., Chandler, T. L., & Baird, G. (2008). Psychiatric disorders in children with autism spectrum disorders: Prevalence, comorbidity, and associated factors in a population-derived sample. *Journal of the American Academy of Child and Adolescent Psychiatry, 47,* 921–929.

Singhi, P. D., Jagirdar, S., & Malhi, P. (2003). Epilepsy in children with cerebral palsy. *Journal of Child Neurology, 18,* 174–179.

Smile, S., Dupuis, A., MacArthur, C., Roberts, W., & Fehlings, D. (2013). Autism spectrum disorder phenotype in children with ambulatory cerebral palsy: A descriptive cross-sectional study. *Research in Autism Spectrum Disorders, 7,* 391–397.

Smits, D. W., Hetelaar, M., Gorter, J. W., van Schie, P., Dallmeijer, A., Jongmans, M., et al. (2011). Development of daily activities in school-aged children with cerebral palsy. *Research in Developmental Disabilities, 32,* 222–234.

Sparrow, S. S., Cicchetti, D. V., & Balla, D. A. (2005). *Vineland adaptive behavior scales: (Vineland-II).* Livonia: Pearson Assessments.

Tarbox, J., Wilke, A. E., Najdowski, A. C., Findel-Pyles, R. S., Balasanyan, S., Caveney, A. C., et al. (2009). Comparing indirect, descriptive, and experimental functional assessments of challenging behavior in children with autism. *Journal of Developmental and Physical Disabilities, 21,* 493–514.

Tomanik, S. S., Pearson, D. A., Loveland, K. A., Lane, D. M., & Shaw, J. B. (2007). Improving the reliability of autism diagnoses: Examining the utility of adaptive behavior. *Journal of Autism and Developmental Disorders, 37,* 921–928.

van Tilburg, M. L., Squires, M. M., Blois-Martin, N. N., Leiby, A. A., & Langseder, A. A. (2013). Test of the child/adolescent Rome III criteria: Agreement with physician diagnosis and daily symptoms. *Neurogastroenterology & Motility, 25,* 302–246.

Valicenti-McDermott, M., McVicar, K., Rapin, I., Wershil, B. K., Cohen, H., & Shinnar, S. (2006). Frequency of gastrointestinal symptoms in children with autistic spectrum disorders and association with family history of autoimmune disease. *Journal of Developmental And Behavioral Pediatrics, 27*(Suppl2), S128-S137.

Vig, S., & Jedrysek, E. (1999). Autistic features in young children with significant cognitive impairment: Autism or mental retardation? *Journal of Autism and Developmental Disorders, 29,* 235–248.

Walker, L. S., Caplan, A., & Rasquin, A. (2000). *Manual for the questionnaire on pediatric gastrointestinal symptoms.* Nashville: Department of Pediatrics, Vanderbilt University Medical Center.

Wechsler, D. (2003). *Wechsler intelligence scale for children-4th edition (WISC-IV).* San Antonio: Harcourt Assessment.

Wechsler, D. (2008). *Wechsler adult intelligence scale-4th edition (WAIS-IV).* San Antonio: Harcourt Assessment.

Wechsler, D. (2012). *Wechsler preschool and primary scale of intelligence-4th edition (WPPSI-IV).* San Antonio: Harcourt Assessment.

Wright, F. V., & Boschen, K. A. (1993). The Pediatric Evaluation of Disability Inventory (PEDI): Validation of a new functional assessment outcome instrument. *Canadian Journal of Rehabilitation, 7,* 41–42.

Yeargin-Allsopp, M., Van Naarden Braun, K., Doernberg, N. S., Benedict, R. E., Kirby, R. S., & Durkin, M. S. (2008). Prevalence of cerebral palsy in 8-year-old children in three areas of the United States in 2002: A multisite collaboration. *Pediatrics, 121,* 547–554.

Zwaigenbaum, L. (2014). The intriguing relationship between cerebral palsy and autism. *Developmental Medicine & Child Neurology, 56,* 7–8.

Chapter 5
Methods and Procedures for Measuring Comorbid Disorders: Motor Movement and Activity

Ting Liu, Casey M. Breslin and Sayed ElGarhy

Part I: Overarching Concerns with Assessment of Autism Spectrum Disorder

As the incidence of children with autism spectrum disorder (ASD) has increased in recent years (CDC 2012, so has the awareness of the unique needs of these children. The clinical diagnosis of ASD focuses on the difficulties in social communication and the repetitive and restrictive stereotypic behaviors (APA 2013). While these are the two hallmarks of the diagnosis, both are impacted by the motor behaviors exhibited by children with ASD (Sacrey et al. 2014). Motor behaviors refer to the muscle actions and movements produced by an individual (Ives 2014). In order to exhibit joint attention, a child must have adequate control over their eye muscles. To hold a meaningful conversation with another child, one must produce motor activity of the mouth, nose, and throat, while interpreting auditory information. Thus, motor behavior may play a large role in the social communicative skills of children with ASD (Bhat et al. 2011; MacDonald et al. 2013).

Recent reports in the literature indicate that a strong moderating relationship may exist between motor skill development and social communicative skills (Bhat et al. 2011; MacDonald et al. 2013). Evidence suggests that contextually inappropriate behaviors such as avoidant, self-injurious, and/or disruptive behaviors may be related to poor fundamental motor skill development (Breslin and Rudisill 2013; MacDonald et al. 2013). On the other hand, cognitive functioning (Piek et al. 2008),

T. Liu (✉)
Department of Health and Human Performance, Texas State University,
San Marcos, TX 78666, USA
e-mail: tingliu@txstate.edu

C. M. Breslin
Temple University, Philadelphia, PA, USA

S. ElGarhy
Fayoum University, Al Fayoum, Faiyum Governorate, Egypt

Johnny L. Matson (ed.), *Comorbid Conditions Among Children with Autism Spectrum Disorders,* Autism and Child Psychopathology Series,
DOI 10.1007/978-3-319-19183-6_5

language development (Hill 2010), social communication (MacDonald et al. 2013), and on-task behaviors (Breslin and Rudisill 2013) are more likely to exist among children with ASD with good motor skill development. Thus, motor skillfulness may play an important role in explaining the symptomology of ASD.

Physical activity participation may also have an impact in moderating the symptomology of ASD (Gordon et al. 1986; Lang et al. 2010; Magnusson et al. 2012; Oriel et al. 2011; Pan et. al. 2011a; Rosenthal-Malek and Mitchell 1997). A growing body of literature suggests that children with ASD, regardless of age, experience positive effects following bouts of exercise. Specifically, after engaging in physical activity, children with ASD exhibit fewer self-injurious and stereotypic behaviors (Gordon et al. 1986; Kern et al. 1982; Levinson and Reid 1993; Petrus et al. 2008; Prupas and Reid 2001; Rosenthal-Malek and Mitchell 1997; Sowa and Meulenbroek 2012), more on-task behaviors (Magnusson et al. 2012; Nicholson et al. 2011), and better academic performance (Oriel et al. 2011). In a study exploring the physical activity habits during middle school physical education, children with ASD who engaged in higher intensity physical activity were found to interact more often with peers than the children who engaged in low-intensity physical activity (Pan et al. 2011b). Furthermore, the development of fundamental motor skills may directly influence a child's physical fitness and physical activity participation (Stodden et al. 2008). Thus, the motor behavior and physical activity of children with ASD are an essential consideration in a therapeutic plan for this population. In this chapter, we will review the literature pertaining to the methods and procedures for measuring motor skill performance and physical activity in children with ASD. We included four parts to this chapter. In the first part, we discuss challenges to motor assessment for children with ASD. Next, we discuss threats to validity and reliability within the measurement of motor skills and physical activity. Then, a review of literature pertaining to motor assessment instruments is presented. In the final part, the physical activity assessments of children with ASD are presented.

Challenges to Motor Assessment of Children with ASD

Administration of standardized motor assessments to children with ASD can be challenging because of deficits in nonverbal communication, social attention, motivation, and imitation, as well as the presence of sensory integration deficits (Chawarska and Bearess 2008). However, there are some procedures that can be used before and during assessment to avoid and minimize these challenges.

Before Assessment Practitioners should obtain the child's background information from parents, teachers, and/or specialists. This information includes the child's age, social skills, method of communication (e.g., spoken language, sign language, or PECS), sensory integration problems, results of other tests (e.g., IQ, receptive and expressive language), and preferred reinforcers. Examiners can use this information to facilitate assessment and help prepare the testing environment.

During Assessment Many aspects need to be taken into consideration during motor assessment such as visual supports, language, attire, environment, paraeducator, and testing equipment (Breslin and Liu 2015; Breslin and Rudisill 2011; Esposito et al. 2014; Liu and Breslin 2013b). Practitioners should use appropriate verbal instructions along with visual supports; repeat the demonstration to make sure the child is attentive; advise children to wear proper assessment attire; provide a paraeducator or a peer tutor during assessment; limit distractions in the testing environment; and use required equipment so that the results of the motor assessment are as accurate and reliable as possible. Practitioners should also use reinforcers to motivate the child during the assessment and to take notes about the child's behavior and responses. If needed, the children may take a break every 2–3 min to help them concentrate on task performance.

In sum, these approaches have been widely employed in educational settings for years, but only recently have been applied in assessment settings (Breslin and Rudisill 2011, 2013; Esposito et al. 2014; Liu and Breslin 2013b). Adopting these strategies may improve validity and reliability, and also help practitioners feel more competent in administering motor skill assessments to children with ASD.

Validity and Reliability

Validity refers to the degree to which a test measures what it intends to measure (Thomas et al. 2011). That is, it is important to match the assessment instrumentation to the characteristics to be measured and the population of interest and be certain that the test instrument does not measure something else. There is concern that some assessments used for children with ASD may not measure the intended construct due to the nature of the disorder. For example, many research studies suggest that children with ASD did not understand instructions during motor skill assessments (Berkeley et al. 2001; Breslin and Buchanan 2014; Breslin and Liu in press; Breslin and Rudisill 2011; Green et al. 2002; Staples and Reid 2010). This may be due to the language used during the assessment instructions (Breslin and Liu 2015) or due to the child misunderstanding the purpose of the action to be completed (Berkeley et al. 2001; Green et al. 2002; Staples and Reid 2010).

Utilizing visual supports during motor skill assessments can improve the validity of scores (Breslin and Rudisill 2011; Esposito et al. 2014; Liu and Breslin 2013b). In these studies, a picture was used to illustrate the action needed to be performed to complete the assessment. It was reported that children with ASD improved their motor performance regardless of whether the assessment utilized a process or product approach. Specifically, two of the studies found that children with ASD earned higher performance scores on the Test of Gross Motor Development-Second Edition (TGMD-2) using picture task cards (Breslin and Rudisill 2011; Esposito et al. 2014). Liu and Breslin (2013b) also showed higher scores on the Movement Assessment Battery for Children-Second Edition (MABC-2) by children with ASD using a picture activity schedule. Therefore, visual supports such as picture task cards may improve the face or logical validity of the motor assessments. Furthermore, each published assessment instrument has undergone rigorous validation procedures to ensure adequate content validity, criterion validity, and predictive validity (Thomas et al. 2011). Practitioners should consult the manual for the validation process describing either assessment administration for the motor skill assessment or device monitoring physical activity.

Reliability refers to repeatability (Thomas et al. 2011). To ensure the measurements are repeatable in motor and physical activity assessments, it is important to build a rapport with the children with ASD and familiarize the child with any instruments to be used during an assessment (Block et al. 2013). This can be done through an acclimation period where the equipment and instruments used in the assessment are available, and the child with ASD is shown how to use the equipment to complete the assessment (Breslin and Rudisill 2011).

When measuring motor performance and physical activity in children with ASD, it is critical to consider how to maximize the assessment's validity and reliability (Breslin and Liu 2015). Practitioners should pay attention to how motor assessments are being administered in order to ensure reliability and reduce barriers towards understanding motor performance of children with ASD.

Concerning Comorbidities

Children with ASD may have comorbid disorders including anxiety, attention deficit hyperactivity disorder (ADHD), gastrointestinal disorders, intellectual disability, obesity, obsessive-compulsive disorder, seizure disorders, sleep disorders, Tourette's syndrome, or difficulties in sensory processing (Bauman 2010; Egan et al. 2013). Although the exact prevalence of these concomitant disorders is unknown, there are reports in the literature suggesting that these disorders may also influence the motor performance and physical activity participation in children with ASD (Bauman 2010).

These children are also at high risk for the co-occurrence of mental health disorders (Stratis and Lecavalier 2013) and there is significant variability in the estimated prevalence rates of mental health disorders among children with ASD (Lainhart 1999). Approximately 70 % of children with ASD meet the criteria for at least one additional psychiatric disorder (Brookman-Frazee et al. 2012; Leyfer et al. 2006; Simonoff et al. 2008). Skokauskas and Gallagher (2010) suggest that children with ASD are more likely to have additional co-occurring psychiatric issues: 0–6 %, schizophrenia; 10–50 %, affective disorders; 5–35 %, generalized anxiety; 10–64 %, simple phobias; 1–37 %, obsessive-compulsive disorder; and 30–39 %, intellectual disability. Thus, children with ASD may have additional psychological or emotional needs that must be accounted for during motor skill assessments.

Beyond psychological and emotional conditions that must be acknowledged in this population, there are physical needs as well. A well-established inverse relationship between physical activity and obesity status exists, and children with disabilities have a higher incidence of being overweight and are twice as likely to be physically inactive as their peers without disabilities (Rimmer et al. 2007; Tsiros et al. 2011). Among children with disabilities, those with ASD have an even higher prevalence of obesity than those who do not have ASD (Egan et al. 2013). The cause of this increase in obesity rates may be due to lifestyle choices similar to ones facing typically developing children. However, certain medications commonly prescribed to children with ASD have weight gain as a documented side effect (McCracken et al. 2002). Additionally, many behavioral and educational interventions used with children with ASD are based on rewards systems using edible products (Cappadocia and Weiss 2011). Finally, these children may have greater challenges than their peers without disabilities in combatting being overweight and obese because of their limited social outlets for recreational activities that promote health and wellness (Johnson 2009). Therefore, children with ASD who are obese may face additional challenges when attempting to engage in enough physical activity because they also require additional resources and support for safe physical activity participation (Hills et al. 2010).

In addition, some children with ASD experience medical conditions that may affect their motor and physical activity participation. For example, gastrointestinal disorders, metabolic disorders, or hormonal dysfunction are prevalent among children with ASD as opposed to typically developing peers. The exact occurrence of these conditions is unclear. Sometimes these disorders may be left rather untreated because of difficulties communicating with medical professionals about symptoms and treatment approaches (Bauman 2010). Thus, it can be problematic to account for these concerns during motor performance and physical activity participation in children with ASD (Bauman 2010). However, identifying more information about these types of medical conditions and their influence on motor behavior can help identify subgroups of children with ASD with common symptoms (Bauman 2010). Specific educational treatments and interventions targeting these symptoms may then be targeted for use with these subgroups in physical activity settings.

Another issue prevalent among children with ASD is sleep disorders. While the exact proportion of children with ASD who also have a sleep disorder is unknown, these children are far more likely to have the disorder than their typically developing peers (Bauman 2010). Sleep disorders can cause far-reaching developmental and behavioral problems and they are often treated through educational interventions targeting sleep hygiene and exercise behaviors. Specifically, it is suggested that moderate-to-vigorous physical activity (MVPA) early in the day combined with a regular nighttime routine incorporating light stretching or yoga can facilitate more restful sleep, which in turn could lead to better daytime outcomes and increased quality of life for children with ASD (Reynolds and Malow 2011).

In summary, children with ASD have additional needs and considerations when assessing their motor skillfulness and physical activity. A review of some common assessment approaches follows, including methods and procedures for measuring motor movement and physical activity in children with ASD, and the strengths and weaknesses of each motor and physical activity assessment technique.

Part II: Motor Assessment Instruments for Children with ASD

It is important that the motor skills of children with ASD are assessed properly. Without proper assessment, children may be placed in educational settings that are inappropriate for their motor abilities. To understand the motor movement and activity of children with ASD, tests and instruments must be used. However, the choice of which test or instrument to use is considered a challenge for many practitioners, especially with the number of assessment instruments available (Staples 2013).

A variety of standardized assessment instruments have been used to examine the fine and gross motor skill performance of children with ASD (Pan et al. 2009). Some instruments focus on assessing individuals' motor skills such as the Bruininks-Oseretsky Test of Motor Proficiency-Second Edition (BOT-2; Bruininks and Bruininks 2005), Movement Assessment Battery for Children-Second Edition (MABC-2; Henderson et al. 2007), Peabody Development Motor Scales-Second Edition (PDMS-2; Folio and Fewell 2000), and TGMD-2 (Ulrich 2000). Others may include subtests on motor skill assessment such as Bayley Scales of Infant and Toddler Development-Third Edition (Bayley-III; Bayley 2006), Mullen Scales of Early Learning (MSEL; Mullen 1995), and Vineland Adaptive Behavior Scales-Second Edition (Vineland-II; Sparrow et al. 2005). Before making decisions on which motor assessment instrument to use for children with ASD, practitioners should have a basic understanding of the discrepancies in these instruments. For example, the TGMD-2 only assesses gross motor skills for children, while the MABC-2, PDMS-2, and BOT-2 can be used to assess a wider range of fine and gross motor skills including stationary balance, locomotion, object manipulation, strength and agility, manual coordination, body coordination, fine manual control, and/or manual dexterity.

In this section, we discuss each of these motor assessment instruments in detail in terms of their targeted skills, age ranges, estimated testing time, subtests, procedures, type of scores, and interpretation. The main emphasis is on the BOT-2, MABC-2, PDMS-2, and TGMD-2 because they are the only instruments that solely focus on motor assessment. We include a case study to compare and contrast the four instruments and then provide recommendations for practitioners on how to choose the appropriate instrument. A detailed comparison of studies using these assessments is presented in Table 5.1.

Motor Assessment Instruments

Bruininks-Oseretsky Test of Motor Proficiency-Second Edition (BOT-2)

The BOT-2 (Bruininks and Bruininks 2005) is designed to measure fine and gross motor skills, manual, body, and limb coordination skills, and strength and agility abilities for children and individuals aged between 4 and 21 years. The BOT-2 can

Table 5.1 A detailed comparison of the studies that used MABC-2, TGMD-2, PDMS-2, and BOT-2 on children with ASD (ordered by publication date)

The Movement Assessment Battery for Children-2 (MABC-2)			
Study	Title	Participants	Results
Liu (2013)	Sensory processing and motor skill performance in elementary school children with autism spectrum disorder	Thirty-two children with ASD (26 boys, 6 girls) aged **5–11 years**	About 78 % of children were in the red zone indicating that they had significant movement delays, 6 % of the children were in the amber zone suggesting that they were at risk of having movement delays, and 16 % of the children were in the green zone and had no movement delays. Furthermore, scores for sensory processing were positively correlated with their motor performance
Liu and Breslin (2013a)	Fine and gross motor performance of the MABC-2 by children with autism spectrum disorder and typically developing children	Thirty children with ASD aged **3–16 years** (males = 25, females = 5) and 30 age-matched typically developing children (males = 16, females = 14)	Children with ASD showed significantly lower MABC-2 percentile scores than typically developing children on manual dexterity, ball skills, and static and dynamic balance
Liu and Breslin (2013b)	The effect of a picture activity schedule on performance of the MABC-2 for children with autism spectrum disorder	Thirty children with ASD (ages **3–16** years) and 30 age-matched typically developing children	Descriptive data showed that all typically developing children were classified in the green zone on MABC-2. However, the majority of children (80 %) with ASD were categorized in the red and amber zones suggesting they experienced motor difficulty or were at risk for motor delay. In addition, children with ASD showed significantly lower MABC-2 percentile scores than typically developing children on manual dexterity, ball skills, and static and dynamic balance
Study	Title	Participants	Participants
Whyatt and Craig (2012)	Motor skills in children aged 7–10 years, diagnosed with autism spectrum disorder	Eighteen children aged between **7 and 10** years, and 19 age-matched receptive vocabulary control group, and 22 age matched nonverbal IQ control group	Children with ASD experienced general motor impairment when compared to typically developing children

Table 5.1 (continued)

Study	Title	Participants	Results
The Movement Assessment Battery for Children-2 (MABC-2)			
Borremans et al. (2009)	Motor skills of young adults with Asperger syndrome: A comparative study	Twenty-one males (mean age was **16.9 years**) and nine females (mean age was **18.0 years**). The control group consisted of 30 children, age and gender matched, young adults (mean age was **16.9 years**)	Results suggested that 60 % of individuals were at risk for motor impairment. Most of the 18 participants with Asperger syndrome who scored below the 15th percentile displayed a range of motor problems across the three subscales. Another five individuals scored on the 16th percentile. These children were more likely to have one or two areas of relative strength, often with one score close to the 50th percentile. Their stronger areas were balance and fine motor skills. Across all abilities, children with ASD earned the lowest scores on ball skills, indicating the greatest impairment in that domain. Individuals in the control group were scored between 16th and 95th percentile putting them in the normal range
Green et al. (2008)	Impairment in movement skills of children with autistic spectrum disorders	One hundred and one children with ASD, aged **10–14 years**, and 101 typical children with wide range of IQ scores (35 IQ < 70 and 66 IQ > 70)	About 79 % of the children with ASD had definite movement impairments on the MABC-2, 10 % were at the risk of motor impairments. Children with an IQ less than 70 were more impaired than those with IQ more than 70
Study	Title	Participants	Results
Hilton et al. (2007)	Relationship between motor skill impairment and severity in children with Asperger syndrome	Fifty-one children with Asperger syndrome aged **6–12 years**, and a control group of 56 typical children	Results showed that 65 % of children have definite levels of motor impairment, and 25 % were at risk of motor impairments. About 82 % were delayed in manual dexterity, 53 % in ball skills, and 33 % in balance. Strong correlations were found between the MABC-2 motor impairment levels and the Social Responsiveness Scaleseverity levels
Miyahara et al. (1997)	Brief report: motor incoordination in children with Asperger syndrome and learning disabilities	Twenty-six children with Asperger syndrome (22 boys, and 4 girls) aged from **6 to 15 years**, and 18 children with learning disabilities (14 boys and 2 girls) aged from 6 to 15 years	All children with Asperger syndrome were impaired on manual dexterity, 96 % impaired on ball skills, and 92 % impaired on balance. A total of 95 % children with learning disabilities were impaired on manual dexterity, 100 % were impaired on ball skills, and 80 % were impaired on balance

Table 5.1 (continued)

The Movement Assessment Battery for Children-2 (MABC-2)			
Test of Gross Motor Development-2 (TGMD-2)			
Study	Title	Participants	Results
Liu et al. (2014)	Gross motor performance by children with autism spectrum disorder and typically developing children on TGMD-2	Twenty-one children with ASD (M=**7.57 years**) and 21 age-matched typically developing children (M=7.38 years)	Concerning the locomotor subtest, about 67 % of the children with ASD received poor standard scores and 40 % of scores were classified very poor. About 60 % of the participants had poor standard scores of ≤5 and 33 % of scores were very poor on object control skills. For overall gross motor quotient scores, 81 % children with ASD were below 79 and classified as poor and about 76 % children scored below 70 and received very poor rating. Overall, gross motor quotient scores revealed significant performance differences between children with ASD and typically developing children
MacDonald et al. (2013)	The relationship of motor skills and social communicative skills in school-aged children with autism spectrum disorder	Thirty-five children with high-functioning ASD aged **6–15 years**	Object control skills can be used to calibrate ASD severity. Children with weaker motor skills also have greater social communicative skill deficits
Staples and Reid (2010)	Fundamental movement skills and autism spectrum disorders	Twenty-five children **(9.1–12.8 years)** with ASD were compared to three typically developing comparison groups, each individually matched on different developmental variables: (a) chronological age, (b) movement skill performance, and (c) mental age	Results showed children with ASD scored significantly lower (16 %) on both locomotor and object control tests than chronologically age-matched and mental age-matched children. When the typically developing children were matched to the children with ASD, the typically developing children were half the age of the children with ASD
Pan et al. (2009)	Fundamental movement skills in children diagnosed with autism spectrum disorders and attention deficit hyperactivity disorder	Children with HFA (**6–10 years**), children with attention deficit hyperactivity disorder (ADHD), and age-matched typically developing children	About 5 % of children with HFA and ADHD had a mean locomotor subtest score that was equal to or more than 1.5 standard deviations below the mean. The gross motor quotient scores placed 16 % of the participants with ASD and ADHD in the very poor and poor performance categories

Table 5.1 (continued)

The Movement Assessment Battery for Children-2 (MABC-2)			
Berkeley et al. (2001)	Locomotor and object control skills of children diagnosed with autism	Fifteen children (10 boys and 5 girls) with high functioning autism (HFA), aged **6–8 years**	It was reported that 80 % of children with HFA (all girls and 7 boys) were placed in the poor and very poor categories for locomotor skills and 53 % children were in the poor and very poor categories on object control skills
Peabody Development Motor Scales-2 (PDMS-2)			
Study	Title	Participants	Results
Provost et al. (2007a)	Levels of gross and fine motor development in young children with autism spectrum disorder	Thirty-eight young children aged **21–41 months**, 19 children with ASD, 19 children with developmental disorders	The levels of gross motor and fine motor development did not differ for the majority (66 %) of children with ASD. Approximately a third of the children had discrepant levels of development between fine and gross motor skills. About 25 % of the children's fine motor skills were more advanced than gross motor skills, an approximately 10 % children with ASD showed gross motor skills that were more advanced than their fine motor skills. The gross and fine motor scores of young children with ASD did not differ when compared to young children with developmental delay
Provost et al. (2007b)	A comparison of motor delays in young children: autism spectrum disorder, developmental delay, and developmental concerns	Fifty-six young children aged **21–41 months** divided into three groups: 19 children with ASD, 19 children without ASD but with developmental delay (DD) including motor delay, and 18 children without ASD who had developmental concerns but without motor delay	All participants were assessed on PDMS-2 and Bayley-II. One child with ASD was classified as average in both the gross motor and total motor areas, and another child was also categorized as average in the fine motor area in PDMS-2. Most children scored below average or lower with 16–26 % scoring in the very poor category. Using the classifications based on the standard scores of Bayley-II Motor Scale, three children with ASD (16 % of the ASD group) were classified as mildly delayed, and 16 children (84 % of the children) were classified as significantly delayed in motor skill performance

Table 5.1 (continued)

The Movement Assessment Battery for Children-2 (MABC-2)			
Study	Title	Participants	Results
Vanvuchelen et al. (2007)	Nature of motor imitation problems in school-aged males with autism: How congruent are the error types?	Eight low-functioning males with autism aged from **5 to 6 years,** IQ ranged from 55 to 79. Thirteen low-functioning comparison males with learning disability, aged 5–6 years, IQ from 55 to 78; 17 high-functioning males with autism aged 7–10 years, IQ 80–124; and 17 typically developing males, age range 7–10 years	The participants were examined using motor tests suitable for their cognitive abilities. The PDMS-2 was used for the low-functioning group and the high-functioning group was assessed with MABC-2. The motor performance of the low-functioning and the high-functioning children with ASD was significantly delayed compared to the typically developing children
Bruininks-Oseretsky Test of Motor Proficiency-2 (BOT-2)			
Study	Title	Participants	Results
Mattard-Labrecque et al. (2013)	Children with autism and attention difficulties: a pilot study of the association between sensory, motor, and adaptive behaviors	Thirty children aged **5–14 years** diagnosed with HFASD (13 children) and ADHD (17 children)	About 62 % of children with high-functioning ASD and ADHD, and 23.5 % of children with ADHD had a total motor performance below 1 standard deviation. The lower total motor performance of children with high-functioning ASD and ADHD was probably due to poorer gross motor skills
Dewey et al. (2007)	Motor and gestural performance in children with autism spectrum disorders, developmental coordination disorder, and/or ADHD	Forty-nine children with ASD, 46 children with DCD, 38 children with DCD and ADHD, 27 with ADHD, and 78 typically developing children	Children with ASD, DCD, and DCD and ADHD were significantly impaired on motor coordination skills when compared to the typically developing children as measured by the BOT-2 short form. Additionally, children with ASD showed impairment on gestural skills
Ghaziuddin and Butler (1998)	Clumsiness in autism and Asperger syndrome: a further report	Twelve children with AS (age average **11.4 years** and IQ 104.9), compared to 12 children with autism disorder (age average **10.3 years** and IQ 78.4), and 12 children with Pervasive Developmental Disorder, Not Otherwise Specified (age average **10.1 years** and IQ 78.2)	While coordination deficits were found in all three groups, children with AS were found to be less impaired than those with autism disorder and PDD-NOS. However, no significant relationship was found between coordination and diagnosis after adjusting for the level of intelligence

be administered in the short form with 14 items and takes between 15 and 20 min, or in the complete form with 53 items takes 45–60 min. The BOT–2 covers four motor areas; each area includes two subtests with a total of eight subtests. The fine manual control area includes the fine motor precision subtest (precise control of finger and hand movements) and the fine motor integration subtest (ability to integrate visual stimuli with motor control). The manual coordination area has the manual dexterity subtest (goal-directed activities that involve reaching, grasping, and bimanual coordination with small objects) and the upper-limb coordination subtest (visual tracking with coordinated arm and hand movement). The body coordination area includes the bilateral coordination subtest (tasks requiring body control, and sequential and simultaneous coordination of the upper and lower limbs) and the balance subtest (motor control skills integral to maintaining posture when standing, walking, or performing activities such as reaching for a cup on a shelf). The strength and agility area has the running speed and agility subtest (running speed and agility) and the strength subtest (trunk and upper and lower body strength).

The score a child receives on the BOT-2 is quantitative. It may be the number of points, correct activities performed, or time in seconds for each item. The BOT-2 raw scores can be converted to point scores, scale scores, standard scores, confidence intervals, five descriptive categories for each subtest (ranging from well below average to well above average), and total motor composite scores. At the end of each subtest, there is an area labeled notes and observations. This empty space is designed for an examiner to record any specific observations during the child's performance such as attitude, effort, behaviors, or strategies that the examinee used to complete the task during assessment. These observations may be included in the assessment report (Bruininks and Bruininks 2005). When used to record assessment modifications and/or behaviors exhibited by the child with ASD, this observation part of the assessment report can help practitioners have a clear understanding of the results.

Procedures The BOT-2 short form can be used as a screening tool. For children with ASD who had problems on the short form, the complete form must be used for detailed assessment. To ensure accurate and/or best performance, the child may perform two trials for each test item. The *BOT-2 Manual* includes images that represent the sequence of steps of each task in color and includes realistic photos. These colored pictures may facilitate the administration of items to children with ASD, as visual supports conveying the task to be completed have been found to lead to higher scores on motor assessments (Breslin and Rudisill 2011, 2013; Liu and Breslin 2013b).

Previous Research The authors only found two studies using BOT-2 on children with ASD (Dewey et al. 2007; Mattard-Labrecque et al. 2013). Mattard-Labrecque et al. (2013) found that children with high functioning autism (HFA) and ADHD performed below one standard deviation and the low total motor performance score was probably due to poor gross motor development. Dewey et al. (2007) reported that children with ASD were impaired on motor coordination skills when compared to the typically developing children. More studies are needed on BOT-2 for children with ASD.

Limitation It takes much more time to administer the BOT-2 complete form to children than other motor assessments such as the MABC-2 and the TGMD-2. Therefore, for better time management, practitioners should assess the child on the short form first. The complete form is more appropriate for assessments in clinical settings than school settings. It may also be difficult to administer testing items that require the child to close his eyes. In the case study presented later in this chapter, we believe the child's difficulty in performance was related to understanding the tasks rather than to closing his eyes. That is, the sensory integration deficits in children with ASD may cause difficulties in sensory processing and performance of these tasks.

Movement Assessment Battery for Children-Second Edition (MABC-2)

The MABC-2 (Henderson et al. 2007) is developed as a screening tool that can be used to identify children who are significantly behind their age-matched peers in motor skill performance. It measures both fine and gross motor skill performance for children in three age bands (3–6, 7–10, and 11–16 years) and takes about 15–20 min to administer. The MABC-2 contains eight tasks for each of the three age bands in three different constructs: manual dexterity, ball skills, and static and dynamic balance. A score can be the number of seconds, steps, throws or catches. An "F" is given if the child failed to perform the task properly, an "R" is recorded when the child refuses to perform the task, and an "I" is noted if the task is inappropriate for the child.

Each task's raw score can be converted to a standard score, and a total test score can be calculated by summing the eight tasks' standard scores. Using the total test score, a percentile score can be found from the norm tables published in the *MABC-2 MANUAL* to determine a child's motor performance difficulty. The test percentile scores are described as a traffic light scoring system including a red zone, amber zone, and green zone. A percentile score ≤5th is classified in the red zone indicating significant movement difficulty, a percentile score between the 5th and 15th is categorized as the amber zone, indicating a risk of movement difficulty, and a percentile score > 15th is classified as the green zone, indicating that no movement difficulty was detected. In addition to quantitative scores, each task has its qualitative observations. These observations are listed in a systematic way, from the distinction of a child's ability to control his or her own body to the extent to which the demands of the task are met, and the examiner may add more notes to the observations. The observations are not part of the quantitative scores and have no normative data. Therefore, the MABC-2 is considered a quantitative oriented motor assessment instrument (Yun and Shapiro 2004).

Procedure Detailed verbal descriptions and demonstrations of motor skills to be performed should be provided to children with ASD prior to the MABC-2 administration. Children should also be given additional instructions and directions if they do not seem to understand when observed during their practice trials or if requested by the children. The children may need to perform two trials to get the best performance for each task.

Previous Research Several studies have used MABC-2 to assess fine and gross motor skills of children with ASD (Borremans et al. 2009; Green et al. 2008, 2002; Hilton et al. 2007; Liu 2013; Liu and Breslin 2013a, b; Miyahara et al. 1997; Whyatt and Craig 2012). Results of these studies were consistent regarding the motor skill impairments for children with ASD. A detailed comparison of the studies that used MABC-2 on children with ASD is presented in Table 5.1.

Limitations The MABC-2 only has eight tasks in each of the three domains (i.e., manual dexterity, ball skills, and static and dynamic balance) for the age band. Performance on one or two motor tasks may or may not provide a true representation of children's capacities for fine and gross motor skill performance in that domain (Staples 2013). Therefore, researchers should use the MABC-2 as a screening tool for motor impairment. This is consistent with the viewpoint of Whyatt and Craig (2012) about the nature of the MABC-2 that it may not be sufficiently sensitive to identify specific mechanisms underlying the impaired motor performance of children with ASD. In part, this lack of sensitivity may be related to how the tasks are scored rather than the assessment itself, especially with the quantitative nature of scoring (Staples 2013). In addition, Borremans et al. (2009) recommend "careful" use of the MABC-2 for young adults, as many participants were identified as being at risk for severe motor impairment because of the limited norm-referenced instruments for those above the age of 16 years.

Peabody Developmental Motor Scales-Second Edition (PDMS-2)

The PDMS-2 (Folio and Fewell 2000) is a norm-referenced instrument containing 249 items. The PDMS-2 is appropriate for children from birth to 5 years of age. It is composed of six subtests examining fine and gross motor domains through reflexes, stationary, locomotion, object manipulation, grasping, and visual-motor integration. The fine motor domain includes two subtests, grasping (ability to use his or her hands), and visual-motor integration (ability to use visual perceptual skills to perform complex eye–hand coordination tasks).The gross motor domain includes the other four subtests, reflexes (for children from birth to 11 months), stationary (ability to sustain control of body within its center of gravity and retain equilibrium), locomotion (ability to move from one place to another), and object manipulation (ability to manipulate balls, for children 12 months and older).

A child may receive a score of 2, 1, or 0 for each motor skill performance. A 2 is given when a child performs the skill according to the criteria, a 1 is recorded when a child's performance shows a clear resemblance to the skill mastery criteria but does not fully meet the criteria, and a 0 is specified if the child cannot or will not attempt the item, or the attempt does not show that the skill is emerging.

The PDMS-2 has five types of scores. Raw scores can be converted to subtest age equivalent scores, percentiles, subtest standard scores, and fine, gross, and total motor quotients. Although the PDMS-2 has a mean motor quotient standard score of 100 and standard deviation of 15, it classifies motor performance primarily into seven categories ranging from very poor to very superior based on 10-point increments (rather than the 15-point standard deviation increments).

Procedures The entry points, basals, and ceiling are used on all testing items. Entry points are determined empirically to allow the examiner to begin testing on an item that 75 % of children in the normative sample at that age passed. The examiner needs to find the age-appropriate tasks for the child before establishing the basal level. The basal is established when the child receives a score of 2 on three items in a row. The last three scores of 2s before 1 or 0 become the basal level. If the child scores 0 or 1 on any of the first three items administered, the examiner should test backward until the child scores 2 on three items in a row. All items below the basal are scored 2 and the ceiling level is established when the child scores 0 on each of three consecutive items in a row. After the ceiling has been established, testing is discontinued.

The examiner may repeat the instructions to the child up to three times. Examiners can administer the item using appropriate adaptive instructions on children with ASD. Testing may be stopped if the child is tired or has lost interest. The remaining items can be tested in another session using the same entry points, basals, and ceiling on all items except the reflexes subtest (i.e., administered only to children less than 1 year old and children with motor or neurological disabilities). This can shorten the time of the second testing (Folio and Fewell 2000). Furthermore, the PDMS-2 contains both qualitative (i.e., how well child performs the skill) and quantitative (i.e., how many skills child is able to perform) aspects of the performance. PDMS-2 also includes the reflexes subtest, which is not included in other testing instruments. This subtest is important to assess infants and toddlers with ASD because they tend to display numerous problems with primitive reflexes (Bildt et al. 2012).

Previous Research Limited studies have used the PDMS-2 on children with ASD (Provost et al. 2007a, b; Vanvuchelen et al. 2007). The findings of these studies agreed that the motor abilities of children with ASD were significantly impaired when compared to those of the typically developing children.

Limitation Although a high degree of reliability for all ages within their normative sample is reported in the PDMS-2 manual (Folio and Fewell 2000), limited research has been reported on the reliability of PDMS-2 motor assessments on young children with ASD (Provost et al. 2007a). Furthermore, the PDMS-2 is only valid for children from birth to 5 years of age. For practitioners who are interested in knowing the motor skill performance of children older than 5 years, the PDMS-2 is inappropriate. There are also some age gaps between items for the two subtests. In the stationary subtest, the age gap is between item 19 "kneeling," and item 20 "standing on one foot" is large (i.e., from 13 months in item 19 to 31–32 months in item 20). Similarly, in the grasping subtests, the age gap between item 21 "grasping marker" and item 22 "grasping marker" is also large (i.e., from 15 to 16 months in item 21 to 41–42 months in item 22). In addition, some testing items' orders may be inconsistent with the children's age and developmental abilities. Those items such as throwing a ball underhand (item 18; 43–44 months old), throwing a ball overhand (item 19; 45–46 months old), should be rearranged in the object manipulation subtest. Children tend to perform better in item 19 than item 18, so item 19 should be listed before 18. The other testing items are cutting a circle (item 65; 49–50 months old) and cutting a square (item 68; 53–54 months old) in the visual integration subtest. Liu and ElGarhy (2014) studied 115 preschool children who completed the PDMS-2 and found that cutting a square was a much easier task for children to acquire than cutting a circle. Therefore, item 68 should be listed before item 65.

Test of Gross Motor Development-Second Edition (TGMD-2)

The TGMD-2 (Ulrich 2000) is a norm- and criterion-referenced test that assesses the gross motor ability of children 3–10 years. The TGMD-2 measures performance of 12 gross motor skills. It includes two subtests: locomotor subtest (run, gallop, hop, leap, jump, and slide) and object-control subtest (strike, dribble, catch, kick, throw, and roll). The TGMD-2 has evidence of validity and reliability among children and takes about 15–20 min to administer (Ulrich 2000). Each motor skill includes 3–5 performance criteria to qualitatively describe the performance. Children are asked to perform two trials. The children's performance is scored as a 1 or 0 to indicate the presence or failure to perform the specific performance criterion. The scores of the two trials are added together to obtain the score for each criterion within each skill, and then summed across the six skills to obtain the subtest raw scores. These raw scores can then be converted to standard scores from the standardized norms, and overall gross motor quotient scores (i.e., combination of all 12 gross motor skills) can be converted by summing up the standard scores on both subtests. The standard scores and quotient scores can be classified into seven categories for the TGMD-2, ranging from very poor to very superior (Ulrich 2000).

Procedures The examiner needs to determine a child's hand and foot preference first. After an accurate demonstration, a practice trial should be provided to the child. Two trials need to be administered and scored, and more than one child can be tested at a time. Therefore, a para-educator or peer buddy can be used to facilitate motor skill performance by children with ASD.

The TGMD-2 uses qualitative aspects of the movement as performance criteria and it highlights potential strategy differences used by the children during skill performance with little regard to movement outcome (Logan et al. 2011; Yun and Shapiro 2004). The inclusion of qualitative information related to how each task is performed is likely to provide further indications about the nature of motor impairment (Staples 2013). One problem raised by the researchers is that each performance criterion in TGMD-2 reflects how children perform the skill, not their motor ability. For example, when catching, the child's hands must be adjusted to the speed, direction, weight, and size of the ball; more points are awarded for the number of properly caught balls rather than the ability to manipulate these variables and catch (Van Waelvelde et al. 2004).

However, Pan et al. (2009) suggested several benefits to using the TGMD-2 to assess gross motor performance of children with ASD. First, the TGMD-2 can be completed in one testing session. Second, all materials needed to complete the TGMD-2 are readily available and can be arranged to keep distractions to a minimum. Third, data are gathered to allow for decisions to be made about the overall need for specialized therapeutic services as well as specific gross motor skill information. Fourth, the TGMD-2 evaluates both locomotor and object control skills, which are prerequisites for successful participation in many sports and games.

Previous Research Many studies have used the TGMD-2 to assess gross motor skill performance on children with ASD (Berkeley et al. 2001; Breslin and Rudisill 2011, 2013; Liu et al. 2014; MacDonald et al. 2013; Pan et al. 2009; Staples and Reid 2010). These studies have found delays in motor skill performance by children with ASD compared to typically developing peers.

Limitations The TGMD-2 is designed to assess gross motor skills for children but it does not provide the whole perspective regarding motor skill performance because fine motor skills are not assessed. For children with ASD, delays in fine motor skills may adversely impact handwriting and/or keyboarding ability, leading to challenges in communication. Therefore, it is important to capture data pertaining to fine motor skills, which is not possible with the TGMD-2. In addition, the age range of 3–10 years is small. The TGMD-2 is not appropriate for practitioners who are interested in evaluating the fundamental motor skill performance of children younger than 3 years and older than 10 years. Furthermore, some of the motor skills included in the TGMD-2 such as striking, kicking, throwing, and dribbling are related to sports. Therefore, those gross motor skills assessed in the TGMD-2 may be directly influenced by the aptitude of practice and training for specific sports such as baseball, soccer, and basketball, and may not reflect the child's true motor capacities.

Instruments That Partially Focus on Motor Assessment

Bayley Scales of Infant and Toddler Development-Third Edition (Bayley-III)

The Bayley-III (Bayley 2006) is designed to identify young children with developmental delays from ages 1 month to 42 months, and to provide information for future interventions. Bayley-III provides developmental risk indicators that may need further evaluations. Bayley-III consists of five subscales: cognitive, language (expressive and receptive), motor (fine and gross motor), social–emotional, and adaptive behavior. Testing time for children ages 1–12 months is estimated at 50 min and testing time for older children 13–42 months is expected to take about 90 min. The Bayley-III motor subscale includes fine and gross motor subtests. The fine motor subtest contains 66 items and measures skills related to eye movements, perceptual-motor integration, motor planning, and motor speed. The gross motor subtest includes 72 items and is designed to measure movements of the limbs and torso. Limited studies have used Bayley-III to assess motor skill performance for children with ASD because it targets infants and very young children. Provost et al. (2007a), for example, found that 3 of 19 children with ASD aged 21–41 months were classified as mildly delayed and 84% of the children were classified as significantly delayed in motor development.

The number of items in Bayley-III that require verbatim directions from the examiner is high. Thus, prior review and rehearsal are necessary. Furthermore, because young children with ASD may need modified instructions to increase understanding of the task at hand (Breslin and Rudisill 2011, Liu and Breslin 2013b), the Bayley-III may be inappropriate for use with this population (Ford et al. 2012).

Mullen Scales of Early Learning (MSEL)

The MSEL (Mullen 1995) is a standardized developmental test designed for young children from birth to 68 months. MSEL assesses the child's development in five domains: gross motor, visual reception, fine motor, receptive language, and expressive language (Mullen 1995). MSEL takes about 15–60 min to administer, depending on the age of the child; younger children take less time to complete the assessment than older ones (Gilliam and Mayes 2004).

The MESL was developed as a cognitive test for children. However, researchers have used MSEL for assessing motor development (Bishop et al. 2011). Children with ASD tend to perform better in the motor subtest than other subtests in the MSEL (Akshoomoff 2006). The children with ASD performed relatively better in the fine motor scale and they showed significantly lower scores on all scales compared to the children in the typically developing group. MSEL has also been used in longitudinal investigations of children with ASD. Barbaro and Dissanayake (2012) reported that children with ASD performed at an age-appropriate level for their fine motor skills at 18 months, although delays were ample between 18 and 24 months. The gross motor subscale was not measured in that study.

One drawback of the MSEL is that the gross motor subscale is only applicable to children from birth to 33 months, and the subscale is not included in the overall early learning composite score (Gilliam and Mayes 2004). This might be the reason some clinicians do not administer the MSEL gross motor subscale in their assessment. Additionally, the MSEL is a developmental test used almost exclusively by psychologists and it is not commonly used by practitioners in the kinesiology or physical therapy domains. In terms of gross motor skill assessment, the MSEL is not as detailed as the other testing instruments mainly focused on motor skill assessment. Therefore, the MSEL is recommended for use in the clinical setting (Lloyd et al. 2011).

Vineland Adaptive Behavior Scales-II (Vineland-II)

The Vineland-II (Sparrow et al. 2005) has been commonly used to assess motor skills in individuals with ASD as well as other social and communication skills

(Gillham et al. 2000; Manohari et al. 2013). The Vincland-II provides a comprehensive assessment from birth to 90 years of age. It has 383 items and covers the three domains of communication (receptive, expressive, and written), daily living skills (personal, domestic, and community), socialization (interpersonal relationship, play, and leisure time-coping skills), and motor skills (gross and fine). The Vineland-II uses survey interview, parent/caregiver rating, teacher rating, and expanded interview forms for supporting the diagnosis of intellectual and developmental disabilities. It has a maladaptive behavior domain to assess problematic behaviors (Sparrow et al. 2005).

Children with ASD and children with the combination of ASD and mental retardation are likely to exhibit higher standard scores on the motor skill performance than their communication and social interaction skills (Sparrow et al. 2005). However, Vineland-II has only been used in two studies in assessing motor skills for children with ASD (Leonard et al. 2013; Lloyd et al. 2011). Leonard et al. (2013) conducted a longitudinal study to assess the development of motor skills of 20 children at increased risk of developing ASD, and reported that early motor difficulties may be a risk factor for later motor impairment. These findings are consistent with Lloyd et al. (2011) in that the gross and fine motor skills of young children with ASD are delayed and become progressively more delayed with age.

Although the VABS-II is an effective assessment for children with ASD, there are two drawbacks while using the adaptive behavior scales. First, by nature of the interview format, ratings are based on the responses provided by the informant. Unless the informant is chosen carefully, "third party" administration can create measurement errors (Manohari et al. 2013). Second, motor skill norms are only available for children under 7 years (Gillham et al. 2000). If the motor deficit is suspected in children aged 7 and older, the children's performance will be estimated using the normative data for 6 years 9 months to 6 years 11 months.

Motor Assessment Perspective

The increasing prevalence of ASD has made the use of motor assessment in understanding the motor skill performance of children with ASD a high priority for researchers and practitioners. Because many motor assessment instruments are available for testing, there is not one gold standard instrument to investigate motor skill performance of children with ASD, especially because none are designed exclusively for this population (Piek et al. 2012). Two types of assessments exist in measuring motor skill performance in children. One is the quantitative assessment such as MABC-2 and BOT-2, and the other is the qualitative assessment such as TGMD-2 and PDMS-2. Each type of assessment provides a different picture of motor competence. Qualitative assessments allow for the description of movement that led to the outcome, while the quantitative assessments do not provide this information but instead provide numeric values of the outcome (Logan et al. 2011). Another way to think of qualitative assessments is that they are process-based assessments, as opposed to the product-based approach used in quantitative assessments.

Yun and Shapiro (2004) stated that the qualitative differences in motor skill performance of individuals with and without mental retardation may reflect different movement strategies and patterns of behavior used to successfully achieve the task. A qualitative performance assessment highlights potential strategy differences used in skill performance with little regard to movement outcome. Most standardized quantitative oriented assessment tools intended to evaluate motor ability items include balance, agility, reaction time, and manual dexterity tests. Although the methods of measuring these variables are product oriented, the intent of these instruments is to measure the underlying construct.

Thus, qualitative assessment provides specific and process-related information that may be valuable to practitioners, clinicians, and researchers. In contrast, quantitative assessment provides the numeric values of performance outcome. Thus, each type of assessment yields scores that may lead to different interpretations of performance (Logan et al. 2011). For example, the jumping task of the TGMD-2 includes four performance criteria that must be met for "successful" jump performance. Each criterion successfully completed yields a score of 1. The success of the jumping task on the MABC-2 is based on the number of consecutive jumps a child performs (up to five), with few qualitative definitions of success or failure. The main definition of success for jumping on the MABC-2 is that children must jump within the boundaries of the mats (provided with the MABC-2 testing kit) and perform one jump per mat. Thus, the maturity of the jumping movement is not measured and a child who can only complete one jump could earn the same scores on both assessments, even if the quality is very different (Logan et al. 2011). Other instruments, such as the PDMS-2 and BOT-2, focus on measuring the distance when jumping from start point (the line) to the point where the back of the nearest heel touches the floor. The score given to the child is based on the distance without paying attention to the strategies used to perform the jump.

Some researchers may not use a qualitative assessment because it requires more time to score performances accurately because of the need to analyze behavioral characteristics (i.e., performance criteria) of each skill. Examiners should go through extensive training and be tested for inter-rater reliability before conducting a qualitative assessment because the scoring of the testing items can be subjective. Meanwhile, scoring of a quantitative assessment is relatively easy and more reliable due to the clear-cut success or failure of performance as indicated by the assessment guidelines. Nonetheless, the type of assessment chosen for a particular research study should be driven by the purpose of assessment, not just the ease of administration (Logan et al. 2011; Yoon et al. 2006).

Case Study

We assessed a child (AL) with ASD to compare and contrast four instruments that are designed for motor skill assessment, the MABC-2, TGMD-2, PDMS-2, and BOT-2, and then provide suggestions for practitioners on how to choose the appropriate motor assessment instrument.

AL is a 5-year-old boy with HFA. He was diagnosed at the age of 4 years. AL was assessed at a local elementary school gym for all of the gross motor skills. A quiet room was used for all the fine motor skills. The school psychologist completed an observation form for AL including information on diagnosis, method of communication, reinforcers, and behavioral and sensory challenges. To provide context to AL's social communicative skills, the school psychologist shared the results of his most recent completion of the Preschool Language Scales-Fifth Edition (PLS-5) and the Developmental Profile-Second Edition (DP-2). AL had performed very poorly on all the subtests within the PLS-5. AL scored at the 5th percentile for auditory comprehension, 1st percentile for expressive communication, and 1st percentile for total language. In addition, AL's profile on the DP-2 was below average on physical, adaptive behavior, and social–emotional subtests. The school psychologist described AL's behavior as impulsive at times, but also that he enjoys interaction with adults and some peers. Sometimes he does not like to stay with too many children in the same center, but no definite behavioral or sensory integration problems were observed. AL likes reinforcers such as eating chips, writing letters, playing with cars, and giving high fives and thumbs ups.

We used a variety of strategies during AL's motor assessments. For example, in addition to performing demonstrations and displaying pictures from the assessment manuals, we used simple and short instructions (Breslin and Rudisill 2011; Liu and Breslin 2013b). Reinforcers were also used to encourage AL to concentrate on testing, and breaks were given every 5–10 min so he did not get tired. AL's standard and total score on the four assessments (MABC-2, TGMD-2, PDMS-2, and BOT-2) and the time he spent in each assessment is presented in Table 5.2.

For the MABC-2, AL was below average in both manual dexterity and balance subtests. His standard score for the aiming and catching subtest was in the average category. Overall, his total test score classified him as having significant movement difficulty. AL's total score of MABC-2 was consistent with his PDMS-2 gross motor quotient and total motor quotient, and his gross motor quotient of TGMD-2. AL's scores were in the 13th and 16th percentile for both MABC-2 and PDMS-2, which classify him within the “below average” category. However, AL's gross motor performance was inconsistent between the PDMS-2 and the TGMD-2. He scored at the 16th percentile on the locomotion subtest in PDMS-2 (below average), but his score was at the 37th percentile on the TGMD-2 (average). In addition, AL's object manipulation score was in the 25th percentile (average) in PDMS-2, but he scored in the 9th percentile in the TGMD-2's object control skills subtest (below average). For fine motor skills, AL was in the 25th percentile for the grasping subtest and the 37th percentile for the visual-motor integration subtest (both were in the average category) in PDMS-2. These scores were consistent with his BOT-2 performance on fine motor precision, fine motor integration, and manual dexterity (average). However, they were inconsistent with the manual dexterity test in the MABC-2. AL scored in the 16th percentile and was classified as below average on the MABC-2. Furthermore, there was a discrepancy between the balance subtests in MABC-2 and BOT-2. AL was classified as below average for MABC-2 balance tests but his performance was average on the BOT-2.

Table 5.2 Case study: AL's scores on the four assessment instruments and the time he spent in each assessment

Comparison aspect	MA B C-2	PDMS-2	TGMD-2	BOT-2
Time spent in testing	25 min	75 min (2 testing sessions)	27 min	120 min for the complete form
Subtests standard scores (SS) Percentile (descriptive category)	*Manual dexterity* SS: 7 Percentile: 16th (below average) *Aiming and catching* SS: 10 Percentile: 50th (average) *Balance* SS: 3 Percentile: 1st (below average)	Reflexes: NA Stationary SS: 7Percentile:16th (below average) Locomotion SS: 7 Percentile:16th (below average) Object manipulation SS: 8 Percentile:25th (average) Grasping: SS: 8 Percentile:25th (average) *Visual- motor integration* SS: 9 Percentile: 37th (average)	*Locomotor* SS: 9 Percentile: 37th (average) *Object control* SS: 6 Percentile: 9th (below average)	*Fine motor precision*: 13 (average) *Fine motor integration*: 15 (average) *Manual dexterity*: 16 (average) Upper-limb coordination: 12 (below average) *Bilateral coordination*: 12 (below average) *Balance*: 10 (average) *Running speed and agility*:13 (average) *Strength*: 11 (well below average)
Quotients, SS, percentile, or total motor composite (descriptive category)	*Total test score: 54* *SS: 5* *Percentile*: 5th (significant movement difficulty)	Gross motor quotient: 83 Percentile: 13th (below average) Fine motor quotient: 91 Percentile:27th (average) Total motor quotient: 85 percentile:16th (below average)	Gross motor quotient: 85 Percentile: 16 (below average)	*Strength and agility:* Percentile: 47th–38th (average) *Manual coordination*: Percentile: 48th–42nd (average) *Body coordination*: Percentile: 39th–14th (below average) *Fine manual control*: Percentile: 43rd–24th (below average) *Total motor composite*: Percentile: 42nd–21st (average) *Short form composite*: Percentile: 42nd–21st (average)

The authors picked two motor tasks (one fine and one gross motor skill) from the four assessments to provide a detailed comparison of these instruments. These comparisons are listed below:

1. *Jumping forward (gross motor skill)*
   The jumping task in TGMD–2 includes four performance criteria. The first criterion is that arms are extended behind the body and knees are flexed during the preparatory phase of the jump (AL scored a 2); the second criterion is that arms extend carefully forward and upward reaching full extension above the head (AL scored a 0); the third criterion is the ability to take off and land on both feet simultaneously (AL scored a 2); and the fourth criterion is arms are thrust downward during landing (AL scored a 1). AL performed the first and third criteria on both trials, and on only one trial did he drive his arms downward, and on no trial did he reach full extension. Thus, the total score for the jump was 5. On the MABC–2, the jumping task is scored by the number of times a participant jumps. AL scored a 4 for the first trial, and made 3 jumps for the second trial. Therefore, AL scored a 4 for jumping on the MABC-2. The PDMS-2 has two items related to jumping forward. AL scored a 2 on jumps forward for 30 in. using a two-footed takeoff and landing and he received a score of 1 on the second forward jump for 36 in. Finally, AL received 3 points for the jumping task in BOT-2. He jumped 27 in. for the first trial (1 point) and jumped 29 in. for the second trial (2 points).
2. *Drawing line through path and filling in shapes (fine motor skill)*
   In the MABC-2 for the drawing trail task, AL had five errors in the first trial as shown in Fig. 5.1, and four errors for the second trial. A qualitative observation was recorded that he was constantly moving during the two drawing trials. AL scored better on the drawing line through crooked paths in the BOT-2. He made only three errors (Fig. 5.2) and for filling in shapes in the same test, he scored 1 point for each shape (Fig. 5.3). AL scored a 0 on coloring between lines in PDMS-2 because he crossed the lines more than four times (Fig. 5.4).

For gross motor assessment (jumping), the TGMD-2 performance criteria are more detailed and focused on the jumping strategies that AL used to perform the tasks,

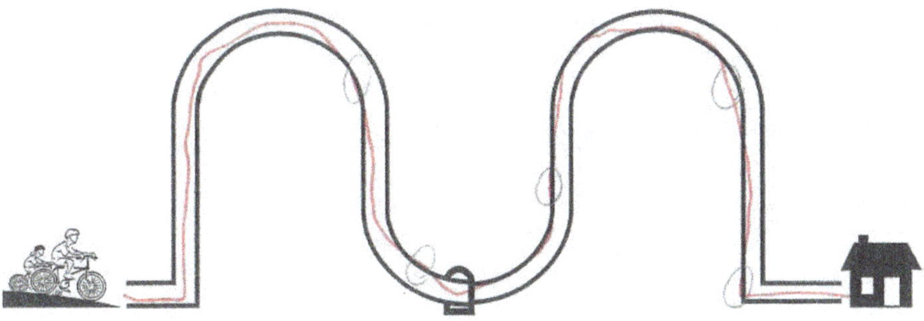

Fig. 5.1 Drawing line through path (manual dexterity subtest MABC-2)

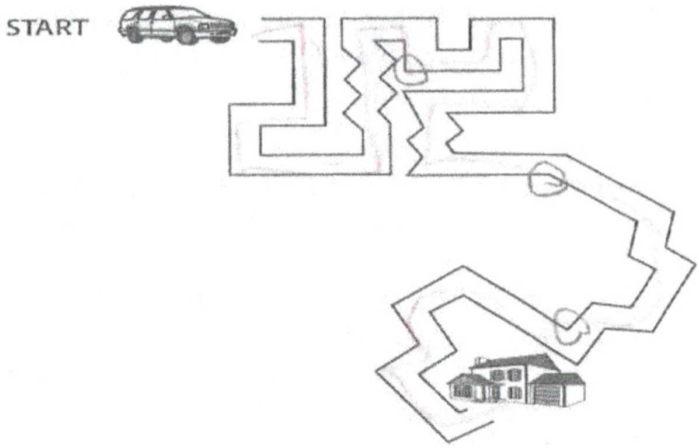

Fig. 5.2 Drawing line through crooked paths (fine motor precision subtest BOT-2)

Fig. 5.3 Filling in shape (fine motor precision subtest BOT-2)

while the MABC-2 focuses on controlling the body during consecutive jumps within the mat borders. However, the PDMS-2 and BOT-2 focus on the jumping distance from the starting line to where the back of the nearest heel touches the floor. Therefore, jumping in MABC-2, PDMS-2, and BOT-2 is measured with strength and maturity of the jump rather than the forms and techniques as in the TGMD-2.

It is interesting to note that AL performed better on the fine motor skill task (through the crooked path) on the BOT-2 than his performance on the curved path in MABC-2. A possible explanation for this contradiction could be that his performance was affected by the size of the two shapes. That is, the smaller size of the crooked path made him more precise and slower while drawing, whereas the bigger size of the path in MABC-2 made him feel comfortable with his hand movement so that he drew faster and made more errors. From the qualitative observations of his constant motion (i.e., inability to sit still in chair) while drawing, we can anticipate

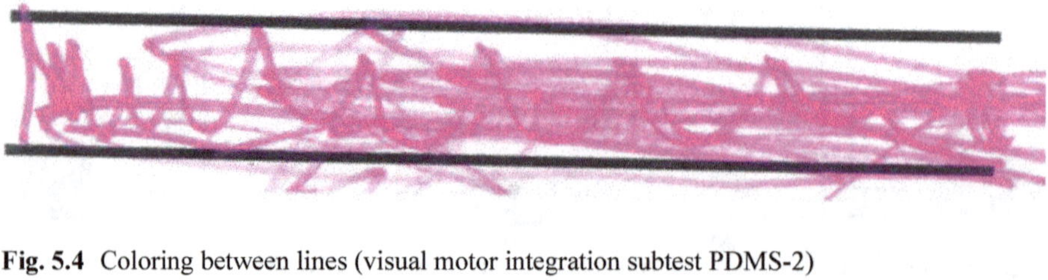

Fig. 5.4 Coloring between lines (visual motor integration subtest PDMS-2)

that AL would not perform well on the coloring between lines and filling in small shapes in PDMS-2 (Fig. 5.4).

Based on this case study, we noticed that AL performed the best on the PDMS-2 out of all four instruments. A possible explanation for this finding is that PDMS-2 has a large number of similar tasks. The repeated items with varying levels of difficulty gave AL the chance to practice and perform better as the assessment progresses. Furthermore, the wide range of tasks and items in PDMS-2 could contribute to his relative success and may serve as objectives for future intervention programs for AL. Though AL scored the highest on the PDMS-2, this does not indicate the other three instruments are inappropriate for AL. Each assessment has its advantages and limitations. In the next section, we will provide some recommendations and suggestions for practitioners on how to select the appropriate motor assessment instrument.

Recommendations to Practitioners on Choosing the Appropriate Instrument

To choose the appropriate motor assessment instrument, practitioners should consider the purpose of the assessment in the six important areas: testing purpose, age range, type of motor skills, motor variables, functioning, and assessment setting.

Testing Purpose If the purpose of testing is to screen a child with ASD for eligibility for special services, a quantitative assessment like MABC-2 or the short form of the BOT-2 may be more suitable for this purpose. If the purpose of testing is to capture and analyze the motor performance of children with ASD, a qualitative assessment such as the PDMS-2 or TGMD-2 would be appropriate. However, even though the complete form of BOT-2 is a quantitative assessment, it can also be a good choice for qualitative assessment because of the variety of skills included in the test.

Age Range The age range is different from one assessment to another. The Vineland-II, MSEL, Bailey-III, TGMD-2, and PDMS-2 may be more appropriate for preschool children with ASD. The MABC-2 and BOT-2 have a wider age range including adolescents. For longitudinal studies, one may choose to use more than one test. In addition, some studies have used two different tests to measure motor and cognitive performance of children with ASD (Vanvuchelen et al. 2007; Provost et al. 2007a).

Type of Motor Skills The TGMD-2 is designed to measure gross motor skills exclusively, while the PDMS-2 assesses fine and gross motor skills separately and yields a separate quotient for fine and gross motor skills as well as total quotient scores. In addition to fine and gross motor skill assessment, the BOT-2 also assesses body coordination and strength and agility whereas the MABC-2 also assesses dynamic and static balance (Piek et al. 2012).

Motor Variables One thing practitioners should also think about is whether the motor skills are the main focus or a secondary factor in the research. For example, if the research purpose is to assess adaptive behaviors and motor skills are considered a secondary variable, a practitioner should choose to use the Vineland-II, Bayley-III, or MSEL. Otherwise, the MABC-2, TGMD-2, PDMS-2, or BOT-2 should be used because these instruments are designed for motor skill assessments.

Functioning The PDMS-2 is suggested for assessing low-functioning children with ASD while the MABC-2 is recommended for use for high-functioning children with ASD. The authors found only one study that used different assessments for measuring motor skills of children with ASD based on their cognitive functioning (Vanvuchelen et al. 2007). Children with ASD were classified as low functioning with an IQ range of 55–79 and high functioning for an IQ between 80 and 124. The low-functioning participants were assessed with the PDMS-2 and the high-functioning group completed the MABC-2.

Assessment Setting Quantitative assessments of shorter duration such as the MABC-2, the TGMD-2, and the short form of the BOT-2 are more appropriate for school settings. Qualitative assessments which require more time such as the PDMS-2 are more appropriate for clinical settings.

Part III: Physical Activity Assessment for Children with ASD

Physical activity is defined as voluntary body movements produced by skeletal muscles resulting in energy expenditure (Caspersen et al. 1985; Cervantes and Porretta 2010). The term "voluntary" is included to eliminate involuntary body movements that may characterize certain disabilities such as cerebral palsy. One can also think that physical activity is when children move their arms and/or legs, their heart beats faster, and they breathe harder. If they do that long enough, they may start sweating. For example, physical activity can be walking, jogging, doing sit-ups, playing soccer, or dancing. Physical activity also includes day-to-day body movements such as climbing stairs, biking for transportation, doing house work, and gardening (Biddle 1994; Obrusnikova and Miccinello 2012).

Although motor deficits are gaining attention in ASD research, limited research has focused on physical activity in children with ASD (MacDonald et al. 2011). Physical activity has been suggested to help children with ASD reduce maladaptive behaviors and improve their overall health (Bandini et al. 2013; Janssen and Leblanc 2010; Magnusson et al. 2012; Pan and Frey 2006; Pan et al. 2011a, 2011c). Participation in physical activity is often a challenge for children with ASD because of their poor motor functioning and low self-esteem. In addition, organized team activities may be hard for some children with ASD because of a lack of social interaction and motor skill competence (Todd and Reid 2006). Therefore, children with ASD are at risk of inactivity due to social and behavioral deficits associated with their disorder, such as difficulties in understanding social cues, making eye contact, playing imaginative and social games, engaging in sharing/turn-taking and reciprocal conversation, and making friends. These deficits could limit their opportunities to participate in physical activity during physical education, and leisure time sports. This is in contrast to typically developing children who are more likely to be physically active with their peers (e.g., by riding a bike to school without supervision or playing tag with peers during recess). Thus, physical activities that do not require a team environment or high skill levels may be more appealing to children with ASD (Fox and Riddoch 2000; Rosser Sandt and Frey 2005; Todd and Reid 2006).

Do Children with ASD Meet Physical Activity Recommendations?

Current physical activity recommendations for youth without disabilities are twofold: (1) children should participate in at least 60 min or more of age and developmentally appropriate physical activity on all or most days of the week; and (2) adolescents should be active every day, including 20 min bouts of continuous MVPA three or more times per week (USDHHS 2002). Physical activity is known to have a wide range of health and psychological benefits for developing a healthy lifestyle for children (Ensel and Lin 2004). That is, regular physical activity participation reduces morbidity and mortality risk associated with chronic diseases such as cardiovascular disease, certain cancers, diabetes, and obesity (USDHHS 2002). In addition to the health-related benefits of physical activity, research indicates that decreased stereotypy and self-stimulating behavior are the most common behavioral improvements following physical activity for children with ASD (Magnusson et al. 2012). Additionally, children with ASD experienced decreases in negative behavior such as stereotypes, and increases in positive behavior such as time on task (Burns and Ault 2009; Levinson and Reid 1993). Elliot et al. (1994) also found that aerobic exercise prior to performing a vocational task reduced maladaptive and stereotypic behaviors in adults with ASD. Rosenthal-Malek and Mitchell (1997) reported that adolescents with ASD decreased self-stimulatory behavior, increased correct responding and task completion following aerobic exercise. Others have shown the viability of exercise training programs for children with ASD (Lochbaum and Crews 2003; Schultheis et al. 2000), including strategies to maintain participation in physical activity (Todd and Reid 2006). Furthermore, Hillier et al. (2011) suggested that physical activity and relaxation could improve symptoms of stress for adolescents and young adults with ASD.

Tan et al. (2013) examined the effects of physical activity on attention span and health-related quality of life for 12 children with ASD aged 2–6 years. Results indicated that as the exercise increased (i.e., exercises included eight sessions of tri-cycling each lasting for 15 min), the children with ASD demonstrated longer duration of attention span. These results extend the findings that physical activity enhances cognition of ASD children and support its consideration in early intervention programs.

Research in physical activity has progressed beyond studying patterns of MVPA and more interest has begun to emerge in measuring sedentary physical activity patterns (MacDonald et al. 2011). Pan and Frey (2006) examined age-related physical activity patterns in 30 youths with ASD aged 10–19 years. Participants were divided into three groups: (1) elementary school (M= 10.67 ± 0.50 years; n= 9), (2) middle school (M= 13.33 ± 1.00 years; n= 9), and (3) high school (M= 15.08 ± 1.38 years, n= 12). Each participant wore an accelerometer and completed an activity questionnaire for 7 consecutive days. The main findings were that elementary school children were more active than the other two groups, regardless of type of day or time period. In addition, 78 % of the elementary school children, 67 % of the middle school children, and 8 % of the high school children accumulated 60 min of daily MVPA. Only 23 % of the participants with ASD in the study met the daily criteria for MVPA. No consistent patterns were found in physical activity for children with ASD according to day or time period. Findings emphasize that interventions for this population should address increasing extracurricular physical activity options during adolescence years.

In another study, MacDonald et al. (2011) examined the physical activity patterns of children with ASD aged 9–18 years (n= 72, males = 55, females = 17). The results clearly showed declines in physical activity as children with ASD aged. Beyond this pattern, as the children grew older, they also experienced an increased pattern of sedentary activity. MacDonald et al. (2011) also stated that children with ASD appeared to be meeting the minimum requirements of physical activity. The observed age-related declines shed light on the lack of physical activity demonstrated in older children with ASD. At the same time, 43 % of the children in this study were overweight (falling within or above the 85th percentile based on gender and age). Todd and Reid (2006) reported that including instructional strategies such as self-monitoring, verbal cueing, and edible reinforcers had a positive association with increased sustained participation in physical activity for 30 min twice a week. These results suggested that interventions can be developed to promote sustained participation in physical activity for individuals with autism.

Rosser Sandt and Frey (2005) compared daily physical education class, recess, and after-school MVPA levels between 15 children with ASD and 13 children without ASD aged 5–12 years. Accelerometer and direct observation were employed to measure physical activity in children for 5 days (4 weekdays and 1 weekend day). The time period of interest was from 10:00 a.m. to 7:00 p.m. There were no differences between children with and without ASD by physical activity setting. Both groups were more active during recess compared to after school, and children with ASD were equally active in recess and physical education class. Although many children with ASD were given 60 min of physical education per day, this quantity of physical activity may decrease with age as opportunities for recess and physical education class are reduced.

Bandini et al. (2013) compared physical activity levels among 53 children with ASD and 58 typically developing children aged 3–11 years. Based on accelerometer measures, the two groups of children had similar levels of physical activity throughout the week. The only difference observed was on weekdays. Children with ASD spent less time in moderate physical activity than the typically developing children.

It is speculated that children with ASD may engage in fewer activities after school than typically developing children. In contrast, based on parent report data, children with ASD spent significantly less time in physical activities and participated in a smaller variety of activities than did the typically developing children. The differences between parent report and accelerometer measures may be because some of the physical activity engaged in by children with ASD was not captured by the questionnaires. Children with ASD may engage in repetitive or self-stimulating activities such as pacing and roaming. For example, children with ASD may engage in more repetitive movement (e.g., rocking) than the typically developing children during television watching. These activities may be captured by an accelerometer but may not be reported as physical activity by parents because they perceive watching television to be a sedentary behavior.

To examine the age-related physical activity patterns in elementary school children with ASD, Pan et al. (2010) used a uniaxial accelerometer to examine physical activity in 35 children with ASD aged 7–12 years (grades 1–2, $n=13$; grades 3–4, $n=13$; grades 5–6, $n=9$) for up to 5 weekdays and 2 weekend days. Younger children were more active during weekend days compared with weekdays, while the opposite was observed in older children. Age variation also exists in children's physical activity levels within a weekday, with this effect being most evident during recess and after school. Weekend days and free time within school days seem appropriate targets when promoting physical activity in older children with ASD.

Measurement Tools

A range of methods and techniques have been used to assess physical activity. These measurements include (a) accelerometers, (b) pedometers, (c) survey-based research, (d) heart rate monitors, and (e) direct observation (Cervantes and Porretta 2010; John 2013). Practitioners should consider the purpose of the physical activity data when selecting appropriate methodology for physical activity measurement. If the intensity of physical activity is desired, perhaps heart rate monitors or survey-based questionnaires might be appropriate. If the goal is to determine how much physical activity is accrued throughout the duration of time, perhaps a workday and/or weekend direct observation plus an accelerometer is the proper choice (Sirard and Pate 2001; Sylvia et al. 2014). However, when examining the physical activity of children with ASD, special consideration should be paid to how the physical activity measurement methodology may interact or exacerbate certain behaviors and performance sensitivities among children with ASD. We will provide details on several types of physical activity measurement next, while Table 5.3 provides a summary of the findings from research on children with ASD using the different types of physical activity measurement included in this chapter.

Accelerometers Accelerometers are objective physical activity monitors that directly measure the duration, intensity, and frequency of movement (Herrmann et al. 2013). They measure physical activity using a sensor that integrates the degree

Table 5.3 A detailed comparison of the studies measuring the physical activity of children with ASD (grouped by instrumentation and ordered by publication date)

Accelerometers

Study	Title	Participants	Results
Memari et al. (2013)	Physical activity in children and adolescents with autism assessed by triaxial accelerometry	Eighty children with ASD between the ages of 7 and 14 years; mean age **9.7 years;** grouped by 2-year age bands (7–8 years, 9–10 years, 11–12 years, 13–14 years)	Significant differences in physical activity (PA) emerged across the age groups, between weekdays and weekends, and after school. Younger children with ASD were more physically active than older children with ASD. PA was higher outside of school than during school, and children from two-parent families engaged in more PA than children from single-parent households. Additionally, an inverse relationship was found between children's preference for sedentary activities and PA. Finally, the best predictors of PA were age, gender, a preference for sedentary activities, household structure, and the presence of comorbid conditions
Bandini et al. (2013)	Comparison of physical activity between children with ASD and typically developing children	Fifty-three children with ASD and 58 typically developing children aged **9–11 years**	Throughout the week, the PA levels of children with ASD and typically developing peers were similar as measured by accelerometers. However, children with ASD were less active on weekdays. The survey completed by parents regarding their child's PA participation yielded data of questionable validity, regardless of ASD status
Study	Title	Participants	Results
MacDonald et al. (2011)	The physical activity patterns of children with autism	Seventy-two children with ASD were grouped by age (**9–11 years and 12–18 years**)	No differences in PA were reported between genders, the severity of ASD, and IQ. Younger children with ASD spent roughly 17 min/day in MVPA, while older children with ASD spent 10 min/day in MVPA. Thus, PA seems to decrease by age, and there is a need for interventions to increase PA for children with ASD
Pan et al. (2011b)	Physical activity and self-determined motivation of adolescents with and without autism spectrum disorders in inclusive physical education	Twenty-five adolescents with ASD (mean age **14.26 years**), 75 children without ASD (mean age **14.08 years**)	Children with ASD engaged in less PA than their typically developing peers. Both groups spent approximately 41 min in physical education lessons, and neither group met target goals for physical activity of at least 50% MVPA engagement during physical education

Table 5.3 (continued)

Accelerometers			
Pan et al. (2011a)	Physical activity correlates for children with autism spectrum disorders in middle school physical education	Eighty-five children (19 boys with ASD, and 76 typical peers), **mean age 14.19 years**	Middle school children are less physically active than elementary school-age children during physical education. Middle school children with ASD on average engaged in MVPA for 40 % of their physical education class, while typically developing peers engaged in MVPA for 45 % of the class
Pan et al. (2011c)	Accelerometer-determined physical activity among elementary school-age children with autism spectrum disorders in Taiwan	Thirty-five boys with ASD aged 7–12 years grouped by grade levels (lower grades **mean age 7.56 years**, middle grades mean age **9.57 years**, and upper grades **11.82 years**)	The inverse relationship between age and PA was reported in this study. Additionally, upper-grade students were more physically active on weekdays than weekends, whereas lower- and middle-grade students were more physically active during the weekend than the weekdays
Obrusnikova and Cavalier (2011)	Perceived barriers and facilitators of participation in after-school physical activity by children with autism spectrum disorders	Fourteen children with ASD (12 boys, 2 girls) **mean age 10.64 years**	Children with ASD spent a majority of their time (nearly 80 %) in sedentary activities. The average engagement in MVPA was about 82 min per day. However, five of the children engaged in less than 60 min of MVPA per day, so there was tremendous variability in activity counts across participants
Study	Title	Participants	Results
Pan (2009)	Age, social engagement, and physical activity in children with autism spectrum disorders	Twenty-five boys with ASD (mean age **9.28 years**)	A positive relationship emerged between age and PA as measured with accelerometers. There was no relationship between social engagement (measured by direct observation) and PA
Pan (2008a)	Objectively measured physical activity between children with autism spectrum disorders and children without disabilities during inclusive recess settings in Taiwan	Forty-eight gender matched children (24 typically developing and 24 with ASD); mean age **9.21 years**	The differences by disability status in the amount of MVPA accrued approached significance, as 27.7 % of the recess was spent in MVPA by children with ASD and typically developing peers spent 36.15 % of recess in MVPA. The differences may be attributed to personal characteristics of the children or due to the sociocultural environment, as the children with ASD may have been afforded less recess time to allow for more academic instruction

Table 5.3 (continued)

Accelerometers			
Pan (2008b)	Schooltime physical activity of students with and without autism spectrum disorders during PE and recess	Twenty-four children with ASD (23 boys, 1 girl in grades 1–6) and 24 boys without ASD **(mean age 9.21 years)**	Children with ASD and their typically developing peers engaged in similar levels of MVPA during physical education. The percentage of time spent in MVPA during physical education exceeds that during recess, regardless of disability status. However, children with ASD accrued significantly less MVPA during recess than their typically developing peers (27.70 % vs. 36.15 % of time)
Pan and Frey (2006)	Physical activity patterns in youth with autism spectrum disorders	Thirty children with ASD, **mean age 13.2 years**	Younger children with ASD were more physically active than older children across recess, physical education, and after-school time. No differences in MVPA emerged between weekdays and weekends. Children accrued the most PA during after-school hours, but the most MVPA was accumulated during school hours
Study	Title	Participants	Results
Rosser Sandt and Frey (2005)	Comparison of physical activity levels between children with and without autistic spectrum disorders	Twenty-eight children (15 with ASD and 13 without) ranging in age from **5 to 12 years**	Using both accelerometer and direct observation, typically developing peers were more physically active than the children with ASD across all time points. There were no significant differences in physical activity during physical education, but during recess and after-school hours, children with ASD obtained significantly less MVPA than their typically developing peers
Pan and Frey (2005)	Identifying physical activity determinants in youth with autistic spectrum disorders	Thirty children with HFA	Forty-seven percent of children with ASD engaged in at least 60 min of PA per day, and the amount of PA accrued was consistent across weekend and weekdays
Pedometers			
Beets and Pitetti (2011)	Using pedometers to measure moderate-to-vigorous physical activity for youth with an intellectual disability	Twenty-eight children with intellectual disability (10 girls, 18 boys); **mean age 11.8 years old**	This study validated the use of a pedometer to determine exercise intensity for children with ID using heart rate reserve calculations. A preliminary calculation is presented to provide the cut-off step counts necessary for MVPA using a pedometer in children with intellectual disabilities

Table 5.3 (continued)

Accelerometers			
Survey-based research			
Ziviani et al. (2006)	Physical activity of young children	Fifty children, mean age 7.74 years	Boys and girls exhibited similar PA participation rates, although girls spent more time on weekends reading and crafting. The greatest predictors of children's PA include parent's perception of PA, family socioeconomic status, and peers' perceptions of PA
Pan and Frey (2005)	Identifying physical activity determinants in youth with autism spectrum disorders	Thirty children with HFA as a part of 29 parent-child dyads (one pair of siblings with ASD)	Children were more physically active than their parents. As children approached adolescence, they felt fewer opportunities for PA exist
Heart rate monitors			
Study	Title	Participants	Results
Breslin et al. (in press)	Heart rate profiles of children with and without ASD in response to physical play: a preliminary investigation	Four typically developing children (two boys, two girls) and three boys with ASD, **mean age 5.31 years**	No children met recommendations for MVPA during physical play time. There were no differences in resting heart rate and all children spent a majority of their time engaged in light to moderate PA. Children without ASD spent more time above PAHR-50, a measure of higher intensity PA
Pitetti et al. (2009)	Physical activity levels of children with intellectual disabilities during school	Fifteen children (nine girls, six boys) with intellectual disabilities (including one with ASD), **mean age 8.8 years**	Nearly 80 % of time spent engaged in adapted physical education lessons and recess time can be classified as MVPA for children with intellectual disabilities. Nearly 40 % of instructional class time can be classified as MVPA according to data collected by heart rate monitors
Direct observations			
Sit et al. (2007)	Physical activity levels of children in special schools	One hundred and seventy-two children enrolled in five schools for children with special needs in Hong Kong. The schools (grouped by disability type) were designed for children with physical disabilities, intellectual disabilities, hearing impairments and visual impairments	Using the SOFIT, it was found that children with special needs do not accrue much MVPA during school hours. Specifically, nearly 42 % of physical education time is spent in MVPA, while 58 % of (an average 15.6 min long) recess is. Furthermore, there was no significant difference in the amount of MVPA accrued by disability type

and intensity of motion and produces a voltage output signal whose magnitude is recorded as activity counts. The devices may be fastened via Velcro closures to an elastic belt that the child wears around his/her waist over either the left or right hip (Bandini et al. 2013).

Accelerometers are a widely used physical activity assessment technique among children with ASD. The literature using this measurement technique overwhelmingly suggests that children with ASD attain lower levels of physical activity than their typically developing peers. This finding is salient across all types of physical activity including structured physical activity, leisure time opportunities afterschool, and recess (MacDonald et al. 2011; Pan 2008b; Pan et al. 2011b, c; Pan and Frey 2006; Rosser Sandt and Frey 2005). Furthermore, it is noted that, like typically developing individuals, the physical activity of individuals with ASD decreases as they age (Bandini et al. 2013; Memari et al. 2013; Pan et al. 2011c).

The basic and critical limitation of accelerometers is that MVPA recorded could be engaged in by the child intermittently. That is, the situations when children with ASD engage in frequent stereotypic and repetitive behaviors such as roaming, rocking, and pacing (Bandini et al. 2013). Furthermore, depending on accelerometer placement and behavioral characteristics of the child, behaviors such as body rocking or hand flapping may be recorded as activity counts but are not considered purposeful physical activity (Albainali et al. 2012; Goodwin et al. 2011).

Pedometers Pedometers are increasingly being used as a surveillance tool to objectively assess ambulatory (walking) activity levels and patterns in different populations because of their low cost, small size, simple, and unobtrusive nature. They enable the accumulative measurement of daily activities, providing a measure of total volume of ambulatory activity (Craig et al. 2010). In addition, pedometers offer a practical and cost-effective method for the objective assessment of physical activity and continue to be an instrument of choice for many practitioners. Additionally, they are a very effective tool for self-monitoring and motivation. Pedometers are easily interpretable and accessible as they provide an immediately visible display of accumulated step counts, a function not available in accelerometers (Clemes and Biddle 2013). However, only one study used the pedometer to assess the physical activity of children with ASD (Kodish et al. 2006). Kodish et al. (2006) concluded that no significant differences were found between physical activity levels in classes that had children with autism and in those that did not.

Survey-based Research Survey-based research involves asking participants to explicitly describe their own attitudes toward and/or participation in physical activity. This technique for measuring attitudes has strong face validity, especially when a Likert scale is used. A Likert scale is a well-known method that contains statements expressing strongly favorable, neutral, or unfavorable positions, and the degree to which a respondent agrees with these statements using a numerical scale (e.g., 1 = strongly agree and 7 = strongly disagree; Pethkar et al. 2010). To effectively use survey-based research, practitioners should identify appropriate questionnaires to use for their settings. The survey needed in a surveillance system would be different than that used in a clinical setting. Recommendations for survey-based research are matching the purpose of the assessment with the type of questionnaire; using the questionnaire as intended; using a questionnaire appropriate for the study population; using the correct scoring and analytic methods, and avoid asking questions that aggregate physical activity domains which are difficult for the respondent to recall (Ainsworth et al. 2012).

Specifically, survey-based research data may not accurately reflect the physical activity engagement. The language or meaning behind the questions on a physical activity questionnaire may be misperceived because some children with ASD have difficulty extracting meaning from text (Bishop and Seltzer 2012). As these questionnaires are subjective in nature, children with ASD may over- or underreport the intensity of engagement in physical activity. This may be due to a receptive language delay such as a lack of understanding or fluency of the language used in the question (Boyle et al. 2010) or because of sensory experiences that manifest during physical activity (Ismael and Lawson 2012). Furthermore, given that children under 9 years of age are unable to reliably report their physical activity habits in terms of frequency, intensity, type, or time (McKenzie 2010) and children with ASD have documented communicative difficulties, survey-based research is probably inappropriate to use with this population. However, a variation of survey-based research that may be more appropriate is parent or caregiver report data. Parents or caregivers could be asked their attitudes towards their child's physical activity participation, as well as their perceived quantity in which their child engages. To date, parent report research has been used in only one study with children with ASD (Pan 2008a). Although surveys utilizing parent report data are reasonably reliable when compared to accelerometer data among children with typically developing children (Dwyer et al. 2011; Ziviani et al. 2006), no validity or reliability studies have been conducted exploring the relationship between accelerometer data and parent report surveys when measuring physical activity in children with ASD. Thus, concerns are raised regarding the validity of this methodology for children with ASD.

Heart Rate Monitor A heart rate monitor is a sophisticated physical activity monitoring technique that estimates physical activity engagement based on the frequency of the heartbeat. However, the issues of reactivity, interpretation, age suitability, technical issues with electrode placement, and fixation still trouble this method. It is not often employed, apart from situations where cardiac function is the primary outcome of concern. There are multiple situations and environments that lead to elevated heart rate beyond that of physical activity. Thus, the attempts to correlate heart rate with energy expenditure further distance this as a measure of physical activity (John 2013).

Only one study utilized heart rate monitors to measure physical activity. Breslin et al. (2015) compared the resting heart rate, the amount of time spent in light physical activity, and the amount of time spent in MVPA between children with and without ASD. Typically developing children spent greater amounts of time in MVPA than the children with ASD; however, both groups had similar resting heart rates and engagement in light physical activity.

Most of the literature utilizing heart rate monitors in children with ASD was not intended to collect physical activity data (Beets and Pitetti 2011; Goodwin et al. 2006). Rather, the purpose of these studies was to measure cardiovascular response at rest or in response to stressful situations (e.g., a stranger's presence or a challenging mental task). It was found that children with ASD had a higher resting heart rate than their typically developing peers (Goodwin et al. 2006). However, the heart rate response in children with ASD during stressful situations was not as expected (Beets and Pitetti 2011; Goodwin et al. 2006). Goodwin et al. (2006) reported that the increase in heart rate for children with ASD was not as high as expected, which may be due to the huge variability in heart rate response among the children with ASD. It may be that the medications or diet consumed by some children may influence their heart rate reading (Beets and Pitetti 2011; Breslin et al. 2015). Furthermore, a child with ASD may have unpleasant sensory responses to the electrodes composed of the heart rate monitors (Breslin et al. 2015; Pitetti et al. 2009). Thus, the heart rate monitor might inaccurately measure the amount of MVPA in this population.

Direct Observation Direct observation is the gold standard tool for establishing the nature, duration, frequency, and relative intensity of physical activity. However, there are limits to the portions of a day that can be observed because researchers or a camera recording activity must be present. Thus, it may fail the practicality of the assessment. In addition, training staff to code behavior is often costly and difficult. Studies using direct observation usually explain physical activity during the school day or at a community program (McKenzie 2010). Therefore, it is presently not used to explain physical activity accrued during the weekends or in solitary activities.

To avoid the limitations of each of the existing physical activity measurements, multiple measurements can be used at the same time to provide a more accurate and comprehensive assessment of physical activity. By using multiple measurements, one technique can compensate for the weakness of another (Bandini et al. 2013). When considering the pediatric population with ASD, there is a dearth of research using several of the methodologies reviewed here. Future researchers should work to explore the reliability, validity, and practicality of these methodologies in children with ASD.

In summary, the extant literature on physical activity in children with ASD is sparse. Most studies are limited by small sample sizes (Breslin et al. 2015; Breslin and Rudisill 2011, 2013; Goodwin et al. 2006; Magnusson et al. 2012; Nicholson et al. 2011; Obrusnikova and Cavalier 2011; Oriel et al. 2011; Pitetti et al. 2009; Rosser Sandt and Frey 2005), lack of a comparison group (MacDonald et al. 2011; Magnusson et al. 2012; Memari et al. 2013; Nicholson et al. 2011; Oriel et al. 2011; Pan 2009; Pan and Frey 2005, 2006; Venkatesan 2005), or have only focused on a particular part of the day. More research is needed to fill the gap in information related to physical activity for children with ASD.

References

Ainsworth, B., Caspersen, C., Matthews, C., Mâsse, L., Baranowski, T., & Zhu, W. (2012). Recommendations to improve the accuracy of estimates of physical activity derived from self-report. *Journal of Physical Activity and Health, 9,* S76–S84.

Akshoomoff, N. (2006). Use of the Mullen scales of early learning for the assessment of young children with autism spectrum disorders. *Child Neuropsychology, 12,* 269–277. doi:10.1080/09297040500473714.

Albainali, F., Goodwin, M. S., & Intille, S. (2012). Detecting stereotypical motor movements in the classroom using accelerometry and pattern recognition algorithms. *Pervasive and Mobile Computing, 8,* 103–114. doi:10.1016/j.pmcj.2011.04.006.

American Psychiatric Association. (2013). *Diagnostic and statistical manual of mental disorders* (5th ed., pp. 50–59). Washington, DC: American Psychiatric Association.

Bandini, L. G., Gleason, J., Curtin, C., Lividini, K., Anderson, S. E., Cermak, S. A., Maslin, M., Must, A. (2013). Comparison of physical activity between children with autism spectrum disorders and typically developing children. *Autism: The International Journal of Research and Practice, 17,* 44–54. doi:10.1177/1362361312437416.

Barbaro, J., & Dissanayake, C. (2012). Developmental profiles of infants and toddlers with autism spectrum disorders identified prospectively in a community-based setting. *Journal of Autism and Developmental Disorders, 42,* 1939–1948. doi:10.1007/s10803-012-1441-z.

Bauman, M. L. (2010). Medical comorbidities in autism: Challenges to diagnosis and treatment. *Neurotherapeutics, 7,* 320–327. doi:10.1016/j.nurt.2010.06.001.

Bayley, N. (2006). *Bayley scales of infant development manual* (3rd ed.). San Antonio: The Psychological Corporation.

Beets, M. W., & Pitetti, K. H. (2011). Using pedometers to measure moderate-to-vigorous physical activity for youth with an intellectual disability. *Disability and Health Journal, 4,* 46–51. doi:10.1016/j.dhjo.2010.02.002.

Berkeley, S. L., Zittel, L. L., Pitney, L. V., & Nichols, S. E. (2001). Locomotor and object control skills of children diagnosed with autism. *Adapted Physical Activity Quarterly, 18,* 405–416.

Bhat, A. N., Landa, R. J., & Galloway, J. C. (2011). Current perspectives on motor functioning in infants, children, and adults with autism spectrum disorders. *Physical Therapy, 91,* 1116–1128. doi:10.2522/ptj.20100294.

Biddle, S. (1994). What helps and hinders people becoming more physically active? In A. Killoran, P. Fentem, & C. Caspersen (Eds.), *Moving on: International perspectives on promoting physical activity* (pp. 110–126). London: Health Education Authority.

Bildt, A., Mulder, E. J., Van Lang, N. D., With, S. A., Minderaa, R. B., Stahl, S. S...., Anderson, G. M. (2012). The visual rooting reflex in individuals with autism spectrum disorders and co-occurring intellectual disability. *Autism Research, 5,* 67–72. doi:10.1002/aur.225.

Bishop, S. L., & Seltzer, M. M. (2012). Self-reported autism symptoms in adults with autism spectrum disorders. *Journal of Autism and Development Disorders, 42,* 2354–2363. doi:10.1007/s10803-012-1483-2.

Bishop, S., Guthrie, W., Coffing, M., & Lord, C. (2011). Convergent validity of the Mullen Scales of Early Learning and the differential ability scales in children with autism spectrum disorders. *American Journal of Intellectual and Developmental Disabilities, 116,* 331–343. doi:10.1352/1944-7558-116.5.331.

Block, M. E., Taliaferro, A., & Moran, T. (2013). Physical activity and youth with disabilities: Barrier and supports. *The Prevention Researcher, 20,* 18–20.

Borremans, E., Rintala, P., & Mc Cubbin, J. (2009). Motor skills of young adults with Asperger syndrome: A comparative study. *European Journal of Adapted Physical Activity, 2,* 21–33.

Boyle, J., McCartney, E., O'Hare, A., & Law, J. (2010). Intervention for mixed receptive-expressive language impairment: A review. *Developmental Medicine and Child Neurology, 52,* 994–999. doi:10.1111/j.1469–8749.2010.03750.x.

Breslin, C. M., & Buchanan, A. M. (2014). A researcher's perceptions of assessing motor skills of children with autism spectrum disorder. *Journal of American Academy of Special Education Professionals, 8*, 201–217.

Breslin, C. M., & Liu, T. (2015). Do you know what I'm saying? Strategies to assess motor skills for children with autism spectrum disorder. *Journal of Physical Education, Recreation, and Dance, 86*, 10–15. doi:10.1080/07303084.2014.978419

Breslin, C., & Rudisill, M. (2011). The effect of visual supports on performance of the TGMD-2 for children with autism spectrum disorder. *Adapted Physical Activity Quarterly, 28*, 342–353.

Breslin, C. M., & Rudisill, M. E. (2013). Relationships among assessment time, time on-task, and motor skill performance in children with autism spectrum disorders. *Adapted Physical Activity Quarterly, 30*, 338–350.

Breslin, C. M., Rudisill, M. E., & Wadsworth, D. D. (2015). Heart rate profiles of children with autism spectrum disorder in response to physical play. *The Physical Educator, 72*(1), 1–19.

Brookman-Frazee, L., Baker-Ericze´n, M., Stadnick, N., & Taylor, R. (2012). Parent perspectives on community mental health services for children with autism spectrum disorders. *Journal of Child Family Study, 21*, 533–544. doi:10.1007/s10826-011-9506-8.

Bruininks, R., & Bruininks, B. (2005). *Bruininks-Oseretsky test of motor proficiency: Manual* (2nd ed.). Minneapolis: Pearson Assessment.

Burns, B., & Ault, R. (2009). Exercise and autism symptoms: A case study. *Journal of Undergraduate Research: The International Honor Society in Psychology, 14*(2), 1089–4136.

Cappadocia, M. C., & Weiss, J. A. (2011). Review in social skills training groups for youth with Asperger syndrome and high functioning autism. *Research in Autism Spectrum Disorders, 5*, 70–78. doi:10.1016/j.rasd.2010.04.001.

Caspersen, C., Powell, K., & Christenson, G. (1985). Physical activity, exercise, and physical fitness: Definitions and distinctions for health-related research. *Public Health Reports, 100*, 126–131.

Centers for Disease Control and Prevention. (2012). *Autism spectrum disorders (ASDs)*. http://www.cdc.gov/ncbddd/autism/research.html.

Cervantes, C., & Porretta, D. (2010). Physical activity measurement among individuals with disabilities: A literature review. *Adapted Physical Activity Quarterly, 27*, 173–190.

Chawarska, K., & Bearess, K. (2008). Assessment of cognitive and adaptive skills. In K. Chawarska, A. Kiln, & F. Volkmar (Eds.), *Autism spectrum disorders in infants and toddlers: Diagnosis, assessment, and treatment* (pp. 50–75). New York: The Guilford Press.

Clemes, S., & Biddle, S. (2013). The use of pedometers for monitoring physical activity in children and adolescents: Measurement considerations. *Journal of Physical Activity and Health, 10*, 249–262.

Craig, C., Tudor-Locke, C., Cragg, S., & Cameron, C. (2010). Process and treatment of pedometer data collection for youth: The Canadian physical activity levels among youth study. *Medicine and Science in Sports and Exercise, 42*, 430–435. doi:10.1249/MSS.0b013e3181b67544.

Dewey, D., Cantell, M., & Crawford, S. (2007). Motor and gestural performance in children with autism spectrum disorders, developmental coordination disorder, and/or attention deficit hyperactivity disorder. *Journal of the International Neuropsychological Society, 13*, 246–256. doi:10.1017/S1355617707070270.

Dwyer, G. M., Hardy, L. L., Peat, J. K., & Baur, L. A. (2011). The validity and reliability of a home environment preschool-age physical activity questionnaire (Pre-PAQ). *International Journal of Behavioral Nutrition and Physical Activity, 8*, 86. doi:10.1186/1479-5868-8-86.

Egan, A. M., Dreyer, M. L., Odar, C. C., Beckwith, M., & Garrison, C. B. (2013). Obesity in young children with autism spectrum disorders: Prevalence and associated factors. *Childhood Obesity, 9*, 125–131. doi:10.1089/chi.2012.0028.

Elliot, R., Dobbin, A., Rose, G., & Soper, H. (1994). Vigorous, aerobic exercise versus general motor training activities: Effects on maladaptive and stereotypic behaviors of adults with both autism and mental retardation. *Journal of Autism and Developmental Disorders, 24*(5), 565–576. doi:10.1007/BF02172138.

Ensel, W. M., & Lin, N. (2004). Physical fitness and the stress process. *Journal of Community Psychology, 32,* 81–101. doi:10.1002/jcop.10079.

Esposito, P., Ulett, O., Staples, K., & Prestesater, H. (2014). Visual supports for TGMD-2 testing in youth with autism. *Research Quarterly for Exercise and Sport, 85*, A60.

Folio, M. R., & Fewell, R. R. (2000). *Peabody developmental motor scales: Examiner's manual* (2nd ed.). Austin: Pro-Ed.

Ford, L., Kozy, M., & Negreiros, J. (2012). Cognitive assessment in early childhood: Theoretical and practice perspectives. In D. P. Flanagan & P. L. Harrison (Eds.), *Contemporary intellectual assessment: Theories, tests, and issues* (pp. 585–622). New York: Guilford press.

Fox, K., & Riddoch, C. (2000). Charting the physical activity patterns of contemporary children and adolescents. *Proceedings of the Nutrition Society, 59,* 497–504. doi:10.1017/S0029665100000720.

Ghaziuddin, M., & Butler, E. (1998). Clumsiness in autism and Asperger syndrome: A further report. *Journal of Intellectual Disability Research, 42,* 43–48. doi:10.1046/j.1365–2788.1998.00065.x.

Gillham, J., Carter, A., Volkmar, F., & Sparrow, S. (2000). Toward a developmental operational definition of autism. *Journal of Autism Developmental Disorders, 30,* 269–278. doi:10.1023/A:1005571115268.

Gilliam, W., & Mayes, L. (2004). Integrating clinical and psychometric approaches—Developmental assessment and the infant mental health evaluation. In R. DelCarmen-Wiggins & A. Carter (Eds.), *Handbook of infants, toddlers, and preschool mental health assessment* (pp. 185–203). Oxford: Oxford University Press.

Goodwin, M. S., Groden, J., Velicer, W. F., Lipsitt, L. P., Baron, M. G., Hofmann, S. G., Groden, G. (2006). Cardiovascular arousal in individuals with autism. *Focus on Autism and Developmental Disabilities, 21,* 100–123. doi:10.1177/10883576060210020101.

Goodwin, M. S., Intille, S. S., Albinali, F., & Velicer, W. F. (2011). Automated detection of stereotypical motor movements. *Journal of Autism and Developmental Disorders, 41,* 770–782. doi:10.1007/s10803-010-1102-z.

Gordon, R., Handleman, J., & Harris, S. (1986). The effects of contingent versus non-contingent running on the out-of-seat behavior of an autistic boy. *Child and Family Behavior Therapy, 8*(3), 37–44. doi:10.1300/J019v08n03_04.

Green, D., Baird, G., & Barnett, A. L. (2002). The severity and nature of motor impairment in Asperger's syndrome: A comparison with specific developmental disorder of motor function. *Journal of Child Psychology and Psychiatry, 43,* 655–668. doi:10.1111/1469-7610.00054.

Green, D., Charman, T., Pickles, A., Chandler, S., Loucas, T., Simonoff, E., Baird, G. (2008). Impairment in movement skills of children with autistic spectrum disorders. *Developmental Medicine and Child Neurology, 51,* 311–316. doi:10.1111/j.1469–8749.2008.03242.x.

Henderson, S., Sugden, D., & Barnett, A. (2007). *Movement assessment battery for children* (2nd ed.). London: Harcourt Assessment.

Herrmann, S., Barreira, T., Kang, M., & Ainsworth, B. (2013). How many hours are enough? Accelerometer wear time may provide bias in daily activity estimates. *Journal of Physical Activity and Health, 10,* 742–749.

Hill, E. (2010). Motor difficulties in specific language impairment: Evidence for the Iverson account?—A commentary on Iverson's 'developing language in a developing body: The relationship between motor development and language development'. *Journal of Child Language, 37*(2), 287–292. doi:10.1017/S0305000909990444.

Hillier, A., Murphy, D., & Ferrara, C. (2011). A pilot study: Short-term reduction in salivary cortisol following low level physical exercise and relaxation among adolescents and young adults on the autism spectrum. *Journal of the International Society for the Investigation of Stress, 27*(5), 395–402. doi:10.1002/smi.1391.

Hills, A. P., Okely, A. D., & Baur, L. A. (2010). Addressing childhood obesity through increased physical activity. *Nature Reviews Endocrinology, 6,* 543–549. doi:10.1038/nrendo.2010.133.

Hilton, C., Wente, L., LaVesser, P., Ito, M., Reed, C., & Herzberg, G. (2007). Relationship between motor skill impairment and severity in children with Asperger syndrome. *Research in Autism Spectrum Disorders, 1,* 339–349. doi:10.1016/j.rasd.2006.12.003.

Ismael, N. T., & Lawson, L. M. (2012). The impact of preschoolers' gender and sensory preferences on physical activity levels during play. *British Journal of Occupational Therapy, 75,* 429–435. doi:10.4276/030802212 × 13470263980874.

Ives, J. C. (2014). *Motor behavior: Connecting mind and body for optimal performance*. Philadelphia: Lippincott Williams & Wilkens.

Janssen, I., & Leblanc, A. (2010). Systematic review of the health benefits of physical activity and fitness in school-aged children and youth. *International Journal of Behavioral Nutrition and Physical Activity, 7,* 40–55. doi:10.1186/1479-5868-7-40.

John, H. (2013). Activity measurement: Not simply child's play. *Pediatric Exercise Science, 25,* 536–547.

Johnson, C. C. (2009). The benefits of physical activity for youth with developmental disabilities: A systematic review. *The Science of Health Promotion, 23,* 157–167. doi:10.4278/ajhp.070930103.

Kern, L., Koegel, R. L., Dyer, K., Blew, P. A., & Fenton, L. R. (1982). The effects of physical exercise on self-stimulation and appropriate responding in autistic children. *Journal of Autism and Developmental Disorders, 12,* 399–419. doi:10.1007/BF01538327.

Kodish, S. R., Hodges-Kulinna, P., Martin, J. J., Pangrazi, R., & Darst, P. (2006). Determinants of physical activity in an inclusive setting. *Adapted Physical Activity Quarterly, 23,* 390–409.

Lainhart, J. (1999). Psychiatric problems in individuals with autism: Their parents and siblings. *International Review of Psychiatry, 11,* 278–298. doi:10.1080/09540269974177.

Lang, R., Koegel, L. K., Ashbaugh, K., Regester, A., Ence, W., & Smith, W. (2010). Physical exercise and individuals with autism spectrum disorders: A systemic review. *Research in Autism Spectrum Disorders, 4,* 565–576. doi:10.1016/j.rasd.2010.01.006.

Leonard, H., Bedford, R., Charman, T., Elsabbagh, M., Johnson, M., & Hill, E. (2013). Motor development in children at risk of autism: A follow-up study of infant siblings. *Autism*. (Advance online publication). doi:10.1177/1362361312470037.

Levinson, L., & Reid, G. (1993). The effects of exercise intensity on the stereotypic behaviors of individuals with autism. *Adapted Physical Activity Quarterly, 10,* 255–268.

Leyfer, O. T., Folstein, S. E., Bacalman, S., Davis, N. O., Dinh, E., Morgan, J., Tager-Flusberg, H., Lainhart, J. E. (2006). Comorbid psychiatric disorders in children with autism: Interview development and rates of disorders. *Journal of Autism and Developmental Disorders, 36,* 849–861. doi:10.1007/s10803-006-0123-0.

Liu, T. (2013). Sensory processing and motor skill performance in elementary school children with autism spectrum disorder. *Perceptual and Motor Skills, 116,* 197–209. doi:10.2466/10.25.PMS.116.1.197–209.

Liu, T., & Breslin, C. M. (2013a). Fine and gross motor performance of the MABC-2 by children with autism spectrum disorder and typically developing children. *Research in Autism Spectrum Disorders, 7,* 1244–1249. doi:10.1016/j.rasd.2013.07.002.

Liu, T., & Breslin, C. M. (2013b). The effect of a picture activity schedule on performance of the MABC-2 for children with autism spectrum disorder. *Research Quarterly for Exercise and Sport, 84,* 206–212. doi:10.1080/02701367.2013.784725.

Liu, T., & ElGarhy, S. (2014). Fine and gross motor skill development of preschool children on PDMS-2. Unpublished raw data.

Liu, T., Hamilton, M., Davis, L., & ElGarhy, S. (2014). Gross motor performance by children with autism spectrum disorder and typically developing children on TGMD-2. *Journal of Child and Adolescent Behaviour, 2,* 123. doi:10.4172/jcalb.1000123.

Lloyd, M., Macdonald, M., & Lord, C. (2011). Motor skills of toddlers with autism spectrum disorders. *Autism, 17,* 1–18.

Lochbaum, M., & Crews, D. (2003). Viability of cardiorespiratory and muscular strength program for the adolescent with autism. *Complementary Health Practice Review, 8,* 225–233, doi:10.1177/1076167503252917.

Logan, W., Robinson, L., & Getchell, N. (2011). The comparison of performances of preschool children on two motor assessments. *Perceptual and Motor Skills, 113,* 715–723. doi:10.2466/03.06.25.PMS.113.6.715–723.

MacDonald, M., Esposito, P., & Ulrich, D. (2011). The physical activity patterns of children with autism. *BMC Research Notes, 4,* 422. doi:10.1186/1756-0500-4-422.

MacDonald, M., Lord, C., & Ulrich, D. (2013). The relationship of motor skills and social communicative skills in school-aged children with autism spectrum disorder. *Adapted Physical Activity Quarterly, 30,* 271–282. doi:10.1186/1756-0500-4-422.

Magnusson, J., Cobham, C., & McLeod, R. (2012). Beneficial effects of clinical exercise rehabilitation for children and adolescents with autism spectrum disorder (ASD). *Journal of Exercise Physiology Online, 15*(2), 71–79.

Manohari, S., Raman, V., & Ashok, M. (2013). Use of Vineland adaptive behavior scales-II in children with autism: An Indian experience. *Journal of Indian Association for Child and Adolescents Mental Health, 9,* 5–12.

Mattard-Labrecque, C., Amor, L., & Couture, M. (2013). Children with autism and attention difficulties: A pilot study of the association between sensory, motor, and adaptive behaviors. *Journal of the Canadian Academy of Child and Adolescent Psychiatry, 22,* 139–146.

McCracken, J. T., McGough, J., Shah, B., Cronin, P., Hong, D., Aman, M. G., et al. (2002). Risperidone in children with autism and serious behavioral problems. *New England Journal of Medicine, 347,* 314–321. doi:10.1056/NEJMoa013171.

McKenzie, T. L. (2010). 2009 C. H. McCloy lecture seeing is believing: Observing physical activity and its contexts. *Research Quarterly for Exercise and Sport, 81,* 113–122.

Memari, A. H., Ghaheri, B., Ziaee, V., Kordi, R., Hafizi, S., & Moshayedi, P. (2013). Physical activity in children and adolescents with autism assessed by triaxial accelerometry. *Pediatric Obesity, 8,* 150–158. doi:10.1111/j.2047–6310.2012.00101.x.

Miyahara, M., Tsujii, M., Hori, M., Nakanishi, K., & Kageyama, H. (1997). Brief report: Motor incoordination in children with Asperger syndrome and learning disabilities. *Journal of Autism and Developmental Disorders, 27,* 595–602. doi:10.1023/A:1025834211548.

Mullen, E. (1995). *Mullen scales of early learning.* Circle Pines: American Guidance Service Inc.

Nicholson, H., Kehel, T. J., Bray, M. A., & van Heest, J. (2011). The effects of antecedent physical activity on the academic engagement of children with autism spectrum disorder. *Psychology in the Schools, 48,* 198–213. doi:10.1002/pits.20537.

Obrusnikova, I., & Cavalier, A. R. (2011). Perceived barriers and facilitators of participation in after-school physical activity by children with autism spectrum disorders. *Journal of Developmental and Physical Disabilities, 23,* 195–211. doi:10.1007/s10882-010-9215-z.

Obrusnikova, I., & Miccinello, D. (2012). Parent perceptions of factors influencing after-school physical activity of children with autism spectrum disorders. *Adapted Physical Activity Quarterly, 29,* 63–80.

Oriel, K. N., George, C. L., Peckus, R., & Semon, A. (2011). The effects of aerobic exercise on academic engagement in young children with autism spectrum disorder. *Pediatric Physical Therapy, 23,* 187–193. doi:10.1097/PEP.0b013e318218f149.

Pan, C. (2008a). School time physical activity of students with and without autism spectrum disorders during PE and recess. *Adapted Physical Activity Quarterly, 25,* 308–321.

Pan, C. (2008b). Objectively measured physical activity between children with autism spectrum disorders and children without disabilities during inclusive recess settings in Taiwan. *Journal of Autism and Developmental Disorders, 38,* 1292–1301. doi:10.1007/s10803-007-0518-6.

Pan, C. (2009). Age, social engagement, and physical activity in children with autism spectrum disorders. *Research in Autism Spectrum Disorders, 3,* 22–31. doi:10.1016/j.rasd.2008.03.002.

Pan, C., & Frey, G. C. (2005). Identifying physical activity determinants in youth with autistic spectrum disorders. *Journal of Physical Activity and Health, 2,* 412–422.

Pan, C., & Frey, G. (2006). Physical activity patterns in youth with autism spectrum disorders. *Journal of Autism Developmental Disorders, 36,* 597–606. doi:10.1007/s10803-006-0101-6.

Pan, C., Tsai, C., & Chu, C. (2009). Fundamental movement skills in children diagnosed with autism spectrum disorders and attention deficit hyperactivity disorder. *Journal of Autism and Developmental Disorders, 39,* 1694–1705. doi:10.1007/s10803-009-0813-5.

Pan, C., Tsai, C., & Hsieh, K. (2011a). Physical activity correlates for children with autism spectrum. *Research Quarterly for Exercise and Sport, 82,* 491–498. doi:10.1080/02701367.2011.10599782.

Pan, C., Tsai, C., Chu, C., & Hsieh, K. (2011b). Physical activity and self-determined motivation of adolescents with and without autism spectrum disorders in inclusive physical education. *Research in Autism Spectrum Disorders, 5,* 733–741. doi:10.1016/j.rasd.2010.08.007.

Pan, C., Tsai, C., Hsieh, K., Chu, C., Li, Y., & Huang, S. (2011c). Accelerometer-determined physical activity among elementary school-aged children with autism spectrum disorders in Taiwan. *Research in Autism Spectrum Disorders, 5,* 1042–1052. doi:10.1016/j.rasd.2010.11.010.

Pethkar, V., Naik, S., & Sonawaane, S. (2010). Attitudes toward physical activity and its measurement. *Journal of Physical Education and Sport, 29,* 30–36.

Petrus, C., Adamson, S. R., Block, L. R., Einarson, S. J., Sharifnejad, M., & Harris, S. R. (2008). Effects of exercise interventions on stereotypic behaviours in children with autism spectrum disorder. *Physiotherapy Canada, 60,* 134–245. doi:10.3138/physio.60.2.134.

Piek, J. P., Dawson, L., Smith, L. M., & Gasson, N. (2008). The role of early fine and gross motor development on later motor and cognitive ability. *Human Movement Science, 27,* 668–681. doi:10.1016/j.humov.2007.11.002.

Piek, J., Hands, B., & Licari, M. (2012). Assessment of motor functioning in the preschool period. *Neuropsychology Review, 22,* 402–413. doi:10.1007/s11065-012-9211-4.

Pitetti, K. H., Beets, M. W., & Combs, C. (2009). Physical activity levels of children with intellectual disabilities during school. *Medicine and Science in Sports and Exercise, 41,* 1580–1586. doi:10.1249/MSS.0b013e31819d4438.

Provost, B., Heimerl, S., & Lopez, B. (2007a). Levels of gross and fine motor development in young children with autism spectrum disorder. *Physical and Occupational Therapy in Pediatrics, 27*(3), 21–36. doi:10.1300/J006v27n03_03.

Provost, B., Lopez, B., & Heimerl, S. (2007b). A comparison of motor delays in young children: Autism spectrum disorder, developmental delay, and developmental concerns. *Journal of Autism and Developmental Disorders, 37,* 321–328. doi:10.1007/s10803-006-0170-6.

Prupas, A., & Reid, G. (2001). Effects of exercise frequency on stereotypic behaviors of children with developmental disabilities. *Education and Training in Mental Retardation and Developmental Disabilities, 36,* 196–206.

Reynolds, A. M., & Malow, B. A. (2011). Sleep and autism spectrum disorders. *Pediatric Clinics of North America, 58,* 685–698. doi:10.1016/j.pcl.2011.03.009.

Rimmer, J., Rowland, J., & Yamaki, K. (2007). Obesity and secondary conditions in adolescents with disabilities: Addressing the needs of an underserved population. *Journal of Adolescent Health, 41,* 224–229. doi:10.1016/j.jadohealth.2007.05.005.

Rosenthal-Malek, A., & Mitchell, S. (1997). The effects of exercise on the self-stimulatory behaviors and positive responding of adolescents with autism. *Journal of Autism and Developmental Disorders, 27,* 193–202. doi:10.1023/A:1025848009248.

Sacrey, L. R., Germani, T., Bryson, S. E., & Zwaigenbaum, L. (2014). Reaching and grasping in autism spectrum disorder: A review of recent literature. *Frontiers in Neurology*. (Advance online publication). doi:10.3389/fneur.2014.00006.

Rosser Sandt, D. D., & Frey, G. (2005). Comparison of physical activity levels between children with and without autistic spectrum disorders. *Adapted Physical Activity Quarterly, 22,* 146–159.

Schultheis, S., Boswell, B., & Decker, J. (2000). Successful physical activity programming for students with autism. *Focus on Autism and Other Developmental Disabilities, 15*(3), 159–163. doi:10.1177/108835760001500306.

Simonoff, E., Pickles, A., Charman, T., Chandler, S., Loucas, T., & Baird, G. (2008). Psychiatric disorders in children with autism spectrum disorders: Prevalence comorbidity and associated factors in a population derived sample. *Journal of the American Academy of Child and Adolescent Psychiatry, 47,* 921–929. doi:10.1097/CHI.0b013e318179964f.

Sirard, J. R., & Pate, R. R. (2001). Physical activity assessment in children and adolescents. *Sports Medicine, 31,* 439–454. doi:10.2165/00007256-200131060-00004.

Sit, C. H. P., McManus, A., McKenzie, T. L., & Lian, J. (2007). Physical activity levels of children in special schools. *Preventative Medicine, 45,* 424–431. doi:10.1016/j.ypmed.2007.02.003.

Skokauskas, N., & Gallagher, L. (2010). Psychosis, affective disorders and anxiety in autistic spectrum disorder: Prevalence and nosological considerations. *Psychopathology, 43,* 8–16. doi:10.1159/000255958.

Sowa, M., & Meulenbroek, R. (2012). Effects of physical exercise on autism spectrum disorders: A meta-analysis. *Research in Autism Spectrum Disorders, 6,* 46–57. doi:10.1016/j.rasd.2011.09.001.

Sparrow, S., Cicchetti, D., & Balla, D. (2005). *Vineland adaptive behavior scales* (2nd ed.). Minneapolis: Pearson Assessment.

Staples, K. (2013). Commentary: The motor skills of 7–10 year old children diagnosed with ASD: Are the comparison groups and assessments being used appropriate for the research questions being asked? *Journal of Autism and Developmental Disorders, 43,* 2732–2736. doi:10.1007/s10803-013-1809-8.

Staples, K., & Reid, G. (2010). Fundamental movement skills and autism spectrum disorders. *Journal of Autism and Developmental Disorders, 40,* 209–217. doi:10.1007/s10803-009-0854-9.

Stodden, D. F., Goodway, J. D., Langendorfer, S. J., Roberton, M. A., Rudisill, M. E., Garcia, C., Garcia, L. E. (2008). A developmental perspective on the role of motor skill competence in physical activity: An emergent relationship. *Quest, 60,* 290–306. doi:10.1080/00336297.2008.10483582.

Stratis, E., & Lecavalier, L. (2013). Restricted and repetitive behaviors and psychiatric symptoms in youth with autism spectrum disorders. *Research in Autism Spectrum Disorders, 7,* 757–766. doi:10.1016/j.rasd.2013.02.017.

Sylvia, L. G., Bernstein, E. E., Hubbard, J. L., Keating, L., & Anderson, E. J. (2014). Practical guide to measuring physical activity. *Journal of the Academy of Nutrition and Dietetics, 114,* 199–207. doi:10.1016/j.jand.2013.09018.

Tan, B., Cohen, L., & Pooley, J. (2013). The implication of physical activity on attention span and quality of life in children with autism spectrum disorders: A pilot study. *Journal of Law and Social Sciences, 2*(2), 121. doi:10.5176/2251-2853_2.2.121#sthash.bvDKjDWY.dpuf.

Thomas, J. R., Nelson, J. K., & Silverman, S. J. (2011). *Research methods in physical activity* (6th edn.). Champaign: Human Kinetics.

Todd, T., & Reid, G. (2006). Increasing physical activity in individuals with autism. *Focus on Autism and Other Developmental Disabilities, 21,* 167–176. doi:10.1177/10883576060210030501.

Tsiros, M. D., Coates, A. M., Howe, P. R. C., Grimshaw, P. N., & Buckley, J. D. (2011). Obesity: The new childhood disability? *Obesity, 12,* 26–36. doi:10.1111/j.1467-789X.2009.00706.x.

Ulrich, D. (2000). *Test of gross motor development (2nd ed.) examiner's manual.* Austin: Pro-Ed Inc.

U. S. Department of Health and Human Services. (2002). *Healthy people 2010: Physical activity and fitness.* http://www.health.gov/healthypeople/Document/HTML/Volume2/22Physical.htm.

Van Waelvelde, H., De Weert, W., De Cock, P., Smits-Engelsman, B., & Peersman, W. (2004). Ball catching performance in children with developmental coordination disorder. *Adapted Physical Activity Quarterly, 21,* 348–363.

Vanvuchelen, M., Roeyers, H., & Weerdt, W. (2007). Nature of motor imitation problems in school-aged males with autism: How congruent are the error types? *Developmental Medicine and Child Neurology, 49,* 6–12. doi:10.1017/S0012162207000047.x.

Venkatesan, S. (2005). Activity log of preschool children with developmental disabilities and autism spectrum disorders. *Asia Pacific Disability Rehabilitation Journal, 16*(1), 68–76.

Whyatt, C. P., & Craig, C. M. (2012). Motor skills in children aged 7-10 years, diagnosed with autism spectrum disorder. *Journal of Autism and Developmental Disorders, 42,* 1799–1809. doi:10.1007/s10803-011-1421-8.

Yoon, D., Scott, K., Hill, M., Levitt, N., & Lambert, E. (2006). Review of three tests of motor proficiency in children. *Perceptual and Motor Skills, 102,* 543–552. doi:10.2466/pms.102.2.543–551.

Yun, J., & Shapiro, D. (2004). A quantitative approach to movement skill assessment for children with mental retardation. *Adapted Physical Activity Quarterly, 21,* 269–228.

Ziviani, J., Macdonald, D., Rodger, S., Batch, J., & Cerin, E. (2006). Physical activity of young children. *OTJR: Occupation Participation and Health, 26,* 1–12, doi: 10.1177/153944920602600102

Part III
Psychological Disorders

Chapter 6
Challenging Behavior

Wendy Machalicek, Tracy Raulston, Christen Knowles, Traci Ruppert, Amarie Carnett and Fahad Alresheed

Introduction

Individuals with autism spectrum disorder (ASD) often engage in challenging behaviors such as aggression, self-injurious behavior, stereotypy, and elopement (Baghdadli et al. 2003; Conroy et al. 2005a; Hartley et al. 2008; Horner et al. 2002; Kanne and Mazurek 2011; Militerni et al. 2002). These behaviors emerge early, and without effective treatment persist over time (Hartley et al. 2008; Matson and Shoemaker 2009). Individuals with ASD are at an increased risk for the development of challenging behavior due to social communication impairments and patterns of rigid and repetitive behaviors and interests that are the core characteristics of ASD (Dominick et al. 2007; Murphy et al. 2005). In addition, individuals with ASD are at an increased risk for comorbid diagnoses, such as anxiety disorders, depression and mood disorders, and attention deficit/hyperactivity disorder (Ghaziuddin et al. 2002; Matson and Williams 2013; Van Steensel et al. 2011). These disorders themselves are often associated with internalizing and externalizing challenging behavior.

Challenging behaviors can present difficult-to-overcome barriers in delivering essential instruction and supported social interactions required to improve adaptive behavior often resulting in worsened educational, social, residential, and vocational outcomes (National Research Council 2001). In addition, caregivers often report increased stress, depression, and burn out (Baker et al. 2002; Bernheimer et al. 1990; Lecavalier et al. 2006; Lucyshyn et al. 2004; Seltzer et al. 2001). Parents of children with ASD report higher levels of stress than typically developing children or children with other disabilities (Hayes and Watson 2013; Keenan et al. 2010;

W. Machalicek (✉) · T. Raulston · C. Knowles · T. Ruppert · F. Alresheed
Department of Special Education and Clinical Sciences, University of Oregon,
Eugene, OR 97403, USA
e-mail: wmachali@uoregon.edu

A. Carnett
Victoria University of Wellington, Wellington, New Zealand

Johnny L. Matson (ed.), *Comorbid Conditions Among Children with Autism Spectrum Disorders,* Autism and Child Psychopathology Series,
DOI 10.1007/978-3-319-19183-6_6

Schieve et al. 2007). The presence and severity of challenging behavior is a higher indicator of parental stress than disability type (Floyd and Gallagher 1997; Walsh et al. 2013). The most common characteristics of ASD associated with parental stress are impairments with social communication (Davis and Carter 2008; Hayes and Watson 2013) and restricted or repetitive behaviors (Hayes and Watson 2013). Chronic parental stress can lead to negative outcomes such as marital distress, depression, coercive parenting, and attrition from parent training and interventions (Walsh et al. 2013). Moreover, both parental stress (Giallo and Gavidia-Payne 2006) and parental satisfaction of caring for a child with a developmental disability (Hesse et al. 2013) has been shown to be a predictor of sibling adjustment for siblings of children with developmental delays.

Purpose of This Chapter

The early identification and treatment of challenging behavior in individuals with ASD has received increasing attention due to the high prevalence, their deleterious effects on the individual with ASD and their caregivers, and due to the amplified probability of maladjustment later in life (Dunlap et al. 2006). The purpose of this chapter is to introduce the reader to the current conceptualization of challenging behavior, its causes and risk factors for development, to review the biobehavioral model that guides our understanding of the assessment and treatment of challenging behavior, and to review the extant literature on assessment practices and behavioral interventions found effective in decreasing challenging behavior in this population. In the first section, *Defining Challenging Behavior*, we define the types of behaviors that have typically exemplified "challenging" behavior. In the second section, *Risk Factors,* we discuss the known risk factors associated with the development of challenging behavior for individuals with ASD. In the third section, *Early Emergence, Prevalence, and Chronicity*, we summarize the field's understanding of the population-based occurrence and the extent to which challenging behaviors persist over time for this population. In the fourth section, *Functional Behavior Assessment (FBA)*, we present an overview of the FBA process. In the fifth section, *Behavioral Intervention*, we review evidence-based, individualized behavioral interventions for both social and nonsocial-mediated challenging behavior. Finally, we conclude the chapter with *Suggestions for Future Research.*

Defining Challenging Behavior

Although the identification of what constitutes a challenging behavior could be categorized as a subjective experience, operational definitions in literature that define challenging behavior demonstrate an analogous schema that has, for the most part, remained consistent. For example, challenging behavior is generally described as behaviors with an intensity (i.e., more than one injury to self or others), frequency (i.e., occurs at least weekly) or duration (i.e., more than 1 h of disruption), which is both culturally unacceptable and threatens the safety of self and others (Emerson 2001; Qureshi and Alborz 1992). An individual's age often determines behaviors classified as developmentally appropriate versus challenging (Campbell et al. 2000; Crnic and Greenberg 1990; Kwon et al. 2013). For example, frequent tantrums exhibited by a 2-year old are not uncommon, yet the same behavior from an older elementary age child would be cause for concern. Indeed, behaviors are determined as challenging based on a variety of contextual, cultural, and developmental factors.

Types of challenging behaviors can vary based on the characteristics of each individual. Challenging behaviors include but are not limited to aggression (Kanne and Mazurek 2011; Murphy et al. 2000), repetitive motor behaviors/stereotypies (Loftin et al. 2008; Matson and Nebel-Schwalm 2007; Reid et al. 2011), noncompliance (Donohue et al. 2012), self-injury (Matson and Turygin 2012; Minshawi et al. 2014), property destruction (Luby 2011), disruptions, (McTiernan et al. 2011), and tantrums (Goldin et al. 2013).

Challenging behaviors can escalate for a variety of reasons yet a behavioral escalation sequence usually begins with a benign behavior and increases in severity into more severe responses (Shukla-Mehta and Albin 2003). Certain challenging behaviors can transition to other, more extreme, behaviors (e.g., stereotypy can transform into self-injury for some individuals over time; Reid et al. 2010). Behaviors may, at first, be caused by a certain factor then, over time, be maintained by other consequences (Felce and Emerson 1996). Likewise, some challenging behaviors are demonstrated as a functional chain for the individual (e.g., yelling to property destruction then property destruction to physical aggression) (Murphy et al. 2000). Not surprisingly, externalizing behaviors are more often described as challenging when compared to internalizing behaviors (Lowe et al. 2007).

Aside from the immediate observable characteristics of challenging behavior, the topography of an individual behavior effects likelihood that it will be interpreted as challenging. Behaviors that present at a high rate or frequency as well as the intensity or severity of it can increase one's perception of the degree of challenge (Matson and Nebel-Schwalm 2007; McTiernan et al. 2011). For example, it is not uncommon for an elementary age child to show aggression towards another child on the playground at some point yet, aggression may be interpreted as challenging amidst reoccurrence.

Finally, challenging behaviors are frequently the subject of experimental inquiry considering the significant impact these behaviors have on the individual, teachers, caregivers, family, and social relationships. As a child demonstrating challenging behavior matures, and the longer these behaviors have been expressed, the more concerning the child's developmental trajectory (Conroy et al. 2005a). The overall conceptual definition of challenging behavior captures the negative impact the behaviors have on the individual and that individual's support network. The detrimental consequences of challenging behavior are commonplace in past and present research (Lowe et al. 2007; McTiernan et al. 2011). These behaviors are first and foremost identified by the impact the behavior has on the physical safety of self or others, environmental damage, or severity intense enough to require multiple interventions or individuals to remedy (Emerson et al. 2001).

Early Emergence, Prevalence, and Chronicity

The estimated prevalence of challenging behavior for individuals with intellectual and developmental disabilities has varied widely from 5.7% to as high as 17% of the intellectual disability (ID) population (Emerson et al. 2001; Emerson and Bromley 1995; Lowe et al. 2007; Qureshi and Alborz 1992). Approximately, 94.3% of the children with ASD engage in one or more topographies of challenging behavior (Matson et al. 2009). Aggression is a commonly occurring topography with Kanne and Mazurek (2011) reporting that 68% of the children and adolescents with ASD had demonstrated aggression towards a caregiver and 49% had aggressed towards a non-caregiver. Although some researchers have reported an association between aggression and lower cognitive functioning, poor expressive language, and worsened adaptive skills (Dominick et al. 2007; Hartley et al. 2008), others have found that aggression presents across individuals with ASD regardless of intellectual functioning, communication abilities, or symptom severity (Kanne and Mazurek 2011). Similarly, individuals with ASD are at increased risk for developing self-injurious behavior such as head banging/hitting and self-biting (Minshawi et al. 2014) and these behaviors can be chronic (Murphy et al. 1993). In addition, recent research examining the rate of aggression in children and adolescents with ASD suggests that challenging behavior is equally common among males and females with ASD (Kanne and Mazurek 2011).

Challenging behaviors tend to emerge early in childhood during the developmental period where challenging behaviors, such as tantrums, noncompliance, repetitive stereotyped movements, and insistence on sameness, are common to children with and without neurodevelopmental disabilities (Hartley et al. 2008; Matson et al. 2010; Murphy et al. 1999; Oliver et al. 1987). However, the challenging behaviors of toddlers and preschools with ASD may be expressed with higher frequency, increased intensity, and across environments. The emergence of challenging behavior during early childhood can introduce complexity into the identification of atypical development, FBA, and behavioral intervention. This delay to effective treatment may indirectly contribute to the worsening of challenging behavior as well-meaning caregivers may inadvertently strengthen challenging behavior when they do not fully understand the maintaining consequences.

Fortunately, research suggests that oftentimes, for some individuals with ASD or ID, abnormal or maladaptive behaviors (e.g., abnormal responses to stimuli, resistance to change, repetitive behaviors, and behavior problems) increase throughout childhood and adolescence and then decrease during adulthood (Murphy et al. 2005; Shattuck et al. 2007). Shattuck and colleagues (2007) found decreased challenging behavior (e.g., unusual or repetitive habits, self injurious behavior, aggression, and property destruction) over a 4½year time period for 241 individuals with

ASD, some of who had comorbid conditions (e.g., seizure disorder and ID). Participants who were in the oldest cohort of the study (ages 31 and older) showed greater decline in maladaptive behavior than those who were ages 10 through 21, and disruptive restricted and repetitive patterns of behavior and interests were found to improve more than other areas (Shattuck et al. 2007). Similarly, Murphy et al. (2005) found that challenging behavior tended to decrease with age, although individuals who presented more challenging behaviors at the first assessment still displayed more challenging behaviors when retested (Matson and Rivet 2008). On the other hand, Matson and Shoemaker (2009) noted that individuals with the highest rates of challenging behavior demonstrate this challenging behavior later in life. Similarly, Kanne and Mazurek (2011) found that children who engaged in aggression were likely to continue engaging in aggression. These findings suggest that, although challenging behavior declines for some individuals with ASD, serious challenging behavior tends to persist, often into adulthood, for a subset of individuals with ASD.

Risk Factors for the Development of Challenging Behavior

Challenging behavior has no singular origin; rather, development springs from biological, social, environmental, and psychological underpinnings (Emerson 2001). Risk factors related to the development and maintenance of challenging behavior are both environmental (i.e., negative interactions with a parent) and biological (i.e., severity of ID; Dunlap et al. 2006; Murphy et al. 2009), amidst many others. Nevertheless, increased autism severity appears to increase the risk for exhibiting challenging behavior (e.g., Matson and Rivet 2008). In this section, we discuss the impact that the core diagnostic characteristics of ASD have on the development and expression of challenging behavior as well as the potential influence that common comorbid diagnoses can have on the development of challenging behavior in individuals with ASD.

Challenging Behavior Associated with Diagnostic Characteristics of Autism Spectrum Disorder

The relationship between social communication impairments and increased rates of maladaptive, challenging behavior has been well documented (Dominick et al. 2007; Mancil 2006). For instance, Murphy et al. (2005) conducted a longitudinal study that tracked the challenging behavior of 166 children with characteristics of ASD and severely impaired functioning. Among other findings not reported here, they found that (a) better language, social and cognitive skills (IQ), and higher chronological age were correlated with lower levels of abnormal behavior at assessment time 1 and that (b) better language and social skills and the absence of ASD were correlated with lowered abnormal behavior at assessment time 2.

Additionally, the presence of restricted and repetitive behaviors and interests appears to contribute to the development of challenging behavior related to access to activities or tangibles associated with this autism spectrum symptom (Boyd et al. 2012; Dominick et al. 2007; Matson and Dempsey 2009; Patterson et al. 2010). One of the core defining features of ASD is the presence of restricted, repetitive patterns of behavior, interests, or activities (American Psychiatric Association 2013, p. 50). Repetitive and Restricted Behaviors and Interests (RRBI) include: (a) stereotyped or repetitive motor movements, use of objects, or speech (e.g., motor stereotypies, lining up objects, echolalia, and idiosyncratic speech), (b) insistence on sameness, inflexible adherence to routines, or ritualized patterns or verbal–nonverbal behavior (e.g., severe distress at minor changes, difficulties during transitions, and rigid patterns of thinking), (c) highly restricted, fixated interests that are abnormal in intensity or focus (e.g., preoccupation with odd objects, exceptionally circumscribed or perseverative interests), and (d) hyper- or hyporeactivity to sensory input or unusual interests in sensory aspects of the environment (e.g., indifference to pain, adverse responses to certain sounds or textures, extreme smelling or touching of objects, and visual attraction to lights or movement; American Psychiatric Association 2013). Restricted and repetitive behaviors and interests can be divided into two types: (a) lower order, which can consist of repetitive movement, object manipulation, and repetitive self-injurious behavior; and (b) higher order, which includes insistence on sameness, repetitive language, circumscribed perseverative interests, and rigid adherence to a rule or mental state (Boyd et al. 2012; Patterson et al. 2010). The characteristics of restricted and repetitive behaviors and interests found in individuals with ASD are very similar to the core characteristics of obsessive compulsive disorder (OCD), which can lead to overdiagnosis of OCD in people with ASD (Paula-Perez 2013). Specifically, both of these disorders have a fixation on routine and rituals, resistance to change, and restricted interests that are of higher intensity (Paula-Perez 2013).

Repetitive behaviors can have negative impacts on learning and have been reported by parents as being the most difficult aspect of ASD (Boyd et al. 2012). For example, it can be a challenge to terminate rituals and other perseverative behaviors in order to begin instruction or other routines in the home and community, and some complex stereotyped behavior is performed in a fixed sequence (Murphy et al. 2000), which means that interrupting that chain of behavior can evoke more challenging behavior. Moreover, individuals with ASD and ID are at a greater risk for communication impairment and increased RRBI than those with only an ASD diagnosis (Deb and Prasad 1994).

Challenging Behavior Associated with Intellectual Disability (ID)

ID has been reported in approximately 10–70 % of the individuals with ASD when measured across European countries and the USA contexts (Berney 2004; Deb et al. 2001; Long et al. 2000; Matson and Shoemaker 2009). Variation in reported prevalence may be explained in part due to instrumentation, diagnostic criteria, sample, co-occurring psychiatric disorders, and diagnostic substitution (Keen and Ward 2004; Shattuck 2006). Similar to individuals with ASD, individuals with intellectual and developmental disability often engage in challenging behavior such as stereotypies, aggression, property destruction, and self-injury; reported prevalence has ranged from 10 to 64 % (Bensen and Brooks 2008; Farmer and Aman 2010; Holden and Gitlesen 2006; Murphy et al. 2009). Moreover, challenging behavior occurs at increased rates in individuals with both ASD and ID diagnoses (Lee et al. 2008; Matson and Rivet 2008; McClintock et al. 2003; Symons et al. 2005; Tenneij et al. 2009). Indeed, a known risk factor increasing the likelihood of challenging behavior is the severity of cognitive impairment or the severity of ASD (Matson and Rivet 2008; Matson and Shoemaker 2009; Reese et al. 2005; Rojahn et al. 2004). In addition, both of these disabilities are characterized by deficits in social skills, adaptive functioning, and communication, which can exacerbate challenging behaviors (Matson et al. 2011). Furthermore, it seems that individuals with ASD and ID are particularly vulnerable to comorbid psychopathologies such as anxiety, depression, and schizophrenia (Matson and Shoemaker 2009).

Challenging Behavior Associated with Psychopathology

Anxiety disorders, depression, and attention deficit disorders (AD/HD) are among the disorders most commonly associated with ASD (Matson and Williams 2013).

Anxiety Anxiety is clinically identified through specific phobias, generalized anxiety, social phobia, and separation anxiety disorder (Leyfer et al. 2006). Prevalence rates have varied from 11 to 84 % (White et al. 2009) and a recent meta-analysis demonstrates nearly 40 % of those with ASD were diagnosed with comorbid anxiety disorder (Van Steelsel et al. 2011). Certain conditions, such as strong communication skills or presence of depressive symptoms, may increase a likelihood of a comorbid diagnosis of anxiety for a child with ASD (Mannion and Leader 2013; Sterling et al. 2008).

A comorbid diagnosis of ASD and anxiety could mean increased risk of exhibiting challenging behavior. Individuals may express more oppositional behavior, aggression, and have worsened interpersonal relationships (Kim et al. 2000). Moreover, symptoms of depression and anxiety can cluster together and potentially contribute to increased impairment (Sterling et al. 2008).

Depression and Related Mood Disorders Clinic-based studies suggest that the prevalence of depression alongside ASD is the most common comorbid psychiatric diagnosis and is more likely to occur in adolescence or adulthood (Ghaziuddin et al. 2002). Among a group of adults with ASD, 43 % demonstrated significant levels of depressive symptoms (Sterling et al. 2008). The rates of depression among individuals with autism and Asperger's syndrome vary widely across studies, with the highest being 34 % percent and as low as 4 % (Stewart et al. 2006). Even taking into consideration methodological differences, research demonstrates increased rates of major depression in children with ASD (Leyfer et al. 2006). Some research demonstrates that having better social skills or being of adolescent age was a specific factor associated with the presence of depressive symptoms in individuals with ASD (Sterling et al. 2008) while other research notes no correlation of either IQ or age (Strand et al. 2012).

With depression, there are two diagnostic forms of related mood disorders: unipolar (i.e., episodes of depression) and bipolar (i.e., episodes of mania or hypomania with depression) depression (DeRubeis, Siegle and Hollon 2008). Diagnosis of depression for an individual with ASD is problematic due to diagnostic overshadowing, when the primary diagnosis and associated symptoms overshadow symptoms to other, less superficial indicators (Simonoff et al. 2008). For example, a child with ASD may demonstrate severe challenging behavior related to frustration with limited functional communication, yet the child's depressive symptoms could be manifested through insomnia. Yet the concern of intervening with challenging behavior likely overshadows an investigation for the cause of insomnia. In relation to comorbidity of ASD and depression, feelings of depression and sadness for individuals with ASD can be superficially expressed differently than neurotypical individuals experiencing depression (Ghaziuddin et al. 2002). For instance, individuals with ASD may not be able to fully communicate their feelings, which is important in the diagnostic process. Likewise, individuals with ASD and a comorbid depressive condition may express a depressed mood through perseverative interest in dark topics (e.g., black holes), fears, crying spells, and appetite or sleep problems (Ghaziuddin et al. 2002). Not surprisingly, a comorbid condition of ASD and depression may change the topography and intensity of challenging behavior. For instance, depression can increase oppositional behavior, aggression, and social withdrawal (Kim et al. 2000; Ghaziuddin et al. 2002). The most common presenting symptoms of depression related to challenging behavior may be increased stereotypies, frequent loss of temper, and aggression (Lainhart and Folstein 1994). Also, during a depressive episode, specific behaviors, such as self-injury, are likely to increase (Stewart et al. 2006). These related symptoms of depression may also increase certain deficits of ASD (Perry et al. 2001). In particular, the onset and natural history of depression was usually, if not always, associated with new onset of maladaptive behaviors, particularly self-injury and aggression (Stewart et al. 2006).

Attention Deficit Disorders Although a comorbid diagnosis was accepted for the first time in the Diagnostic and Statistical Manual of Mental Disorders, Fifth Edition (DSM-V) (American Psychiatric Association 2013), AD/HD are among one of the most common disorders associated with ASD (Matson and Williams 2013). Research reports varied comorbid prevalence rates of ASD and AD/HD ranging from 17.6% (Hanson et al. 2013) to over 80% of a sample of those with ASD and comorbid AD/HD symptoms (Frazier et al. 2001). Regardless of the varying statistics reported in research, generally prevalence is listed at around 50% (Leyfer et al. 2006; Murray 2010; Sinzig et al. 2009). On it's own AD/HD is categorized, according to the DSM-V as "a persistent pattern of inattention and/or hyperactivity-impulsivity that interferes with functioning or development" (American Psychiatric Association 2013, p. 59). Symptoms of AD/HD include inattention, hyperactivity, and impulsivity. Although many of these symptoms appear in individuals with ASD, a child with ASD is more likely to have comorbid AD/HD than vice versa (Sinzig et al. 2009). In addition, many individuals with ASD demonstrate symptoms of inattention or hyperactivity without cause for a comorbid diagnosis. According to the DSM-V, abnormalities in attention are common in ASD yet a comorbid diagnosis should be considered when attention and/or hyperactivity difficulties exceed that of others of the same developmental age/level (American Psychiatric Association 2013). Although inattention and social difficulties are found in both children with ASD and those with AD/HD, it is not uncommon for children with an ASD to first be diagnosed with AD/HD (Matson and Williams 2013). The presence of AD/HD could also increase the expression of deficits common to ASD including communication, motor, and social development (American Psychiatric Association 2013).

The literature on challenging behavior as it relates to a dual diagnosis of ASD and AD/HD suggests an overall increase of challenging behavior. Specific increases in challenging behavior include a higher rate of tantrums, anger, and struggle to finish tasks (Goldin et al. 2013). Defiance and losing one's temper are rated as more significant in children with comorbid ASD and AD/HD compared to only a singular presence of one of the disorders (Guttmann-Steinmetz, Gadow and DeVincent 2009). Likewise, a higher score of hyperactivity for children with ASD is associated with an increased impairment in communication (Sinzig et al. 2009), which commonly can attribute to increased challenging behavior.

Tantrums appear to be the most common challenging behavior of a comorbid occurrence in literature regarding a dual diagnosis (Goldin et al. 2013; Konst et al. 2013). As reported by research from Goldin and colleagues (2013) AD/HD increases related symptoms of ASD therefore producing more tantrums when comparing comorbidity to a singular diagnosis.

It is important to note that even though there are many similar crossovers of challenging behaviors found in AD/HD and ASD alone, the mechanism for the challenging behavior can be different based on the expression of the disability. A child with ASD may throw a tantrum due to difficulty with change while a child with AD/HD may tantrum because of impulsivity or issues with self-control (American Psychiatric Association 2013).

Approach to Intervention

Although the prescription of psychotropic medications has increased in an attempt to treat the challenging behavior presented by some individuals with ASD and ID (Aman et al. 2005; Langworthy-Lam et al. 2002; Witwer and Lecavalier 2005), their use is associated with limited success and potentially serious negative side effects (Aman et al. 2005; Emerson et al. 2000; Matson and Boisjoli 2009a; Matson and Neal 2009). A review of the use of psychopharmacological agents to treat challenging behavior is outside the scope of the current chapter but the reader is referred to Handen and Lubetsky (2005) and Malone et al. (2005) for further reading.

The current best practice for treating challenging behavior includes a FBA to identify the social consequence(s) maintaining challenging behavior and the subsequent development of a behavior intervention plan based on the assessment results (Anderson, Freeman and Scotti 1999; Didden et al. 1997). In the sections that follow we will provide an overview of the FBA process.

Functional Behavior Assessment (FBA)

Functional behavioral assessment (FBA) is a process designed to maximize the effectiveness and efficiency of behavioral support by identifying the antecedents and consequences that influence the occurrence of challenging behavior (O'Neill et al. 1997). The FBA process identifies (a) an operational definition of the challenging behavior(s), (b) antecedent conditions under which the challenging behavior is most and least likely to occur, (c) consequence(s) that are most likely maintaining that behavior, and (d) a function-based behavior support plan for minimizing reinforcement for challenging behavior and increasing appropriate behavior (Gresham et al. 2001; O'Neill et al. 1997). The major assumption underlying FBA is that, to change challenging behavior, one must first understand the behavior's operant or communicative function in meeting a specific need for the individual (e.g., gaining attention, escaping a demand, getting access to a tangible item or activity, and automatic reinforcement; Frea and Hepburn 1999). When that need is identified through the FBA processes, an adaptive, alternative means of satisfying the need can be taught. By teaching a functionally equivalent alternative response, the challenging behavior can be reduced (Horner and Carr 1997). The primary purpose of the FBA process is to develop an effective behavior support plan that directly addresses the operant function of an individual's challenging behavior. FBA has long been recognized as a vital component in designing interventions to change behavior (Carr 1977; Frea and Hepburn 1999; Iwata et al. 1982/1994). Moreover, function-based interventions and supports designed based on FBA information are the most effective method for supporting children who exhibit challenging behaviors (Carr et al. 1999; Didden et al. 1997; Heckaman et al. 2000). Intervention strategies that are not derived from FBA findings are less effective at decreasing challenging behavior and may inadvertently reinforce the target behavior, resulting in an increase in challenging behavior (Ingram et al. 2005; Newcomer and Lewis 2004).

There are two distinct types of the FBA process, the indirect and direct process. Both processes include an assessment and development of a plan. The direct FBA process is a comprehensive assessment process that is appropriate when the target behavior is severe in duration, frequency, and intensity (Gresham et al. 2001). The process is also appropriate when critical decisions are being made with regard to verifying a disability, making placement decisions, or choosing intervention methods that are intensive or intrusive. The term *functional analysis* was used by

Skinner (1953) to denote empirical demonstrations of "cause-and-effect relations" between environment and behavior; however, behavior analysts have extended the term to describe procedures and operations (Hanley et al. 2003). Direct FBA uses rating scales, interviews and other documented information, direct observation of the behavior, and an experimental design (e.g., functional analysis [FA; Iwata et al. 1982/1994] or structured descriptive assessment [SDA; Freeman et al. 2000]). Experimental functional analysis (i.e., FA, brief FA) involves manipulation of one or more environmental variables (specific establishing operations, discriminative stimuli, and programmed contingencies) under test and control conditions meant to serve as analogues to social situations in natural settings. Traditional social conditions usually include a control play condition and test conditions that manipulate attention, tangibles (materials or food), and task demands (i.e., escape). However, conditions can be designed to capture relevant, idiosyncratic establishing operations, discriminative stimuli, and consequences thought to maintain challenging behavior. FA conditions are typically conducted in a systematic fashion using a single-subject research design (e.g., reversal, multi-element, or pairwise design) and therefore allow for comparison of rates of challenging behavior across conditions and thus experimental demonstration of a causal relation between environmental events and challenging behavior (Anderson et al. 2006). A large body of literature exists documenting the utility of this experimental approach to assessing challenging behavior of individuals with developmental disabilities including ASD (e.g., Hagopian et al. 2013). Making a strong statement regarding behavioral function is the strength of experimental functional analysis, but there are limitations regarding the amount of time, resources, and expertise required to conduct a valid FA (Scott et al. 2000).

The indirect FBA is a shortened version of the assessment and is most appropriate when the behavior is less serious and/or occurs infrequently, and when only a small group of individuals are involved (i.e., parent and child; Gresham et al. 2001). Indirect FBA consists of verbal or written interviews or rating forms completed by stakeholders (e.g., teachers, family, parents, and child) to identify the target challenging behavior(s), circumstances that prevent the challenging behavior(s) and promote positive appropriate behaviors, and the possible function(s) of the behavior. For instance, Functional Assessment Interview (FAI; O'Neill et al. 1997) or Questions About Behavioral Function (QABF; Paclawskyj et al. 2000) are both questionnaires used to gather information to develop a hypothesis about the function of the behavior. Importantly, results obtained using the QABF have been shown to reliably identify the function of challenging behavior identified by an experimental FA (e.g., Healy et al. 2013; Paclawskyj et al. 2001; Watkins and Rapp 2013); these findings suggest that in some cases the QABF may serve as an efficient substitute for conducting a more time intensive experimental FA. Direct observation should be used to confirm the information obtained from the indirect assessment procedures. Descriptive assessments typically are conducted in the natural environment, and environmental variables are not manipulated (Anderson et al. 2006). Instead, descriptive assessments involve recording instances of the target behavior and environmental events that precede or follow the behavior. The most common method of descriptive assessment is Antecedent–Behavior–Consequence (A–B–C) recording (Bijou et al. 1968). In using this procedure, the child's behavior is observed in the relevant setting and the events occurring immediately prior to and following the behavior are recorded. The A–B–C procedure can lead to a determination of the plausible function of behavior. Based on this information, a hypothesis is developed and a written plan can be formulated. Follow-up interviews and other data are used to determine the success of the intervention or if a direct FBA needs to occur. A strength of the indirect FBA method is it provides a practical way to develop a hypothesis related to function and design interventions in a natural setting, but direct observation in the natural environment can be a limitation. Natural environments can be complex where children can engage in a variety of competing behaviors or demonstrate low frequencies of target behaviors, both may limit the clear determination of behavioral function.

A complete discussion of FBA methods and the creation of an individualized, function-based behavior intervention plan is beyond the scope of this chapter. However, a number of exceptional resources exist for further coverage of this essential topic (e.g., Bambera and Kern 2005; Crone and Horner 2003; Knoster and McCurdy 2002; Lucyshyn et al. 2002; Sigafoos et al. 2003). The remainder of this chapter seeks to familiarize the reader with the most commonly used evidence-based strategies to prevent and decrease challenging behavior in individuals with ASD.

Behavioral Intervention

The primary aim of conducting a comprehensive functional behavior assessment is to identify the antecedent stimuli (i.e., motivating operations (MO) and discriminative stimuli for reinforcement) that commonly precede challenging behavior, the most common times and places for the challenging behavior to occur, and the operant function(s) of a challenging behavior so that an appropriate, effective treatment can be implemented. Challenging behavior can be (a) positively reinforced (i.e., the delivery of adult or peer attention, a preferred tangible, or access to sensory stimulation following instances of challenging behavior that results in future increased challenging behavior) or (b) negatively reinforced (i.e., removal of adult or peer attention, removal or limited access to a preferred tangible, or the removal of aversive stimuli following instances of challenging behavior that result in future increased challenging behavior). In the case of children with ID and ASD, FBA research findings suggest that challenging behaviors are often maintained by escape from aversive events, access to attention, or the retention of preferred tangible items (e.g., Reese et al. 2005). Effective behavior support plans (BSPs) include function-based interventions that serve to match the same consequence(s) that maintains the individual's challenging behavior. In this section, we introduce evidence-based interventions by the operant function thought to maintain the challenging behavior.

Interventions for Challenging Behavior Maintained by Social Positive Reinforcement

Research has investigated various interventions (e.g., functional communication training (FCT), noncontingent reinforcement (NCR), and differential reinforcement of other behavior (DRO)) and a combination of intervention strategies that can be used to address challenging behavior maintained by positive reinforcement (i.e., positive social reinforcement) in individuals with autism.

Antecedent Interventions Antecedent manipulation strategies have been evaluated in the research and found to be an effective intervention for reducing challenging behavior maintained by positive reinforcement. Several studies have evaluated the use of antecedent interventions with attention to MO to increase the effectiveness of behavior interventions (e.g., Call and Lomas Mevers 2014; Rispoli et al. 2011b; O'Reilly et al. 2008). Rispoli and colleagues (2011a) evaluated the use of presession noncontingent access to tangibles (i.e., antecedent manipulation) on problem behavior in a school setting. This study reported a decrease in challenging behavior and increases in academic engagement in conditions with presession access to tangibles. Research has also investigated antecedent communication interventions for tangibly maintained behavior. O'Reilly and colleagues (2012) compared conditions with and without antecedent communication intervention and found greater decreases in challenging behavior in conditions with the antecedent intervention. Both studies suggest that presession access to tangibles can act as an abolishing operation (AO). Although antecedent strategies can be successful in decreasing challenging behavior they may be more successful when combined with consequence strategies, thus further research would be beneficial.

Noncontingent Reinforcement (NCR) Another commonly used intervention to address challenging behavior maintained by positive reinforcement is noncontingent reinforcement (NCR; Carr et al. 2009). This approach involves providing reinforcement on a frequent fixed time reinforcement schedule, regardless of an individual's behavior (i.e., response-independent basis). One benefit of NCR is that it addresses the response–reinforcement relationship. For example, attention can easily be provided prior to the onset of challenging behavior, which essentially makes engaging in the challenging behavior unnecessary (e.g., Sigafoos and Tucker 2000).

The use of NCR as a treatment for challenging behavior dates back to the late 1970s when Boe (1977) used a variable schedule of food reinforcers to decrease aggression. Over time it has transformed into a commonly used intervention that is often combined with other treatments to more effectively decrease challenging behavior in individuals with autism. For example, Marcus and Vollmer (1996) used a reversal design to compare treatment effects using NCR, DRO, and differential reinforcement of an alternative behavior (DRA; i.e., mands). These findings indicate that the use of NCR did not impede the participant's motivation to mand.

Recently, studies have investigated the use of signals (i.e., use of a timer) and schedule density of NCR in the treatment of tangibly maintained aggression (e.g.,

Ringdahl et al. 2010). The results of this study suggest that the use of signaled NCR schedules had greater reduction in challenging behavior than conditions without the signaled NCR. Although NCR is reported as an effective approach for the treatment of challenging behavior, there are a few limitations that should be considered. First, there is potential for inadvertent reinforcement of the challenging behavior if it occurs at the end of an interval. Research has investigated the use a variation of NCR which incorporates the use of a stimulus delay procedure to address this limitation. For example, Britton et al. (2000) evaluated reinforcer delivery rates by comparing the effects of an NCR with a stimulus-delay procedure and DRO. Findings of this study indicated that participants accessed more reinforcement with NCR than DRO. These findings also suggest that the mechanisms responsible for the decrease in challenging behavior were satiation and extinction. Similarly, results reported by Hagopian and colleagues (2000) suggested that the initial reduction in challenging behavior was correlated to the use of NCR; however, the findings also suggested that the use of extinction is a necessary component to thinning schedules. Based on the findings discussed above there are several proposed benefits of NCR, (a) lower possibility of extinction-induced responding, (b) potential increased rate of reinforcer delivery, and (c) ease of implementation (Britton et al. 2000). Although combining NCR with extinction may be necessary, more research is needed to assess the effects of NCR variations.

Functional Communication Training (FCT) One of the most commonly used and most effective approaches to decrease challenging behavior maintained by positive social reinforcement is functional communication training (FCT; Carr and Durand 1985; Casey and Merical 2006; Durand 1999; Durand and Carr 1991; Fisher et al. 1993; Schmidt et al. 2014). FCT utilizes DRA to increase an appropriate communication behavior to replace and decrease challenging behavior. Emission of the appropriate, socially valid communication response by the individual is reinforced with the reinforcer that previously maintained the target challenging behavior. Successful FCT intervention considers the following variables in selection of the alternative communication response (a) the newly trained communication response must result in the *same* maintaining consequence as the target challenging behavior; (b) the alternative communication response must require less physical effort than the challenging behavior, result in the same or increased quantity and quality of reinforcement, and (c) the alternative communication response must be recognized by stakeholders and socially acceptable (Durand and Merges 2001). In addition, FCT often requires the use of extinction (Braithwaite and Richdale 2000; Jarmolowicz et al. 2009) or other decelerative procedures (Durand and Carr 1992; Fisher et al. 2000) to decrease challenging behavior.

For individuals with tangibly maintained challenging behavior FCT typically includes an extinction component, which has the potential to incite extinction induced challenging behavior. Davis and colleagues (2009) investigated this issue by comparing presession exposure and nonexposure during FCT training. The results of this study showed lower rates of challenging behavior and higher rates of independent communication during FCT sessions that followed 15 min of continuous toy access. Although these findings are preliminary, it warrants further investigation to evaluate antecedent combinations for FCT interventions.

Other treatment combinations of FCT include chained schedules of reinforcement to treat challenging behavior maintained by activity interruptions (e.g., Falcomata et al. 2012a). Research has also evaluated response preference within an FCT intervention (e.g., Danov et al. 2010). Findings indicate that preference of response modality during FCT training should be assessed when considering the topography of targeted communication response.

Research continues to explore factors related to the effectiveness of FCT interventions (for a review see Hagopian et al. 2011). The current body of work indicates this intervention can yield effective results for the reduction of challenging behavior (Tiger and Hanley 2008); however, issues related to training duration and thinning of reinforcement can warrant the use of combining other differential reinforcement strategies for more effective results (Betz et al. 2013).

Differential Reinforcement of other Behavior (DRO) Differential reinforcement of other behavior (DRO) involves contingent reinforcement for the absence of challenging behavior during a specific time. Some limitations associated with the use of DRO include the continuous monitoring that is required of this intervention, low rates of reinforcement, and undesirable extinction-induced effects (e.g., aggression). Procedural variations of DRO (i.e., fixed, variable, or momentary) have been investigated to address these limitations. Hammond et al. (2011) evaluated the use of signals verses unsignaled fixed momentary (FM) DRO for problem behavior maintained by access to tangible. Specifically, this study aimed to evaluate the potential benefit of unsignaled reinforcer delivery that is often associated to the benefits of using a momentary DRO. These findings were consistent with other research in that FM DRO can be an effective treatment for decreasing problem behavior. However, the authors also reported that signals correlated with interval termination might have aversive effects because they facilitate discrimination of the momentary contingency. DRO is more commonly used in combination with other interventions to reduce challenging behavior. For example, Matson et al. (2008) used a treatment package, which included DRO, compliance training, extinction, and functional communication to decrease aggressive behaviors in an 11-year-old girl with autism.

Research in the treatment of challenging behavior maintained by positive reinforcement in individuals with autism continues to evaluate effective methods for treatment. The most commonly used interventions discussed by the literature involve the use of FCT and NCR. Although research indicates these interventions can be effective in treating challenging behavior maintained by positive reinforcement, there is a need for further evaluation of the various dimensions of reinforcement, such as reinforcement schedules, quality, and delay to reinforcement.

Challenging Behavior Maintained by Social Negative Reinforcement

For some individuals with autism, challenging behavior may be maintained by negative reinforcement (i.e., negative social reinforcement). This type of behavior is commonly seen in a demand-related situation where an individual engages in challenging behavior in order to escape aversive stimuli. If the aversive demand being removed increases the likelihood of the challenging behavior to occur under similar conditions in the future, the challenging behavior is negatively reinforced (i.e., escape maintained). Research has discussed a number of effective interventions that result in a decrease in challenging behavior that is negatively reinforced.

Antecedent Interventions Antecedent based strategies have been used, often in combination with other interventions, to decrease challenging behavior maintained by negative reinforcement. Antecedent strategies rely on altering common antecedents that occur just before challenging behavior and temporarily make it less likely that the individual will engage in challenging behavior. Common antecedents that may occasion challenging behavior include prompts (e.g., the teacher asks the child to write their name), a change in the setting (e.g., preferred toy is temporarily not available or broken), the difficulty of the task at hand, or the presence (or absence) of a favorite toy, activity, or person. For example, studies have investigated the effects on challenging behavior maintained by escape by providing choices of activity (e.g., DeLeon et al. 2001; Rispoli et al. 2013). Rispoli and colleagues (2013) evaluated the use of within and across-activity choices for reducing challenging behavior maintained by escape. Results of this study highlight the potential benefits of providing frequent choice making as an intervention for challenging behavior and the importance of interventions that can motivate individuals with ASD to engage in academics or other non-preferred tasks. Further, the authors reported across-activity choices were more effective in reducing challenging behavior, but also notes that within-activity choices can still be beneficial in regard to motivation. Other research has investigated the use of noncontingent reinforcement as an AO (e.g., Ingvarsson et al. 2008; Lomas et al. 2010) that temporarily decreased the rate of challenging behavior and the value of the reinforcer. Lomas and colleagues (2010) reported that the use of a variable-time delivery of noncontingent food and praise (i.e., antecedent manipulation) was effective in the reduction of challenging behavior and increases in compliance behavior. The studies highlighted in this section suggest that positive reinforcement, as an antecedent intervention, may be a valuable method for reduction of challenging behavior. However, it is important to note that the effects of MO are transient, thus using antecedent interventions to decrease challenging behavior may be more effective when combined with other procedures (Smith and Iwata 1997).

Functional Communication Training (FCT) Functional Communication Training (FCT) has been used to treat challenging behavior maintained by negative reinforcement or escape. FCT, when addressing negatively reinforced behavior, involves training an individual to request the removal of the aversive stimulus. For example, an individual may be taught to temporarily lessen the aversiveness of the task at hand by requesting a break or help or using a break or help symbol to replace their challenging behavior. Several studies within the research on FCT involve teaching individuals to request for escape (e.g., Casey and Merical 2006; DeLeon et al. 2001; Falcomata et al. 2013, 2012; Fisher et al. 2005; Hagopian et al. 2001; Neidert et al. 2005). FCT has also been used to teach appropriate responses to terminate nonpreferred items (e.g., Yi et al. 2006; Martin et al. 2005).

Aside from the value of increasing communication skills, there are additional benefits to the use of FCT as an intervention for negatively reinforced behavior. For example, FCT has been reported to be effective when conducted in natural environments. Casey and Merical (2006) found that FCT alone decreased challenging behavior maintained by escape from demands in a school setting. FCT has also been effective when conducted by parents at home. Wacker and colleagues (2013) evaluated FCT conducted by 17 parents of children with autism as an intervention for challenging behavior. The majority of FCT interventions used in this study targeted escape maintained behavior (i.e., 13 children treated for escape, 5 for tangible, and 2 for multiple functions). Behavior consultants used video conferencing and/or telephone to provide parent training. The average reduction in challenging behavior was reported at 90% reduction for the majority of children. Additionally, parents rated the acceptability of treatment procedures at 6.47 out of 7, indicating a high level of acceptability.

Although FCT has been reported to be an effective reductive treatment for challenging behaviors, it is not without limitations. For example, there is potential for the individual to overuse the mand (Fisher et al. 1993), natural situations require a thinner reinforcement schedule, and as such there is limited effectiveness in natural settings with parents and teachers (Fisher et al. 2000). However, despite these limitations, FCT provides the individual with an appropriate way for the individual with ASD to gain reinforcement for appropriate adaptive behavior, which is an important aspect of any behavioral reduction intervention. Several strategies for overcoming these limitations have been examined including signaling the availability of reinforcement to assist with stimulus control (e.g., Betz et al. 2013; Ringdahl et al. 2010; Rispoli et al. 2014) and using a multiple schedule of reinforcement to systematically fade reinforcement following FCT training (Hanley, Iwata and Thompson 2001).

Combined Treatments Differential reinforcement of alternative behavior (DRA) has also been evaluated in the research as an intervention for challenging behavior maintained by negative reinforcement (sometimes called differential negative reinforcement of alternative behavior or DNRA). This type of intervention is used to reduce challenging behavior maintained by escape such as escape from a task or demand. DRA is often paired with other procedures such as escape extinction and/or demand fading. For example, Piazza et al. (1996) investigated the use of DRA with escape extinction and demand fading to decrease escape maintained problem behavior and reported a decrease in challenging behavior to near-zero levels.

Other research has investigated the use of DRA with and without demand fading procedures and found greater decreases in challenging behavior with the use of demand fading (e.g., Ringdahl et al. 2002). Additionally, research has investigated the effects of fixed-time and contingent reinforcement schedules with DNRA treatment packages. Reed et al. (2005) reported lower rates of challenging and higher rates of desirable behavior were observed in conditions when fixed-time was lean and when fixed-time schedules were dense low rates of both types of behavior were reported. Research has further investigated the use of DRA without extinction and found that behavior was more sensitive to manipulations in dimensions of reinforcement, such as density, quality, and delay (Athens and Vollmer 2010). These findings suggest some support for the use of DRA without the need for extinction procedures. Although using DRA can be effective to reduce challenging behavior, further research is needed to investigate the effects of this intervention with and without the combination of other reductive strategies.

DRO is often combined with other treatments when creating interventions to decrease challenging behavior maintained by negative reinforcement. For example, Call et al. (2011) reported that the use of DRO alone was not effective in the treatment of elopement when compared to DRO with response blocking. Similarly, Waters et al. (2009) found more effective results with using DRO with extinction, which indicates further support for combined approaches.

Another intervention discussed in current research is noncontingent escape (NCE), which is a variation of NCR where the aversive stimulus is removed. A limited number of studies have evaluated the effects of NCE on decreases in challenging behavior and reported favorable outcomes (e.g., Butler and Luiselli 2007; Kodak et al. 2003). NCE has been compared with differential negative reinforcement of other behavior (DNRO), where escape from the aversive stimulus is made contingent upon the absence of challenging behavior. Kodak and colleagues (2003) found both methods decreased challenging behavior and increased compliance. However, because the authors report it is unclear what behavioral mechanism led to increases in compliance, further research is needed to investigate the effects of NCE and DNRO on increases in compliance.

NCE has also been combined with other procedures, such as demand fading (e.g., Butler and Luiselli 2007). This approach involves using a fixed time schedule for escape with gradual increases in the amount of session time as challenging behavior decreases. NCE has also been compared to noncontingent tangible reinforcement (NCT) as a treatment for multiply-controlled challenging behavior (i.e., escape and tangible; Rispoli et al. 2013). In this study authors reported greater reduction in challenging behavior during NCT, however, an increase in compliance occurred under both NCT and NCE. Research should continue to investigate NCE in comparison to other types of differential reinforcement to further explore potential benefits and limitations for the treatment of challenging behavior.

Escape extinction has been used in several studies as a treatment component for decreasing challenging behavior maintained by negative reinforcement. Escape extinction involves preventing an individual from gaining escape as a consequence for their challenging behavior and is often used in combination with other types of differential reinforcement such as DRA (e.g., Athens and Vollmer 2010; Piazza et al. 1996; Najdowski et al. 2003), DRO (e.g., Pabico et al. 2011; Progar et al. 2001; Matson et al. 2008; Waters et al. 2009) or Differential Reinforcement of Incompatible Behavior (DRI) (e.g., Ricciardi 2003). Although escape extinction can be an effective approach for treatment of challenging behavior maintained by negative reinforcement, there are some ethical considerations that should be considered prior to the use of this intervention. The level of intensity of the challenging behavior should be assessed prior to using escape extinction as an intervention for challenging behavior. For example, if the challenging behavior has potential of causing harm to the individual or therapist by prompting the continuation of the aversive stimuli, the use of escape extinction may not be feasible without protective equipment and thus other differential reinforcement may be more practical for some situations (e.g., Athens and Vollmer 2010).

Interventions for Challenging Behavior Maintained by Automatic Reinforcement Although repetitive, stereotypic movements including self-injury have been shown to serve both social and nonsocial positive and negative reinforcement functions (Cunningham and Schreibman 2008; Hutt and Hutt 1965; Rispoli et al. 2014; Zentall and Zentall 1983), they are commonly thought to be maintained through nonsocial consequences; that is they are often automatically reinforced (Rapp and Vollmer 2005; Vollmer 1994). Nonetheless, this particular subset of challenging behavior can be difficult to treat due to the inherent difficulty in identifying the idiosyncratic variables maintaining the challenging behavior. Few interventions exist and those that do often lack inclusion of a FBA. Treatments regarding both lower and higher order RRBIs can be described by two different overarching categories: (a) antecedent-based interventions that involve manipulating the environment to reduce the likelihood of the challenging behavior and (b) consequence-based interventions. Further, some multicomponent interventions combine both antecedent and consequence-based interventions.

Antecedent-based interventions for lower-order RRBs include strategies such as: (a) environmental enrichment strategies including noncontingent access to competing sources of reinforcement (NCR), (b) visual or verbal cues to foreworn an individual of a change in activity (stimulus control procedures as in Conroy et al. 2005b), (c) physical exercise (Prupas and Redi 2001), and (d) skills enrichment strategies aimed to teach adaptive alternative behaviors to decrease the need for the restricted and repetitive behaviors (Boyd et al. 2012; Patterson et al. 2010).

Environmental enrichment (EE) has a large literature base providing evidence of its effectiveness to decrease automatically maintained stereotypy (Piazza et al. 2000; Rapp et al. 2004; Vollmer et al. 1994; Sigafoos et al. 1997, 2009; Sigafoos and Kerr 1994). EE involves providing access to stimuli (usually preferred and/or competing stimuli identified through systematic preference assessments (Fisher et al. 1992) and conducting a competing items assessment (Groskreutz et al. 2011) in order to increase the availability of alternative sources of reinforcement (Rapp and Vollmer 2005). However, research evaluating EE as a treatment for stereotypy suggests the potential for less than positive outcomes. For instance, previous research has demonstrated that for some individuals, EE may actually lead to an increase in stereotypy. Rapp (2004) found that a young boy with Down syndrome engaged in higher levels of stereotypy in the presence of music, the EE treatment. Van Camp and colleagues (2000) identified components of stimuli that occasioned challenging behavior for two young children. Both participants engaged in challenging behavior in the presence of specific stimuli (toys, attention) in the absence of programmed social consequences for challenging behavior during alone conditions of a FA where access to preferred items varied. Results revealed higher levels of challenging behavior in the presence of tangible items. These results suggest that specific stimuli may have functioned as establishing operations (EOs) by increasing the value of automatic reinforcement. In each of these studies, idiosyncratic stimuli may have served as an EO for stereotypy by temporarily increasing the reinforcing value of automatically maintained behavior and thus the frequency of stereotypy.

Rapp (2007) reported that NCR for vocal stereotypy that incorporated matched sensory stimulation (i.e., audio stimulation from toys) was effective in reducing repetitive language. However, Patterson and colleagues (2010) pointed out that NCR used alone was found to be ineffective in significantly reducing restricted and repetitive behaviors; however, in combination with consequence-based strategies (e.g., response interruption) it was found to be effective, although not more effective than response interruption alone. Overall, the literature base for treatment for lower-order RRBs suggests that antecedent strategies produce greater treatment effects when used in combination with consequence-based strategies (Boyd et al. 2012; Hall et al. 2003; Patterson et al. 2010).

Consequence-based interventions that have been studied for lower-order restricted and repetitive behaviors include (a) response interruption and redirection (RIRD)/response blocking involving physically or verbally blocking the repetitive behavior, (b) DRO, (c) response cost procedures involve removing a desirable item or activity contingent upon the challenging behavior, and (d) extinction (Boyd et al. 2012; Rincover et al. 1979). Although interruption of a repetitive behavior is often effective in reducing the behavior, the use of physical or mechanical interruption alone often occasions other more serious forms of challenging behavior such as aggression (Hagopian and Adelinis 2001; Hagopian et al. 2007; Kuhn et al. 2009; Murphy et al. 2000).

In addition, FCT has been used as a multicomponent intervention that involves teaching a socially appropriate alternative behavior used by the individual to access the same reinforcer as the restricted and repetitive behavior, while simultaneously removing reinforcements for the challenging behavior (i.e., extinction; Boyd et al. 2012). Although interventions such as FCT have been considered less likely to be successful in achieving a positive outcome for nonsocially mediated challenging behavior (see Vollmer 1994, for a review), a growing number of studies suggest that FCT may be an effective intervention for this topography of behavior (e.g., Hanley et al. 2001; Hagopian et al. 2011; Kuhn et al. 2009; Rispoli et al. 2014).

Treatment for higher-order RRBs (e.g., perseverative interests, resistance and insistence on sameness) include antecedent-based interventions such as embedding the perseverative interest into the task which is hypothesized to increase the individual's motivation to complete the task and consequence-based strategies that involve delivering the perseverative interest (e.g., item and activity) contingent on the occurrence of appropriate behavior (Boyd et al. 2012). For example, Carnett et al. (2014) implemented a perseverative interest-based token (i.e., foam puzzle pieces) within a token economy intervention and found that the perseverative interest-based token reduced escaped-maintained challenging behavior to lower levels when compared to a regular token (i.e., a penny) during an elementary literacy activity for a boy with autism. In addition, antecedent events may be altered to minimize the impact of establishing operations that temporarily increase the value of the reinforcers (escape from interruption/access to sensory stimulation) and make challenging behavior more likely. For example, a child may compulsively tear pages out of magazines. When interrupted (e.g., child is asked to put the magazine down), the child may engage in challenging behavior (e.g., screaming and hitting) to obtain access to the magazine so that they may resume tearing pages from the magazine. Antecedent events that may make it temporarily more likely that the child engages in this challenging behavior may include non-preferred or frustrating interactions (e.g., a difficult school schedule on Mondays), a relatively long time having passed without access to the RRBI, or the absence of desired social interaction (e.g., adult is reading a magazine and not paying attention to child). By modifying antecedent events, this type of intervention works by lessening the chance that the child will need to engage in challenging behavior. For instance, a child might engage in challenging behavior when a restricted and repetitive behavior (e.g., lining up markers, rather than drawing) is interrupted. As an intervention, the child may be allowed to first engage in lining up markers, but will be provided with an auditory and visual warning that they should get ready to stop lining up markers so that they can draw. This warning may help prevent the child from being surprised by the change in activity and give them time to get used to the idea of doing something less preferred. Alternatively, a moderately preferred activity might be inserted between the problematic situation and the non-preferred activity (drawing, rather than lining up markers).

Future Research

A variety of focused behavioral intervention strategies are effective in eliminating or reducing problem behavior maintained by social and nonsocial positive and negative reinforcement in individuals with ASD. Research continues to explore the dimensions of differential reinforcement and various treatment combinations in order to find more effective ways to treat the challenging behavior common to individuals with ASD and to sustain positive outcomes. The current literature suggests several avenues for future research to inform clinical practice and research.

Future research should develop and evaluate focused, individualized interventions to treat restricted and repetitive behavior as this is lacking in the literature (Boyd et al. 2012) and should continue to investigate whether and in what cases restricted and repetitive behavior should be minimized in individuals with ASD or used as a strengths-based component to an intervention (Paula-Perez 2013). Additionally, ways for parents and practitioners to differentiate between restricted and repetitive behavior and obsessions and compulsions, as are present in OCD, would help better inform treatment decisions.

Additionally, future research is warranted to identify additional practices for assessing and treating challenging behavior exhibited by individuals with ASD who have comorbid diagnoses such as OCD, AD/HD, anxiety, or depression. For instance, intervention research addressing challenging behavior associated with comorbid ASD/OCD is relatively limited (Boyd et al. 2012; Lehmkuhl et al. 2008; Russell et al. 2013). The most common treatments available are pharmaceutical therapy (e.g., selective serotonin reuptake inhibitors) and cognitive behavior therapy (CBT) including exposure and response prevention (Boyd et al. 2012; Lehmkuhl et al. 2008; Paula-Perez 2013). CBT is a promising therapy for young people and adults with comorbid ASD/OCD that has been shown to have significant effects on obsessions (Russell et al. 2009; Vasa et al. 2014). Further, in a recent randomized control trial both a modified CBT and anxiety management therapy produced significant reductions in OCD symptoms for young people and adult with comorbid ASD/OCD (Russell et al. 2013). CBT particularly shows promise for those with high functioning ASD (Van Steelsel et al. 2011). The effectiveness of these treatments by themselves or in conjunction with behavioral intervention for restricted and repetitive behavior should be examined.

Relatedly, there are effective behavioral and pharmaceutical treatments that may provide relief to those with both depression and ASD. Such treatments include antidepressants used to treat a variety of symptoms (e.g., depressed mood, sleep disturbance, self-injurious behavior, psychomotor agitation, weight loss, reduced communication, tearfulness, and loss of interest) with generally positive results (Perry et al. 2001). Overall, research demonstrates that the most common treatment for a comorbid case of depression was medication. Pharmacological therapy includes antidepressants such as tricyclics and selective serotonin reuptake inhibitors (SSRIs), mood stabilizers, antipsychotics, and hypnotics (Stewart et al. 2006). There is no question that continued research related to comorbidity of depression and ASD is critical to reducing the frequency, occurrence, and intensity of challenging behavior. Future studies, should seek to dissect the mechanisms of the comorbidity in relation to environmental versus genetic factors related to the expression and occurrence of depressive symptoms (Ghaziuddin et al. 2002). Also, there is a need for more studies to investigate the relationship between one's level of social skills or intellectual functioning in relation to depressive symptoms in adults with ASD (Sterling et al. 2008). As with any comorbid condition, continued development and nuances of tools for the assessment and measurement of depression for those with ASD is critical (Stewart et al. 2006). Finally, the most crucial area of future research should investigate appropriate treatment options for those with ASD, depression, and challenging behavior by means of comparing evidenced-based interventions for neurotypical individuals with depression and discovering appropriate adaptations, if any, needed to support and improved the quality of life of these individuals.

Furthermore, some research demonstrates that having better social skills or being of adolescent age was a specific factor associated with the presence of depressive symptoms in individuals with ASD (Sterling et al. 2008) while other research notes no correlation of either IQ or age (Strand et al. 2012). Still, treatment could include instruction in specific social skills and the development of higher-level social navigation strategies. Likewise, suicide prevention may help reduce symptom significance and population mortality rates. Professionals should recognize that individuals with ASD suffering from depression and related difficulties might have thoughts related to suicide and intentionally harm themselves (Sterling et al. 2008). Therefore, mental health and medical professionals should work treatment options similar to neurotypical individuals with depression into an overall treatment plan for an individual who presents with depression, ASD, and challenging behavior.

References

Aman, M. G., Arnold, E., McDougle, C. J., et al. (2005). Acute and long-term safety and tolerability of risperidone in children with autism. *Journal of Child and Adolescent Psychopharmacology, 15,* 869–884.

American Psychiatric Association. (2013). *Diagnostic and statistical manual of mental disorders* (5th ed.). Arlington: American Psychiatric Publishing.

Anderson, C. M., Freeman, K. A., & Scotti, J. R. (1999). Evaluation of the generalizability (reliability and validity) of analog functional assessment methodology. *Behavior Therapy, 30*(1), 31–50.

Anderson, C. M., English, C. L., & Hedrick, T. M. (2006). Use of the structured descriptive assessment with typically developing children. *Behavior Modification, 30*(3), 352–378.

Athens, E. S., & Vollmer, T. R. (2010). An investigation of differential reinforcement of alternative behavior without extinction. *Journal of Applied Behavior Analysis, 43*(4), 569–589.

Baghdadli, A., Pascal, C., Grisli, S., & Aussilloux, C. (2003). Risk factors for self-injurious behaviours among 222 young children with autistic disorders. *Journal of Intellectual Disabilities Research, 47*(8), 622–627.

Baker, B. L., Blacher, J., Crnic, K. A., & Edelbrock, C. (2002). Behavior problems and parenting stress in families of three-year-old children with and without developmental delays. *Journal Information, 107*(6).

Bambera, L., & Kern, L. (2005). *Individualized supports for students with problem behaviors.* New York: The Guilford Press.

Benson, B. A., & Brooks, W. T. (2008). Aggressive challenging behaviour and intellectual disability. *Current Opinion in Psychiatry, 21,* 454–458.

Berney, T. (2004). Autism—An evolving concept. *British Journal of Psychiatry, 176*(2004), 20–25.

Bernheimer, L. P., Gallimore, R., & Weisner, T. S. (1990). Ecocultural theory as a context for the individual family service plan. *Journal of Early Intervention, 14*(3), 219–233.

Betz, A. M., Fisher, W. W., Roane, H. S., Mintz, J. C., & Owen, T. M. (2013). A component analysis of schedule thinning during functional communication training. *Journal of Applied Behavior Analysis, 46,* 219–241.

Bijou, S. W., Peterson, R. F., & Ault, M. H. (1968). A method to integrate descriptive and experimental field studies at the level of data and empirical concepts. *Journal of Applied Behavior Analysis, 1*(2), 175.

Boe, R. B. (1977). Economical procedures for the reduction of aggression in residential setting. *Mental Retardation, 15,* 25–28.

Boyd, B., McDonough, S. G., & Bodfish, J. W. (2012). Evidence-based behavioral interventions for repetitive behaviors in autism. *Journal of Developmental Disorders, 42,* 1236–1248.

Braithwaite, K. L., & Richdale, A. L. (2000). Functional communication training to replace challenging behaviors across two behavioral outcomes. *Behavioral Interventions, 15*(1), 21–36.

Britton, L. N., Carr, J. E., Kellum, K. K., Dozier, C. L., & Weil, T. M. (2000). A variation of noncontingent reinforcement in the treatment of aberrant behavior. *Research in Developmental Disabilities, 21*(6), 425–435.

Butler, L. R., & Luiselli, J. K. (2007). Escape-maintained problem behavior in a child with autism antecedent functional analysis and intervention evaluation of noncontingent escape and instructional fading. *Journal of Positive Behavior Interventions, 9*(4), 195–202.

Call, N. A., & Lomas Mevers, J. E. (2014). The relative influence of motivating operations for positive and negative reinforcement on problem behavior during demands. *Behavioral Interventions, 29,* 4–20.

Call, N. A., Pabico, R. S., Findley, A. J., & Valentino, A. L. (2011). Differential reinforcement with and without blocking as treatment for elopement. *Journal of Applied Behavior Analysis, 44*(4), 903–907.

Campbell, S. B., Shaw, D. S., & Gilliom, M. (2000). Early externalizing behavior problems:Toddlers and preschoolers at risk for later maladjustment. *Development and Psychopathology, 12*(03), 467–488.

Carnett, A., Raulston, T., Lang, R., Tostanoski, A., Lee, A., Sigafoos, J., et al. (online-2014). Effects of a perseverative interest-based token economy on challenging and on-task behavior in a child with autism. *Journal of Behavioral Education, 23*(3), 368–377.

Carr, E. G. (1977). The motivation of self-injurious behavior: A review of some hypotheses. *Psychological Bulletin, 84,* 800–816.

Carr, E. G., & Durand, V. M. (1985). Reducing behavior problems through functional communication training. *Journal of Applied Behavior Analysis, 18,* 111–126.

Carr, E. G., Langdon, N. A., & Yarbrough, S. C. (1999). Hypothesis-based intervention for severe problem behavior. In A. C. Repp & R. H. Horner (Eds.), *Functional analysis of problem behavior: From effective assessment to effective support* (pp. 9–31). Belmont: Wadsworth.

Carr, J. E., Severtson, J. M., & Lepper, T. L. (2009). Noncontingent reinforcement is an empirically supported treatment for problem behavior exhibited by individuals with developmental disabilities. *Research in Developmental Disabilities, 30,* 44–57.

Casey, S. D., & Merical, C. L. (2006). The use of functional communication training without additional treatment procedures in an inclusive school setting. *Behavioral Disorders, 32*(1), 46–54.

Conroy, M. A., Dunlap, G., Clarke, S., & Alter, P. J. (2005a). A descriptive analysis of positive behavioral intervention research with young children with challenging behavior. *Topics in Early Childhood Special Education, 25*(3), 157–166.

Conroy, M. A., Asmus, J. M., & Sellers, J. A. (2005b). The use of an antecedent based intervention to decrease stereotypic behavior in a general education classroom: A case study. *Focus on Autism and Developmental Disorders, 20*(4), 223–230.

Crnic, K. A., & Greenberg, M. T. (1990). Minor parenting stresses with young children. *Child Development, 61*(5), 1628–1637.

Crone, D. A., & Horner, R. H. (2003). *Building positive behavior support systems in schools: Functional behavioral assessment.* New York: Guilford Press.

Cunningham, A., & Schreibman, L. (2008). Stereotypy in autism: The importance of function. *Research in Autism Spectrum Disorders, 2,* 469–479.

Danov, S. E., Hartman, E., McComas, J. J., & Symons, F. J. (2010). Evaluation of two communicative response modalities for a child with autism and self-injury. *Journal of Speech-Language Pathology & Applied Behavior Analysis, 5*(1), 70–79.

Davis, N. O., & Carter, A. S. (2008). Parenting stress in mothers and fathers of toddlers with autism spectrum disorders: Associations with child characteristics. *Journal of Autism and Developmental Disorders, 38,* 1278–1291.

Davis, T. N., O'Reilly, M. F., Kang, S., Rispoli, M., Lang, R. B., Machalicek, W., et al. (2009). Impact of presession access to toys maintaining challenging behavior on functional communication training: a single case study. *Journal of Developmental and Physical Disabilities, 21*(6), 515–521.

Deb, S., & Prasad, K. B. G. (1994). The prevalence of autistic disorder among children with a learning disability. *British Journal of Psychiatry, 165,* 395–399.

Deb, S., Thomas, M., & Bright, C. (2001). Mental disorder in adults with intellectual disability. I: Prevalence of functional psychiatric illness among a community-based population aged between 16 and 64 years. *Journal of Intellectual Disability Research Mental Health and Intellectual Disability, 45*(6), 495–505.

DeLeon, I. G., Neidert, P. L., Anders, B. M., & Rodriguez-Catter, V. (2001). Choices between positive and negative reinforcement during treatment for escape-maintained behavior. *Journal of Applied Behavior Analysis, 34,* 521–525.

DeRubeis, R. J., Siegle, G. J., & Hollon, S. D. (2008). Cognitive therapy versus medication for depression: treatment outcomes and neural mechanisms. *Nature Reviews Neuroscience, 9*(10), 788–796.

Didden, R., Duker, P. C., & Korzilius, H. (1997). Meta-analytic study on treatment effectiveness for problem behaviors with individuals with mental retardation. *American Journal on Mental Retardation, 101,* 387–399.

Dominick, K. C., Davis, N. O., Lainhart, J., Tager-Flusberg, H., & Folstein, S. (2007). Atypical behaviors in children with autism and children with a history of language impairment. *Research in Developmental Disabilities, 28*(2), 145–162.

Donohue, M. M., Baylot Casey, L., Bicard, D. F., & Bicard, S. E. (2012). Effects of differential reinforcement of short latencies on response latency, task completion, and accuracy of an adolescent with autism. *Education and Training in Autism and Developmental Disabilities, 47*(1), 97–108.

Dunlap, G., Strain, P. S., Fox, L., Carta, J. J., Conroy, M., Smith, B. J., et al. (2006). Prevention and intervention with young children's challenging behavior: perspectives regarding current knowledge. *Behavioral Disorders, 32*(1), 29–45.

Durand, V. M. (1999). Functional communication training using assistive devices: Recruiting natural communities of reinforcement. *Journal of Applied Behavior Analysis, 32,* 247–267.

Durand, V. M., & Carr, E. G. (1991). Functional communication training to reduce challenging behavior: Maintenance and application in new settings. *Journal of Applied Behavior Analysis, 24*(2), 251–264.

Durand, V. M., & Carr, E. G. (1992). An analysis of maintenance following functional communication training. *Journal of Applied Behavior Analysis, 25,* 777–794.

Durand, V. M., & Merges, E. (2001). Functional communication training a contemporary behavior analytic intervention for problem behaviors. *Focus on Autism and Other Developmental Disabilities, 16*(2), 110–119.

Emerson, E. (2001). *Challenging behaviour: Analysis and intervention in people with severe intellectual disabilities*. New York: Cambridge University Press.

Emerson, E., & Bromley, J. (1995). The form and function of challenging behaviours. *Journal of Intellectual Disability Research, 39,* 388–398.

Emerson, E., Robertson, J., Gregory, N., et al. (2000). Treatment and management of challenging behaviours in residential settings. *Journal of Applied Research in Intellectual Disabilities, 13,* 197–215.

Emerson, E., Kiernan, C., Alborz, A., Reeves, D., Mason, H., Swarbrick, R., et al. (2001). The prevalence of challenging behaviors: A total population study. *Research in Developmental Disabilities, 22*(1), 77–93.

Falcomata, T. S., Roane, H. S., Muething, C. S., Stephenson, K. M., & Ing, A. D. (2012a). Functional communication training and chained schedules of reinforcement to treat challenging behavior maintained by terminations of activity interruptions. *Behavior Modification, 36*(5), 630–649.

Falcomata, T. S., White, P., Muething, C. S., & Fragale, C. (2012b). A functional communication training and chained schedule procedure to treat challenging behavior with multiple functions. *Journal of Developmental and Physical Disabilities, 24*(6), 529–538.
Falcomata, T. S., Muething, C. S., Gainey, S., Hoffman, K., & Fragale, C. (2013). Further evaluations of functional communication training and chained schedules of reinforcement to treat multiple functions of challenging behavior. *Behavior Modification, 37*(6), 723–746.
Farmer, C. A., & Aman, M. G. (2010). Aggressive behavior in a sample of children with autism spectrum disorders. *Research in Autism Spectrum Disorders, 5*(1), 317–323.
Felce, D., & Emerson, E. (1996). Realities and challenges. *Journal of Applied Research in Intellectual Disabilities, 9*(3), 284–288.
Fisher, W. W., Piazza, , Bowman, L. G., Hagopian, L. P., Owens, J. C., & Slevin, I. (1992). A comparison of two approaches for identifying reinforcers for persons with severe and profound disabilities. *Journal of Applied Behavior Analysis, 25*(2), 491–498.
Fisher, W. W., Piazza, C., Cataldo, M., Harrell, R., Jefferson, G., & Conner, R. (1993). Functional communication training with and without extinction and punishment. *Journal of Applied Behavior Analysis, 26,* 23–36.
Fisher, W. W., Thompson, R. H., Hagopian, L. P., et al. (2000). Facilitating tolerance of delayed reinforcement during functional communication training. *Behavior Modification, 24,* 3–29.
Fisher, W. W., Adelinis, J. D., Volkert, V. M., et al. (2005). Assessing preferences for positive and negative reinforcement during treatment of destructive behavior with functional communication training. *Research in Developmental Disabilities, 26,* 153–168.
Floyd, F. J., & Gallagher, E. M. (1997). Parental stress, care demands, and use of support services for school-age children with disabilities and behavior problems. *Family Relations,* 359–371.
Frazier, J. A., Biederman, J., Bellordre, C. A., Garfield, S. B., Geller, D. A., Coffey, B. J., et al. (2001). Should the diagnosis of attention-deficit/hyperactivity disorder be considered in children with pervasive developmental disorder?. *Journal of Attention Disorders, 4*(4), 203–211.
Frea, W. D., & Hepburn, S. L. (1999). Teaching parents of children with autism to perform functional assessments to plan interventions for extremely disruptive behaviors. *Journal of Positive Behavior Interventions, 1*(2), 112–122.
Freeman, K. A., Anderson, C. M., & Scotti, J. R. (2000). A structured descriptive methodology: Increasing agreement between descriptive and experimental analyses. *Education and Training in Mental Retardation and Developmental Disabilities, 35,* 55–66.
Ghaziuddin, M., Ghaziuddin, N., & Greden, J. (2002). Depression in persons with autism: Implications for research and clinical care. *Journal of Autism and Developmental Disorders, 32*(4), 299–306.
Giallo, R., & Gavidia-Payne, S. (2006). Child, parent, and family factors as predictors of adjustment for siblings of children with a disability. *Journal of Intellectual Disability Research, 50,* 937–948.
Goldin, R. L., Matson, J. L., Tureck, K., Cervantes, P. E., & Jang, J. (2013). A comparison of tantrum behavior profiles in children with ASD, ADHD and comorbid ASD and ADHD. *Research in Developmental Disabilities, 34*(9), 2669–2675.
Gresham, F. M., Watson, T. S., & Skinner, C. H. (2001). Functional behavioral assessment: Principles, procedures, and future directions. *School Psychology Review, 30*(2), 156–172.
Groskreutz, N. C., Groskreutz, M. P., & Higbee, T. S. (2011). Effects of varied levels of treatment integrity on appropriate toy manipulation in children with autism. *Research in Autism Spectrum Disorders, 5*(4), 1358–1369.
Guttmann-Steinmetz, S., Gadow, K. D., & DeVincent, C. J. (2009). Oppositional defiant and conduct disorder behaviors in boys with autism spectrum disorder with and without attention-deficit hyperactivity disorder versus several comparison samples. *Journal of Autism and Developmental Disorders, 39*(7), 976–985.
Hagopian, L. P., & Adelinis, J. D. (2001). Response blocking with and without redirection for the treatment of pica. *Journal of Applied Behavior Analysis, 34*(4), 527–530.

Hagopian, L. P., Crockett, J. L., van Stone, M., et al. (2000). Effects of noncontingent reinforcement on problem behavior and stimulus engagement: The role of satiation, extinction, and alternative reinforcement. *Journal of Applied Behavior Analysis, 33,* 433–449.

Hagopian, L. P., Wilson, D. M., & Wilder, D. A. (2001). Assessment and treatment of problem behavior maintained by escape from attention and access to tangible items. *Journal of Applied Behavior Analysis, 34,* 229–232.

Hagopian, L. P., Bruzek, J. L., Bowman, L. G., & Jennett, H. K. (2007). Assessment and treatment of problem behavior occasioned by interruption of free-operant behavior. *Journal of Applied Behavior Analysis, 40*(1), 89–103.

Hagopian, L. P., Boelter, E. W., & Jarmolowicz, D. P. (2011). Reinforcement schedule thinning following functional communication training. Review and recommendations. *Behavior Analysis in Practice, 4,* 4–16.

Hagopian, L. P., Rooker, G. W., Jessel, J., & DeLeon, I. G. (2013). Initial functional analysis outcomes and modifications in pursuit of differentiation: A summary of 176 inpatient cases. *Journal of applied behavior analysis, 46*(1), 88–100.

Hall, S., Thorns, T., & Oliver, C. (2003). Structural and environmental characteristics of stereotyped behaviors. *American Journal on Mental Retardation, 108,* 391–402.

Hammond, J. L., Iwata, B. A., Fritz, J. N., & Dempsey, C. M. (2011). Evaluation of fixed momentary DRO schedules under signaled and unsignaled arrangements. *Journal of Applied Behavior Analysis, 44*(1), 69–81.

Handen, B. L., & Lubetsky, M. (2005). Pharmacotherapy in Autism and Related Disorders. *School Psychology Quarterly, 20,* 155–171.

Hanley, G. P., Iwata, B. A., & Thompson, R. H. (2001). Reinforcement schedule thinning following treatment with functional communication training. *Journal of Applied Behavior Analysis, 34*(1), 17–38.

Hanley, G. P., Iwata, B. A., & McCord, B. E. (2003). Functional analysis of problem behavior: A review. *Journal of Applied Behavior Analysis, 36*(2), 147–185.

Hanson, E., Cerban, B. M., Slater, C. M., Caccamo, L. M., Bacic, J., & Chan, E. (2013). Brief report: Prevalence of attention deficit/hyperactivity disorder among individuals with an autism spectrum disorder. *Journal of Autism and Developmental Disorders, 43*(6), 1459–1464.

Hartley, S. L., Sikora, D. M., & McCoy, R. (2008). Prevalence and risk factors of maladaptive behaviour in young children with autistic disorder. *Journal of Intellectual Disability Research, 52,* 1–11.

Hayes, S. A., & Watson, S. L. (2013). The impact of parenting stress: A meta-analysis of studies comparing the experience of parenting stress in parents of children with and without autism spectrum disorder. *Journal of Autism and Developmental Disorders, 43,* 629–642.

Healy, O., Brett, D., & Leader, G. (2013). A comparison of experimental functional analysis and the Questions About Behavioral Function (QABF) in the assessment of challenging behavior of individuals with autism. *Research in Autism Spectrum Disorders, 7*(1), 66–81.

Heckaman, K., Conroy, M., Fox, J., & Chait, A. (2000). Functional assessment based intervention research on students with or at risk for emotional and behavior disorders in school settings. *Behavioral Disorders, 25*(3), 196–210.

Hesse, T. L., Danko, C. M., & Budd, K. S. (2013). Siblings of children with autism: Predictors of adjustment. *Research in Autism Spectrum Disorders, 7,* 1323–1331.

Holden, B., & Gitlesen, J. P. (2006). A total population study of challenging behaviour in the county of Hedmark, Norway: Prevalence, and risk markers. *Research in Developmental Disabilities, 27,* 456–465.

Horner, R. H., & Carr, E. G. (1997). Behavioral support for students with severe disabilities: Functional assessment and comprehensive intervention. *Journal of Special Education, 31,* 84–104.

Horner, R. H., Carr, E. G., Strain, P. S., Todd, A. W., & Reed, H. K. (2002). Problem behavior interventions for young children with autism: A research synthesis. *Journal of Autism and Developmental Disorders, 32*(5), 423–446.

Hutt, C., & Hutt, S. J. (1965). Effects of environmental complexity on stereo-typed behaviors of children. *Animal Behavior, 13,* 1–4.

Ingram, K., Lewis-Palmer, T., & Sugai, G. (2005). Function-based intervention planning: Comparing the effectiveness of FBA function-based and non-function-based intervention plans. *Journal of Positive Behavior Interventions, 7*(4), 224–236.

Ingvarsson, E. T., Kahng, S., & Hausman, N. L. (2008). Some effects of noncontingent positive reinforcement on multiply controlled problem behavior and compliance in a demand context. *Journal of Applied Behavior Analysis, 41*(3), 435–440.

Iwata, B. A., Pace, G. M., Dorsey, M. F., Zarcone, J. R., Vollmer, T. R., Smith, R. G., et al. (1982/1994). The functions of self-injurious behavior: An experimental-epidemiological analysis. *Journal of Applied Behavior Analysis, 27*(2), 215–240.

Jarmolowicz, D. P., DeLeon, I. G., & Contrucci-Kuhn, S. A. (2009). Functional communication during signaled reinforcement and/or extinction. *Behavioral Interventions, 24,* 265–273.

Kanne, S. M., & Mazurek, M. O. (2011). Aggression in children and adolescents with ASD: prevalence and risk factors. *Journal of Autism and Developmental Disorders, 41*(7), 926–937.

Keen, D., & Ward, S. (2004). Autism spectrum disorder: A child population profile. *Autism: International Journal of Research and Practice, 8,* 39–48.

Keenan, M., Dillenburger, K., Doherty, A., Byrne, T., & Gallagher, S. (2010). The experiences of parents during diagnosis and forward planning for children with autism spectrum disorder. *Journal of Applied Research in Intellectual Disabilities, 23*(4), 390–397.

Kim, J. A., Szatmari, P., Bryson, S. E., Streiner, D. L., & Wilson, F. J. (2000). The prevalence of anxiety and mood problems among children with autism and Asperger syndrome. *Autism, 4*(2), 117–132.

Knoster, T. P., & McCurdy, B. (2002). Best practices in functional behavioral assessment for designing individualized student programs. *Best practices in school psychology IV*, 2, 1007–1028.

Kodak, T., Miltenberger, R. G., & Romaniuk, C. (2003). The effects of differential negative reinforcement of other behavior and noncontingent escape on compliance. *Journal of Applied Behavior Analysis, 36,* 379–382.

Konst, M. J., Matson, J. L., & Turygin, N. (2013). Comparing the rates of tantrum behavior in children with ASD and ADHD as well as children with comorbid ASD and ADHD diagnoses. *Research in Autism Spectrum Disorders, 7*(11), 1339–1345.

Kuhn, D. E., Hardesty, S. L., & Sweeney, N. M. (2009). Assessment and treatment of excessive straightening and destructive behavior in an adolescent diagnosed with autism. *Journal of Applied Behavior Analysis, 42*(2), 355–360.

Kwon, K. A., Han, S., Jeon, H. J., & Bingham, G. E. (2013). Mothers' and fathers' parenting challenges, strategies, and resources in toddlerhood. *Early Child Development and Care, 183*(3–4), 415–429.

Lainhart, J. E., & Folstein, S. E. (1994). Affective disorders in people with autism: A review of published cases. *Journal of Autism and Developmental Disorders, 24*(5), 587–601.

Langworthy-Lam, K. L., Aman, M. G., & Van Bourgondiem, M. E. (2002). Prevalence and patterns of use of psychoactive medicines in individuals with autism in the Autism Society of North Carolina. *Journal of Child and Adolescent Psychopharmacology, 12,* 311–321.

Lecavalier, L., Leone, S., & Wiltz, J. (2006). The impact of behaviour problems on caregiver stress in young people with autism spectrum disorders. *Journal of Intellectual Disability Research, 50*(3), 172–183.

Lee, L. C., Harrington, R. A., Chang, J. J., & Conners, S. L. (2008). Increased risk of injury in children with developmental disabilities. *Research in Developmental Disabilities, 29,* 247–255.

Lehmkuhl, H. D., Storch, E. A., Bodfish, J. W., & Geffken, G. R. (2008). Brief report: Exposure and response prevention for obsessive compulsive disorder in a 12-year-old with autism. *Journal of Developmental Disorders, 38,* 977–981.

Leyfer, O. T., Folstein, S. E., Bacalman, S., Davis, N. O., Dinh, E., Morgan, J., et al. (2006). Comorbid psychiatric disorders in children with autism: Interview development and rates of disorders. *Journal of Autism and Developmental Disorders, 36*(7), 849–861.

Loftin, R. L., Odom, S. L., & Lantz, J. F. (2008). Social interaction and repetitive motor behaviors. *Journal of Autism and Developmental Disorders, 38*(6), 1124–1135.

Lomas, J. E., Fisher, W. W., & Kelley, M. E. (2010). The effects of variable-time delivery of food items and praise on problem behavior reinforced by escape. *Journal of Applied Behavior Analysis, 43*(3), 425–435.

Long, K., Wood, H., & Holmes, N. (2000). Presentation, assessment and treatment of depression in a young woman with learning disability and autism. *British Journal of Learning Disabilities, 28,* 102–108.

Lowe, K., Allen, D., Jones, E., Brophy, S., Moore, K., & James, W. (2007). Challenging behaviours: Prevalence and topographies. *Journal of Intellectual Disability Research, 51*(8), 625–636.

Luby, J. (2011). An examination of the use of the token economy in reducing behaviors in an adolescent with autism spectrum disorder (Doctoral dissertation, Wichita State University).

Lucyshyn, J. M., Horner, R. H., Dunlap, G., Albin, R. W., & Ben, K. R. (2002). Positive behavior support with families. In J. M. Lucyshyn, G. Dunlap & R. W. Albin (Eds.), *Families and positive behavior support: Addressing problem behavior in family contexts* (pp. 3–43). Baltimore: Paul H. Brookes Publishing Co.

Lucyshyn, J. M., Irvin, L. K., Blumberg, E. R., Laverty, R., Horner, R. H., & Sprague, J. R. (2004). Validating the construct of coercion in family routines: Expanding the unit of analysis in behavioral assessment with families with children with developmental disabilities. *Research & Practices for Persons with Severe Disabilities, 29,* 104–121.

Malone, R. P., Gratz, S. S., Delaney, M. A., & Hyman, S. B. (2005). Advances in drug treatments for children and adolescents with autism and other pervasive developmental disorders. *CNS drugs, 19,* 923–934.

Mancil, G. (2006). Functional communication training: A review of the literature related to children with autism. *Education and Training in Developmental Disabilities, 41,* 213–224.

Mannion, A., & Leader, G. (2013). An analysis of the predictors of comorbid psychopathology, gastrointestinal symptoms and epilepsy in children and adolescents with autism spectrum disorder. *Research in Autism Spectrum Disorders, 7*(12), 1663–1671.

Marcus, B. A., & Vollmer, T. R. (1996). Combining noncontingent reinforcement and differential reinforcement schedules as treatment for aberrant behavior. *Journal of Applied Behavior Analysis, 29*(1), 43–51.

Martin, C. A., Drasgow, E., Halle, J. W., & Brucker, J. M. (2005). Teaching a child with autism and severe language delays to reject: Direct and indirect effects of functional communication training. *Educational Psychology, 25*(2–3), 287–304.

Matson, J. L., & Boisjoli, J. A. (2009a). An overview of developments in research on persons with intellectual disabilities. *Research in Developmental Disabilities, 30,* 587–591.

Matson, J. L., & Demsey, T. (2009). The nature and treatment of compulsions, obsessions, and rituals in people with developmental disabilities. *Research in Developmental Disabilities, 30,* 603–611.

Matson, J. L., & Neal, D. (2009). Psychotropic medication use for challenging behaviors in persons with intellectual disabilities: An overview. *Research in Developmental Disabilities, 30,* 572–586.

Matson, J. L., & Nebel-Schwalm, M. (2007). Assessing challenging behaviors in children with autism spectrum disorders: A review. *Research in Developmental Disabilities, 28*(6), 567–579.

Matson, J. L., & Rivet, T. T. (2008). The effects of severity of autism and PDD-NOS symptoms on challenging behaviors in adults with intellectual disabilities. *Journal of Developmental and Physical Disabilities, 20,* 41–51.

Matson, J. L., & Shoemaker, M. (2009). Intellectual disability and its relationship to autism spectrum disorders. *Research in Developmental Disabilities, 30*(6), 1107–1114.

Matson, M. L., Matson, J. L., & Beighley, J. S. (2011). Comorbidity of physical and motor problems in children with autism. *Research in Developmental Disabilities, 32*(6), 2304–2308.

Matson, J. L., & Turygin, N. C. (2012). How do researchers define self-injurious behavior? *Research in Developmental Disabilities, 33*(4), 1021–1026.

Matson, J. L., & Williams, L. W. (2013). Differential diagnosis and comorbidity: distinguishing autism from other mental health issues. *Neuropsychiatry, 3*(2), 233–243.

Matson, J. L., LoVullo, S. V., Boisjoli, J. A., & Gonzalez, M. L. (2008). The behavioral treatment of an 11-year-old girl with autism and aggressive behaviors. *Clinical Case Studies, 7*(4), 313–326.

Matson, J. L., Wilkins, J., & Macken, J. (2009). The relationship of challenging behaviors to severity and symptoms of autism spectrum disorders. *Journal of Mental Health Research in Intellectual Disabilities, 2*(1), 29–44.

Matson, J. L., Mahan, S., Hess, J. A., Fodstad, J. C., & Neal, D. (2010). Progression of challenging behaviors in children and adolescents with autism spectrum disorders as measured by the autism spectrum disorders–problem behaviors for children (PBC). *Research in Autism Spectrum Disorders, 4*, 400–404.

McClintock, K., Hall, S., & Oliver, C. (2003). Risk markers associated with challenging behaviours in people with intellectual disabilities: A meta-analytic study. *Journal of Intellectual Disability Research, 47*(6), 405–416.

McTiernan, A., Leader, G., Healy, O., & Mannion, A. (2011). Analysis of risk factors and early predictors of challenging behavior for children with autism spectrum disorder. *Research in Autism Spectrum Disorders, 5*(3), 1215–1222.

Militerni, R., Bravaccio, C., Falco, C., Fico, C., & Palermo, M. T. (2002). Repetitive behaviors in autistic disorder. *European Child & Adolescent Psychiatry, 11*(5), 210–218.

Minshawi, N. F., Hurwitz, S., Fodstad, J. C., Biebl, S., Morriss, D. H., & McDougle, C. J. (2014). The association between self-injurious behaviors and autism spectrum disorders. *Psychological Research and Behavior Management, 12*(7), 125–136.

Murphy, G. H., Oliver, C., Corbett, J., Crayton, L., Hales, J., & Head, D. (1993) Epidemiology of self-injury, characteristics of people with severe self-injury and initial treatment outcome. In C. Kiernan (Eds.), *Research to practice? Implications of research on challenging behaviour of people with learning disability* (pp. 1–35). Kidderminster: British Institute of Learning Disabilities, Avon.

Murphy, G., Hall, S., Oliver, C., & Kissi-Debra, R. (1999). Identification of early self-injurious behavior in young children with intellectual disability. *Journal of Intellectual Disability Research, 43*(3), 149–163.

Murphy, G., Macdonald, S., Hall, S., & Oliver, C. (2000). Aggression and the termination of "rituals": A new variant of the escape function for challenging behavior? *Research in Developmental Disabilities, 21*(1), 43–59.

Murphy, G., Beadle-Brown, J., Wing, L., Gould, J., Shah, A., & Holmes, N. (2005). Chronicity of challenging behaviours in people with severe intellectual disabilities and/or autism: A total population sample. *Journal of Autism and Developmental Disorders, 35*, 405–418.

Murphy, O., Healy, O., & Leader,G (2009). Risk factors for challenging behaviors among 157 children with autism spectrum disorders in Ireland. *Research in Autism Spectrum Disorders, 3*, 474–482.

Murray, M. J. (2010). Attention-deficit/hyperactivity disorder in the context of autism spectrum disorders. *Current Psychiatry Reports, 12*(5), 382–388.

Najdowski, A. C., Wallace, M. D., Doney, J. K., & Ghezzi, P. M. (2003). Parental assessment and treatment of food selectivity in natural settings. *Journal of Applied Behavior Analysis, 36*(3), 383–386.

National Research Council. (2001). *Educating children with autism (committee on educational interventions for children with autism, division of behavioral and social sciences and education)*. Washington, DC: National Academy Press.

Neidert, P. L., Iwata, B. A., & Dozier, C. L. (2005). Treatment of multiply controlled problem behavior with procedural variations of differential reinforcement. *Exceptionality, 13*(1), 45–53.

Newcomer, L. L., & Lewis, T. J. (2004). Functional behavioral assessment: An investigation of assessment reliability and effectiveness of function-based interventions. *Journal of Emotional and Behavioral Disorders, 12*, 168–181.

O'Neill, R. E., Horner, R. H., Albin, R. W., Sprague, J. R., Storey, K., & Newton, J. S. (1997). *Functional assessment and program development for problem behaviors: A practical handbook* (2nd ed.). Pacific Grove: Brooks/Cole.

O'Reilly, M. F., Sigafoos, J., Lancioni, G., Rispoli, M., Lang, R., Chan, J., et al. (2008). Manipulating the behavior-altering effect of the motivating operation: Examination of the influence on challenging behavior during leisure activities. *Research in Developmental Disabilities, 29*(4), 333–340.

O'Reilly, M., Fragale, C., Gainey, S., Kang, S., Koch, H., Shubert, J., et al. (2012). Examination of an antecedent communication intervention to reduce tangibly maintained challenging behavior: A controlled analog analysis. *Research in Developmental Disabilities, 33*(5), 1462–1468.

Oliver, C., Murphy, G. H., & Corbett, J. A. (1987). Self injurious behaviour in people with mental handicap: A total population study. *Journal of Mental Deficiency Research, 31,* 147–162.

Paclawskyj, T. R., Matson, J. L., Rush, K. S., Smalls, Y., & Vollmer, T. R. (2000). Questions about behavioral function (QABF): A behavioral checklist for functional assessment of aberrant behavior. *Research in Developmental Disabilities, 21,* 223–229.

Paclawskyj, T. R., Matson, J. L., Rush, K. S., Smalls, Y. Y., & Vollmer, T. R. (2001). Assessment of the convergent validity of the Questions About Behavioral Function scale with analogue functional analysis and the Motivation Assessment Scale. *Journal of Intellectual Disability Research, 45,* 484–494.

Patterson, S. Y., Smith, V., & Jelen, M. (2010). Behavioural intervention practices for stereotypic and repetitive behavior in individuals with autism spectrum disorder: A systematic review. *Developmental Medicine & Child Neurology, 52,* 318–327.

Paula-Perez, I. (2013). Differential diagnosis between obsessive compulsive disorder and restrictive and repetitive behavioural patterns, activities, and interests in autism spectrum disorders. *Revista de Psiquiatria y Salud Mental, 6,* 178–186.

Perry, D. W., Marston, G. M., Hinder, S. A. J., Munden, A. C., & Roy, A. (2001). The phenomenology of depressive illness in people with a learning disability and autism. *Autism, 5*(3), 265–275.

Piazza, C. C., Moes, D. R., & Fisher, W. W. (1996). Differential reinforcement of alternative behavior and demand fading in the treatment of escape-maintained destructive behavior. *Journal of Applied Behavior Analysis, 29*(4), 569–572.

Piazza, C. C., Adelinis, J. D., Hanley, G. P., Goh, H., & Delia, M. D. (2000). An evaluation of the effects of matched stimuli on behaviors maintained by automatic reinforcement. *Journal of Applied Behavior Analysis, 33,* 13–27.

Progar, P. R., North, S. T., Bruce, S. S., et al. (2001). Putative behavioral history effects and aggression maintained by escape from therapists. *Journal of Applied Behavior Analysis, 34,* 69–72.

Prupas, A., & Reid, G. (2001). Effects of exercise frequency on stereotypic behaviors of children with developmental disabilities. *Education and Training in Mental Retardation and Developmental Disabilities, 36*(2), 196–206.

Qureshi, H., & Alborz, A. (1992). Epidemiology of challenging behaviour. *Mental Handicap Research, 5*(2), 130–145.

Rapp, J. T. (2004). Effects of prior access and environmental enrichment on stereotypy. *Behavioral Interventions, 19,* 287–295.

Rapp, J. T. (2007). Further evaluation of methods to identify matched stimulation. *Journal of Applied Behavior Analysis, 39,* 137–140.

Rapp, J. T., & Vollmer, T. R. (2005). Stereotypy I: A review of behavioral assessment and treatment. *Research in Developmental Disabilities, 26,* 527–547.

Rapp, J. T., Vollmer, T. R., St. Peter, C., Dozier, C. L., & Cotnoir, N. M. (2004). Analysis of response allocation in individuals with multiple forms of stereotyped behavior. *Journal of Applied Behavior Analysis, 37*(4), 481–501.

Reed, G. K., Ringdahl, J. E., Wacker, D. P., Barretto, A., & Andelman, M. S. (2005). The effects of fixed-time and contingent schedules of negative reinforcement on compliance and aberrant behavior. *Research in Developmental Disabilities, 26*(3), 281–295.

Reese, R. M., Richman, D. M., Belmont, J. M., & Morse, P. (2005). Functional characteristics of disruptive behavior in developmentally disabled children with and without autism. *Journal of Autism and Developmental Disorders, 35,* 419–428.

Reid, D. H., Parsons, M. B., & Lattimore, L. P. (2010). Designing and evaluating assessment-based interventions to reduce stereotypy among adults with autism in a community job. *Behavior Analysis in Practice, 3*(2), 27.

Ricciardi, J. N., Luiselli, J. K., Terrill, S., & Reardon, K. (2003). Alternative response training with contingent practice as intervention for pica in a school setting. *Behavioral Interventions, 18*(3), 219–226.

Rincover, A., Newsom, R., & Carr, E. (1979). Sensory extinction and sensory reinforcement principles for programming multiple adaptive behavior change. *Journal of Applied Behavior Analysis, 12,* 221–233.

Ringdahl, J. E., Kitsukawa, K., Andelman, M. S., et al. (2002). Differential reinforcement with and without instructional fading. *Journal of Applied Behavior Analysis, 35,* 291–294.

Ringdahl, J. E., Call, N. A., Christensen, T., & Boelter, E. W. (2010). Brief report: Signals enhance the suppressive effects of noncontingent reinforcement. *Journal of Autism and Developmental Disorders, 40*(3), 378–382.

Rispoli, M., O'Reilly, M., Lang, R., Machalicek, W., Davis, T., Lancioni, G., et al. 2011a). Effects of motivating operations on problem and academic behavior in classrooms. *Journal of Applied Behavior Analysis, 44*(1), 187–192.

Rispoli, M. J., O'Reilly, M. F., Sigafoos, J., Lang, R., Kang, S., Lancioni, G., & Parker, R. (2011b). Effects of presession satiation on challenging behavior and academic engagement for children with autism during classroom instruction. *Education and Training in Autism and Developmental Disabilities, 46*(4), 607.

Rispoli, M., Ganz, J., Neely, L., & Goodwyn, F. (2013). The effect of noncontingent positive versus negative reinforcement on multiply controlled behavior during discrete trial training. *Journal of Developmental and Physical Disabilities, 25*(1), 135–148.

Rispoli, M., Camargo, S., Machalicek, W., Lang, R., Ninci, J., *trickland, E., & Sigafoos, J. (2014). Functional communication training in the treatment of problem behaviors maintained by access to rituals. *Journal of Applied Behavior Analysis, 47,* 580–593.

Rojahn, J., Matson, J. L., Naglieri, J. A., & Mayville, E. (2004). Relationships between psychiatric conditions and behavior problems among adults with mental retardation. *American Journal on Mental Retardation, 109*(1), 21–33.

Russell, A. J., Mataix-Cols, D., Anson, M. A., & Murphy, D. G. (2009). Psychology treatment for obsessive compulsive disorder in people with autism spectrum disorders: A pilot study. *Psychotherapy and Psychosomatics, 78,* 59–61.

Russell, A. J., Jassi, A., Fullana, M. A., Mack, H., Johnston, K., Heyman, I., et al. (2013). Cognitive behavior therapy for comorbid obsessive-compulsive disorder in high-functioning autism spectrum disorders: A randomized controlled trial. *Depression and Anxiety, 30,* 697–708.

Schieve, L. A., Blumberg, S. J., Rice, C., Visser, S. N., & Boyle, C. (2007). The relationship between autism and parenting stress. *Pediatrics, 119*(Supplement 1), S114-S121.

Schmidt, J. D., Drasgow, E., Halle, J. W., Martin, C. A., & Bliss, S. A. (2014). Discrete-trial functional analysis and functional communication training with three individuals with autism and severe problem behavior. *Journal of Positive Behavior Interventions, 16*(1), 44–55.

Scott, T. M., Meers, D. T., & Nelson, C. M. (2000). Toward a consensus of functional behavioral assessment for students with mild disabilities in public school contexts: A national survey. *Education and Treatment of Children, 23,* 265–285.

Seltzer, M. M., Greenberg, J. S., Floyd, F. J., et al. (2001). Life course impacts of parenting a child with a disability. *American Journal Mental Retardation, 106,* 265–286.

Shattuck, P. T. (2006). The contribution of diagnostic substitution to the growing administrative prevalence of autism in US special education. *Pediatrics, 117*(4), 1028–1037.

Shattuck, P. T., Seltzer, M. M., Greenberg, J. S., Orsmond, G. I., Bolt, D., Kring, S., et al. (2007). Change in autism symptoms and maladaptive behaviors in adolescents and adults with an autism spectrum disorder. *Journal of Autism and Developmental Disorders, 37*(9), 1735–1747.

Shukla-Mehta, S., & Albin, R. W. (2003). Twelve practical strategies to prevent behavioral escalation in classroom settings. *The Clearing House, 77*(2), 50–56.

Sigafoos, J., & Kerr, M. (1994). Provision of leisure activities for the reduction of challenging behavior. *Behavioral Interventions, 9*(1), 43–53.

Sigafoos, J., & Tucker, M. (2000). Brief assessment and treatment of multiple challenging behaviors. *Behavioral Interventions, 15*(1), 53–70.

Sigafoos, J., Tucker, M., Bushell, H., & Webber, Y. (1997). Practical strategy to increase participation and reduce challenging behavior during leisure skills programming. *Mental Retardation, 35*(3), 198–208.

Sigafoos, J., Arthur, M., & O'Reilly, M. F. (2003). *Challenging behavior and developmental disability*. London: Whurr Publishers.

Sigafoos, J., Green, V. A., Payne, D., O'Reilly, M. F., & Lancioni, G. E. (2009). A classroom-based antecedent intervention reduces obsessive-repetitive behavior in an adolescent with autism. *Clinical Case Studies, 8*(1), 3–13.

Simonoff, E., Pickles, A., Charman, T., Chandler, S., Loucas, T., & Baird, G. (2008). Psychiatric disorders in children with autism spectrum disorders: prevalence, comorbidity, and associated factors in a population-derived sample. *Journal of the American Academy of Child & Adolescent Psychiatry, 47*(8), 921–929.

Sinzig, J., Walter, D., & Doepfner, M. (2009). Attention deficit/hyperactivity disorder in children and adolescents with autism spectrum disorder symptom or syndrome?. *Journal of Attention Disorders, 13*(2), 117–126.

Skinner, B. F. (1953). *Science and human behavior*. New York: Free Press.

Smith, R. G., & Iwata, B. A. (1997). Antecedent influences on behavior disorders. *Journal of Applied Behavior Analysis, 30*(2), 343–375.

Sterling, L., Dawson, G., Estes, A., & Greenson, J. (2008). Characteristics associated with presence of depressive symptoms in adults with autism spectrum disorder. *Journal of Autism and Developmental Disorders, 38*(6), 1011–1018.

Stewart, M. E., Barnard, L., Pearson, J., Hasan, R., & O'Brien, G. (2006). Presentation of depression in autism and Asperger syndrome A review. *Autism, 10*(1), 103–116.

Strand, J. F., Kenworthy, L., Daniolos, P., Case, L., Wills, M. C., Martin, A., et al. (2012). Depression and anxiety symptoms in children and adolescents with autism spectrum disorders without intellectual disability. *Research in Autism Spectrum Disorders, 6*(1), 406–412.

Symons, F. J., Sperry, L. A., Dropik, P. L., & Bodfish, J. W. (2005). The early development of stereotypy and self-injury: a review of research methods. *Journal of Intellectual Disability Research, 49*(2), 144–158.

Tenneij, N. H., Didden, R., Stolker, J. J., & Koot, H. M. (2009). Markers for aggression in inpatient treatment facilities for adults with mild to borderline intellectual disability. *Research in Developmental Disabilities, 30*(6), 1248–1257.

Tiger, J. H., & Hanley, G. P. (2008). Functional communication training: A review and practical guide. *Behavior Analysis in Practice, 1,* 16–23.

Van Camp C. M., Lerman, D. C., Kelley, M. E., Roane, H. S., Contrucci, S. A., & Vorndran, C. M. (2000). Further analysis of idiosyncratic antecedent influences during the assessment and treatment of problem behavior. *Journal of Applied Behavior Analysis, 33,* 207–221.

van Steensel, F. J., Bogels, S. M., & Perrin, S. (2011). Anxiety disorders in children and adolescents with autistic spectrum disorders: A meta-analysis. *Clinical Child Family Psychological Review, 14,* 302–317.

Vasa, R. A., Carroll, L. M., Nozzolillo, A. A., Mahajan, R., Mazurek, M. O., Bennett, A. E., et al. (2014). A systematic review of treatments for anxiety in youth with autism spectrum disorders. *Journal of Autism and Developmental Disorders, 44*(12), 3215–3229.

Vollmer, T. R. (1994). The concept of automatic reinforcement: Implications for behavioral research in developmental disabilities. *Research in Developmental Disabilities, 15,* 187–207.

Vollmer, T. R., Marcus, B. A., & LeBlanc, L. (1994). Treatment of self-injury and hand mouthing following inconclusive functional analysis. *Journal of Applied Behavior Analysis, 27*(2), 331–344.

Wacker, D. P., Lee, J. F., Dalmau, Y. C. P., Kopelman, T. G., Lindgren, S. D., Kuhle, J., et al. (2013). Conducting functional communication training via telehealth to reduce the problem behavior of young children with autism. *Journal of Developmental and Physical Disabilities, 25*(1), 35–48.

Walsh, C., Mulder, E., & Tudor, M. E. (2013). Predictors of parent stress in a sample of children with ASD: Pain, problem behavior, and parental coping. *Research in Autism Spectrum Disorders, 7,* 256–264.

Waters, M. B., Lerman, D. C., & Hovanetz, A. N. (2009). Separate and combined effects of visual schedules and extinction plus differential reinforcement on problem behavior occasioned by transitions. *Journal of Applied Behavior Analysis, 42*(2), 309–313.

Watkins, N., & Rapp, J. T. (2013). The convergent validity of the questions about behavioral function and functional analysis for problem behavior displayed by individuals with autism spectrum disorder. *Research in Developmental Disabilities, 34,* 11–16.

White, S. W., Oswald, D., Ollendick, T., & Scahill, L. (2009). Anxiety in children and adolescents with autism spectrum disorders. *Clinical Psychology Review, 29,* 216–229.

Witwer, A., & Lecavalier, L. (2005). Treatment incidence and patterns in children and adolescents with autism spectrum disorders. *Journal of Child and Adolescent Psychopharmacology, 15,* 671–681.

Yi, J. I., Christian, L., Vittimberga, G., & Lowenkron, B. (2006). Generalized negatively reinforced manding in children with autism. *The Analysis of Verbal Behavior, 22,* 21–33.

Zentall, S. S., & Zentall, T. R. (1983). Optimal stimulation: A model of disordered activity and performance in normal and deviant children. *Psychological Bulletin, 94,* 446–471.

Chapter 7
Psychopathology

Vincent Pandolfi and Caroline I. Magyar

Overview of the Problem

Reports on psychopathology in individuals with autism spectrum disorder (ASD) have appeared since the first descriptions of ASD, dating back to the mid-1950s (see Clarke et al. 1999 for a review). Historically, debate among clinical researchers focused on whether specific psychopathologies contained in the Diagnostic and Statistical Manual of Mental Disorders (DSM) could occur in children with ASD and be reliably diagnosed using DSM criteria (see Volkmar and Klin 2005 for a discussion). One group favored the view that symptoms of some of the most common psychopathologies, such as anxiety and mood disorders, were part and parcel of the child's ASD and did not necessarily reflect a distinct co-occurring condition. Others asserted that children with ASD can present with one or more psychopathological conditions but that symptom presentation can be difficult to assess because of ASD and other co-occurring developmental conditions and impairments (e.g., intellectual disability, language impairment). The "gold standard" clinical interview approach typically used in psychiatric assessment may not be sufficient to accurately identify psychopathology in this population, particularly in those with co-occurring intellectual disability (e.g., see Deprey and Ozonoff 2009). Recent changes to the ASD diagnostic criteria, as defined in the DSM-5, aligns with the position that individuals with ASD can present with one or more emotional and behavioral psychopathologies and therefore, each disorder requires specification when rendering a diagnosis (APA 2013).

These changes to the ASD nosology align with clinical research indicating that a relatively high percentage of children with ASD evidence one or more

V. Pandolfi (✉)
Psychology Department, Rochester Institute of Technology, Rochester, NY, USA
e-mail: vxpgla@rit.edu

C. I. Magyar
Department of Pediatrics, University of Rochester Medical Center, Rochester, NY, USA

Johnny L. Matson (ed.), *Comorbid Conditions Among Children with Autism Spectrum Disorders,* Autism and Child Psychopathology Series,
DOI 10.1007/978-3-319-19183-6_7

emotional psychopathologies, with anxiety and mood disorders among the most common (Lainhart and Folstein 1994; MacNeil et al. 2009; Simonoff et al. 2008; van Steensel Bogels and Perin 2011) and they often co-occur with one or more behavior disorders (Simonoff et al. 2008; Weissman and Bates 2010). While research is accumulating within the area of co-morbid psychopathologies, considerably more work is needed to inform clinical practice. This is particularly relevant given the current prevalence estimate of 1 in 68 children in the USA are affected by ASD (Blumberg et al. 2013) and the consistent finding that the presence of one or more emotional psychopathologies can cause additional functional impairment over and above that caused by the ASD alone and may moderate a child's response to ASD-specific treatment (Kim et al. 2000). Collectively, these findings indicate the need for us to improve our understanding of the clinical presentation of psychopathology in ASD and to ascertain the most reliable assessment approach to improve early identification in order to inform treatment planning. This requires a conceptual approach to understand psychopathology in children with ASD and related conditions. Such a conceptualization should include consideration of the ongoing interaction of developmental and contextual factors over time that gives rise to emotional dysregulation and problem behaviors. This can allow professionals to more reliably diagnose psychopathology when facing a myriad of symptoms that can be related to ASD, other developmental problems, and/or psychopathology across the pediatric age span.

In this chapter, we present an overview of what is known about anxiety and mood disorders in children with ASD aged 5–21 years. These represent the two most common and best studied of the psychopathologies in this population. The chapter begins with a brief overview of the DSM-defined anxiety and mood disorders in the general pediatric population. This enables the reader to critically evaluate how the presence of ASD and related developmental conditions requires one to adopt a developmental psychopathology framework (see Cicchetti and Toth 2009) to understand how these disorders manifest in this population. A concise review of the empirical literature pertaining to anxiety and mood disorders in children with ASD follows, and the chapter ends with considerations for practice and directions for future research.

DSM-5 Anxiety and Mood Disorders in Children: Brief Overview

Anxiety and mood disorders are reported to be some of the most common emotional psychopathologies affecting children and they often co-occur with one another (APA 2013). Approximately 2–21 % of the children are reported to suffer from an anxiety disorder, with the prevalence rising with increasing amounts of time over which anxiety symptoms are counted (Foa et al. 2005). Approximately 1–3 % of children and 5–6 % of adolescents are reported to be affected by major depressive disorder (Klein et al. 2005). A diagnosis of either an anxiety or mood disorder elevates a child's risk for other co-occurring emotional and behavioral psychopathologies as well as for social, family, academic, and occupational problems (see AACAP 2007a, b). Early diagnosis and intervention are the keys to better outcomes. However, accurate identification of anxiety and mood disorders can be challenging especially in younger children because many lack the ability to identify and communicate personal phenomenology, an important component of the diagnostic assessment process. Similar issues are present when evaluating children with ASD, particularly if the child presents with intellectual disability (ID) and language impairment, regardless of chronological age.

Anxiety Disorders

The DSM-5 (APA 2013) specifies 11 anxiety disorders that share similar defining features including excessive anxiety, fear, and avoidance behavior. *Anxiety* refers to an unpleasant feeling state that occurs in anticipation of a future threat which includes cognitive, emotional, physiological, and behavioral symptoms. Cognitive characteristics can include catastrophic thinking, thoughts of self-doubt, self-criticism, overestimation of threat, and underestimation of one's ability to cope. Emotional symptoms include fear and trepidation. *Fear* refers to a feeling state related to a real or perceived imminent danger. It is recognized as an adaptive response to a realistic threat to one's well-being but is considered to be a *phobia* and part of an anxiety disorder when the level of one's fear is disproportionate to the threat that the fear source actually poses. Physiological features include hyperarousal, tension, stress, fatigue, restlessness, panic, and disturbed sleep. Behavioral symptoms include hypervigilance, frequent attempts at reassurance, and other behaviors that serve the function of avoiding or escaping from anxiety-producing situations such as tantrums and withdrawal. The anxiety disorders are distinguished from one another by the source of anxiety or fear, as well as the content of anxious thinking (APA 2013). These disorders are distinguished from normal variation in anxiety by their excessive and persistent nature and the effect they have on the child's functioning.

The DSM-5 arranges the anxiety disorders according to the typical age of onset. Separation anxiety disorder, selective mutism, and specific phobia typically appear in early and middle childhood. Social anxiety disorder, panic disorder, agoraphobia, generalized anxiety disorder, and substance/medication-induced anxiety disorder are more likely to appear during adolescence. Several other anxiety disorders are included in the DSM such as anxiety disorder due to another medical condition, other specified anxiety disorder, and unspecified anxiety disorder. A diagnosis of a specific anxiety disorder is made if a minimum number of symptoms are endorsed or observed for each of the disorders and if functional impairment and/or significant personal distress are present or reported.

Mood Disorders

Mood disorders are described across two categories within the DSM-5: bipolar and related disorders, and depressive disorders. Bipolar disorders include bipolar-I and bipolar-II and several other related disorders, including other specified and unspecified bipolar and related disorders. Bipolar-I is defined by at least one manic episode that may precede or follow a major depressive episode (APA 2013). The DSM-5 requires specification of the current or most recent episode, the severity/remission status, and other related difficulties that are not coded (e.g., with anxious distress, with mixed features). Bipolar-II is distinguished from bipolar-I by the experience of a hypomanic episode preceding or following a major depressive episode, but there cannot be a manic episode in the patient's history. Bipolar-II requires the specification of the current or most recent episode as hypomanic or depressed, severity specifiers, and additional non-coded specifiers similar to bipolar-I.

Depressive disorders share a common core set of clinical features including a sad or irritable mood accompanied by somatic and cognitive changes that impact the person's functioning (APA 2013). Depressive disorders include major depressive disorder, disruptive mood dysregulation disorder, persistent depressive disorder (Dysthymia), and several other disorders, including other specified and unspecified depressive disorders. The various depressive disorders are distinguished by their timing, duration, and presumed etiology. A diagnosis of major depressive disorder requires five or more symptoms to be present during a 2-week period that represents a change from the child's previous baseline level of functioning (APA 2013). Symptoms include depressed or irritable mood, markedly diminished interest or pleasure in activities, failure to make expected weight gain, agitation or psychomotor slowing, fatigue or lack of energy most days, feelings of worthlessness or guilt, difficulty thinking and concentrating or difficulty making a decision, and recurrent thoughts of death or suicidal ideation.

Correlates and Risk Factors

A variety of correlates and risk factors associated with developing one or more anxiety and mood disorders have been identified (see AACAP 2007a, b). These include: (a) biological factors such as genetics and brain abnormalities; (b) child specific factors such as a history of psychopathology, neurocognitive functioning, temperament, and adequacy of coping skills; and (c) contextual factors such as parent–child interactions, parental psychopathology, and significant life events. Considerations for assessing children within a developmental framework can assist clinicians in distinguishing age-typical anxiety and mood variations that may occur across contexts from psychopathology, and for identifying disorders across the pediatric age span (see AACAP 2007a; Albano et al. 2003; Hammen and Rudolph 2003). A child's ability to recognize and report on their personal phenomenology such as anxious and depressive cognitions and feelings is critical for accurate diagnosis. However, a child's ability to identify his or her emotions, cognitions, and the effect his or her behavior has on self and others depends on the child's age and the extent to which his or her cognitive, language, and communication skills are sufficiently developed. These developmental considerations for assessment are promulgated through numerous practice guidelines (e.g., AACAP 2007a, b).

Anxiety and Mood Disorders in Children with ASD

Prevalence

Prevalence rates for anxiety disorders in ASD range from 11 to 84 % (see White et al. 2009 for a review) with specific phobia, obsessive compulsive disorder, and social anxiety disorder among the most common (see van Steensel et al. 2011 for a review). Mood disorders are reported to occur in children with ASD with estimates ranging from around 1 % (Simonoff et al. 2008) to 38 % (Lainhart and Folstein 1994), with most studies examining depressive disorders and few investigating bipolar disorders (e.g. Joshi et al 2013; Weissman and Bates 2010).

Several challenges exist in ascertaining more accurate prevalence estimates for both anxiety and mood disorders in ASD. These include few population-based studies with adequate numbers representing the continuum of ASD impairments (Magnuson and Constantino 2011; Stewart et al. 2006; White et al. 2009). Most studies have included clinical samples. Relatively few studies used assessment protocols that included multiple methods of ascertainment (MacNeil et al. 2009; Magnuson and Constantino 2011) and reliable and valid measures of anxiety and mood disorders in ASD (e.g., see MacNeil et al. 2009; Mannion and Leader 2013; White et al. 2009). Other studies reported on "symptoms" of psychopathology or included case history reports that were not confirmed through a comprehensive diagnostic evaluation (e.g., Hess et al. 2010; White et al. 2009).

Correlates and Risk Factors

Various correlates and risk factors for anxiety and mood disorders have been examined with most studies examining one or more child and family factors. Child factors commonly investigated include age, cognitive level, and ASD severity. Family factors have included parental mental health problems (e.g., see Gadow et al. 2008) and parent–child interactions. Few studies have investigated contextual factors. Collectively, results are inconclusive within each area studied. With respect to rates of anxiety disorders, mixed findings have been reported for the most common variables studied and include age (cf. Hallett et al. 2013; Mayes et al. 2011a;

Strang et al. 2012; Ung et al. 2013; van Steensel et al. 2011; Vasa et al. 2013), IQ (cf. Eussen et al. 2012; Hallett et al. 2013; Mayes et al. 2011b; Mayes et al. 2011a; Mazurek and Kanne 2010; Strang et al. 2012; van Steensel et al. 2011; Vasa et al. 2013; Witwer and Lecavalier 2010), and ASD severity (cf. Eussen et al. 2012; Hallett et al. 2013; Mayes et al. 2011a; Mazurek and Kanne 2010; van Steensel et al. 2011). A few recent studies, however, have examined the relationship between anxiety and insistence on sameness (e.g., routines, rituals, hoarding, dislike of change, and circumscribed or restricted interests) and repetitive motor behaviors (e.g., pacing, spinning). Higher levels of anxiety were found to be related to higher levels of insistence on sameness (Lidstone et al. 2014; Rodgers et al. 2012) and symbolic expression of restricted interests through play, but not restricted interests manifest through the accumulation of facts, verbal memory, and learning (Spiker et al. 2012).

For mood disorders, age (e.g., Mayes et al. 2011; Vickerstaff et al. 2007), IQ (e.g., Mayes et al. 2011), ASD severity (e.g., Kanne et al. 2009; Mayes et al. 2011) and family history of mood disorders (e.g., Gadow et al. 2008; Ghaziuddin and Greden 1998; Joshi et al. 2013) have received the most attention, though the research in this area is much less relative to anxiety in ASD. Collectively, findings are also mixed and generally inconclusive. This appears to be related to various methodological issues within and across studies.

The methodological issues are numerous and apply to research on both anxiety and mood disorders in children with ASD. They include small sample sizes, recruitment bias, restricted ranges for various factors studied (particularly for IQ and age), use of one or more measures not validated in ASD samples for the dependent variable (i.e., mood disorder; van der Gaag et al. 1995) and predictors (risk/correlates; e.g., Gadow et al. 2008); and wide variability in how ASD severity has been defined (e.g., Kim et al. 2000), including type of repetitive behavior (Stratis and Lecavalier 2013), and receipt of special education services (e.g., Gadow et al. 2008). Moreover, the definition of anxiety and mood disorder varied widely across studies, ranging from DSM defined disorders to “mood symptoms” or “anxiety symptoms” defined in various ways. For example, some studies have considered a mood or anxiety disorder to be an elevation on one or two items on a scale measuring a wide variety of other emotional and behavioral problems (e.g., Mayes et al. 2011a). Others have considered an anxiety or mood disorder to be an elevation on a single measure that may or may not have been validated on ASD samples (e.g., see MacNeil et al. 2009 for a review; van der Gaag et al. 1995) or self-report of depressive symptoms as indicators of a mood disorder (e.g., Mazzone et al. 2013), with no independent confirmation by an experienced clinician using multiple valid methods of assessment (e.g., Kim et al. 2000).

The specific role of contextual factors in psychopathology in children with ASD has not received much attention. However, many have been considered for youth with ID and appear relevant to children with ASD. These include trauma, abuse, deprivation, accidents, life transitions such as changes in residence and school placements, stressful life events such divorce or the death of loved ones, limited opportunities for socialization and play, limited freedom to make choices, and bullying (see

Cooray et al. 2007; Stavrakaki and Lunsky 2007; Zablotsky et al. 2013). Contextual factors may result in temporary changes in affect and mood particularly for those children with limited or poorly developed functional communication, coping, and social problem-solving skills (Magnuson and Constantino 2011). These temporary changes should be monitored because without adequate family and professional supports, children with ASD with or without ID often have difficulty dealing with contextual factors that increase the risk for psychopathology.

Conceptualizing Anxiety and Mood Disorders in ASD

The developmental psychopathology framework is useful for assisting clinicians in conceptualizing the nature of anxiety and mood disorders in children with ASD. It provides guidance for evaluating the relative risk for psychopathology in the presence of the various neurodevelopmental and contextual factors associated with ASD. The problems related to social-communication and language impairments and co-occurring ID are well known to those who work regularly with this population. However, co-occurring medical problems such as hypothyroidism, seizure disorders, gastrointestinal disorders, and pain, as well as medication side effects may also be related to the onset of emotional problems (Hurley et al. 2007; Tonge 2007). These neurodevelopmental and medical factors may moderate the presentation of anxiety and mood symptoms and make it hard for clinicians to ascertain the nature of the child's problem. They may even attribute problems to the ASD and not a co-occurring emotional disorder, a situation referred to as diagnostic overshadowing (Reiss et al. 1982).

Numerous examples of how developmental and related factors are related to the risk, onset, and maintenance of psychopathology are evident. For example, impaired social-communication and cognition can challenge the child's ability to identify and report on feelings and personal problems. The presence of ID within the context of ASD can compromise the child's ability to understand his/her personal phenomenology and expectations regarding conventional standards of behavior. ID limits one's ability to solve the problems and apply coping skills to regulate emotions and behavior. In those children with higher full scale IQ's (i.e., ≥ 70) uneven cognitive profiles can similarly affect functioning. Language impairments can compromise the child's ability to use language to alleviate anxiety and mood symptoms (e.g., using self-instructions, coping statements), and articulation problems related to oral-motor impairments can prevent a child from effectively communicating his or her needs. Finally, children with ID may present with behaviors that are atypical for their chronological age but may reflect a typical developmental progression or stage in younger children without ID (e.g., separation anxiety, poor attention span, understanding of right versus wrong, fantasy play, self-talk; Hurley et al. 2007). This may challenge the child's ability to function well among same age peers, and to meet school- and community-based expectations for behavior.

Clinical Presentation of Anxiety and Mood Disorders in Children with ASD

The presentation of anxiety in children with ASD may differ from its presentation in the general pediatric population because of the previously noted developmental factors. Signs and symptoms may be moderated by the child's age, cognitive level, and ASD symptom severity. Children with mild to moderate ID are more likely to present symptoms of anxiety similarly to those in the general population (Tonge 2007). The clinical presentation of those with severe to profound ID may differ from the DSM criteria to a greater extent because these children may not be able to identify and communicate subjective symptoms, or express anxious thinking in a manner that is understandable to others (see also Matson and Nebel-Schwalm 2007).

The extent to which any child's symptoms will be moderated by neurodevelopmental factors is hard to predict; however, the ways in which they might be moderated have been identified. Symptoms related to anxiety may be nonspecific, characterized in part by behavior problems such as aggression, self-injury, agitation, sleep problems, and changes in baseline levels of ASD symptoms such as stereotypies. Such behaviors are often the main reason for referral to mental health professionals. Although some have advocated for using behavioral equivalents for DSM criteria, this remains a controversial topic. Indeed, Witwer and Lecavalier (2010) recently found little support for the use of behavioral equivalents when assessing for psychopathology in youth with ASD.

Some evidence suggests that children with ASD may differ from the general population with respect to the fear sources of specific phobia (Evans et al. 2005). For example, children with ASD may fear loud noises, thunderstorms, medical settings/visits, or specific objects (e.g., toilet bowls) to a greater extent than same-age non-ASD peers. In generalized anxiety disorder, one displays chronic and persistent worry about a number of life issues or events and often worries about more than one thing at a time. Because of their executive dysfunction, children with ASD and co-occurring generalized anxiety disorder may focus on their anxiety-related issues sequentially, or one at a time, rather than focusing on many issues simultaneously. Symptoms may not be age-typical, such as emotional "meltdowns" or tantrums by teenagers under acute stress. An exaggeration of baseline symptoms often coincides with the onset of psychopathology in children with ASD and should be seen as a reason for a diagnostic evaluation.

Finally, there may be apparent symptom overlap between ASD and the anxiety disorders even though recent statistical analyses indicated that anxiety and ASD represent two independent constructs (Renno and Wood 2013). For example, distinguishing between obsessive-compulsive disorder (OCD) and ASD is a difficult diagnostic challenge. Although it is not placed in the DSM-5 anxiety disorders section, OCD is often accompanied by anxiety. When considering a diagnosis of OCD, the clinician needs to discriminate between: (a) OCD-related obsessions and ASD-related preoccupations and interests, and (b) OCD-related compulsions and ASD-related repetitive behaviors. In OCD, obsessions are generally perceived as intrusive and are anxiety provoking. Compulsions are performed specifically to alleviate the anxiety. The ASD-related preoccupations and intense interests are usually perceived as positive, stimulating, and often entertaining. The repetitive behaviors are not necessarily performed to relieve anxiety, but are often automatically reinforcing and have a "feel good" quality so there may be no desire to stop or control them. One can see how neurodevelopmental problems can make differential diagnosis very difficult.

The clinical features of a mood disorder in children with ASD are reported to be similar to the general population, but ASD and related impairments may moderate some symptom expression (e.g., Joshi et al. 2013; Lainhart 1999). Affective changes may include increased irritability and labile mood (Magnuson and Constantino 2011). The child may present with changes in the frequency, intensity, duration, and topography of ASD symptoms (Lainhart 1999). Examples may include increased agitation and repetitive behavior (e.g., Lainhart and Folstein 1994) and shifts in circumscribed interests to negatively themed content (e.g., death, violence; McPheeters et al. 2011). In addition, the presence of a mood disorder has been associated with other emotional disorders (e.g., anxiety disorders), with various behavioral disorders (e.g., ADHD; e.g., Simonoff et al. 2008; Weissman and Bates 2010), with regression in functioning (e.g., Bradley and Bolton 2006), and with the onset or worsening of behavior problems such as aggression (e.g., Bradley and Bolton 2006; Magnuson and Constantino 2011). These findings highlight the importance of evaluating the child relative to his/her personal baseline (Magnuson and Constantino 2011) and within the context of the child's ASD symptom and developmental profile.

Considerations for Assessment

The complex neurodevelopmental characteristics of children with ASD, and our need for more research in psychopathology within this population present diagnostic challenges. Traditionally, these anxiety and mood disorders are identified through clinical interview which is considered best practice in the assessment of these conditions (AACAP 2007a, b). The neurodevelopmental characteristics of ASD such as impaired communication skills and difficulty with self-awareness can compromise the child's ability to participate in a diagnostic interview, and to recognize and convey feelings of anxiety, fear, worry, sadness, hopelessness, and guilt. Moreover, a lack of or impaired facial expression often observed in individuals with ASD can make ascertainment of mood and affect difficult upon clinical observation. Additionally, given the relative paucity of reliable and valid measures for evaluating emotional disorders in children with ASD and the lack of evidence-based assessment guidelines for assisting clinicians in differential diagnosis, anxiety and mood disorders may be under-identified or delayed in identification and therefore, warrant a high degree of vigilance, particularly during adolescence when some with ASD may start to show symptoms as they begin to understand the extent of their disability (Tantam 2003). Until specific evidence-based assessment guidelines for children with ASD are adopted by the clinical community, general best practice assessment guidelines seem appropriate.

Pandolfi and Magyar (2014) and Magyar and Pandolfi (2012) discuss a framework for assessment which should include surveillance, screening, and progress monitoring. The protocol includes multiple methods and informants, including record review, interviews of the primary caregivers and other involved third parties (e.g., teachers), child interview (where appropriate), direct clinical observation, and rating scales that have adequate psychometric support for use in ASD samples. Data collection should target all relevant contexts in which the child functions (i.e., home, school, and community) to identify both baseline and current levels of both ASD-related and psychopathology-related signs and symptoms. Functional behavioral assessment (FBA) is particularly warranted if behavior problems such as aggression and self-injury are present as these may represent nonspecific indicators of the child's personal distress. Regardless of whether such behaviors are related to the presence of an underlying anxiety or mood disorder, they would be additional targets for intervention.

Because children with ASD receive primary intervention in the school setting, with ancillary care from one or more community professionals, each provider will play an important role in identifying an emerging problem early in order to intervene accordingly. This home-school-community collaborative model is consistent with the basic premise of the medical home (American Academy of Pediatrics 2002) and with recommended practice in the educational setting (Magyar and Pandolfi 2012). Children with ASD will need to be routinely monitored by school personnel and primary care providers specifically for changes in baseline that may signal the onset of an anxiety or mood disorder. Specifically for mood disorders, Magnuson and Constantino 2011 suggested monitoring for increasingly negative affect and/or an increase in sadness, tearfulness, and apathy. A loss of or diminished interest in preferred activities may also indicate changes in mood, particularly if coupled with an increase in the frequency or duration of repetitive behaviors and nonfunctional routines. Changes in sleep from the child's typical baseline should also be noted, and any regression in skills or decline in performance should be monitored. The same general approach applies to anxiety disorders, monitoring for anxiety-specific symptoms should also be accompanied by assessment for changes in nonspecific and ASD-related symptoms. Multiple informants using validated rating scales and diagnostic interviews is again recommended which can be helpful in resolving discrepancies between child and parent report, and to determine the extent to which anxiety symptoms are related to specific contexts (see White, Schry and Maddox 2012). As noted earlier in this chapter, clinicians should be familiar with the fact that the sources of fear and anxiety, as well as anxiety expression may not be age-typical.

Considerations for Treatment

A review of the treatment literature indicates little investigation into psychosocial treatments for both anxiety and mood disorders in ASD. For anxiety disorders, a recent meta-analysis indicated that cognitive-behavioral therapy (CBT) may be effective for children with ASD (see Sukhodolsky et al. 2013). It was noted that only eight studies were reviewed of children aged 7–17 years who were mostly boys and with IQ's of 70 or higher. Successful application of CBT will likely require modifications that take into account child developmental factors and learning styles. Addressing both anxiety and ASD symptoms (such as functional communication impairment, social skills deficits), incorporating visual supports, parent involvement, and modifications to the format and pace of therapy should all be considered (see Selles and Storch 2013). More research is also needed to evaluate the efficacy of medication for the treatment of anxiety disorders. Although Selective serotonin Reuptake Inhibitors (SSRI's) have demonstrated efficacy for the treatment of anxiety in the general pediatric population, no medications have FDA approval specifically for the treatment of anxiety in children with ASD (Selles and Storch 2013). Most evidence for the treatment of anxiety was derived through case studies, chart reviews, and open label trials (Selles and Storch 2013).

Psychopharmacological treatment has received the most attention with respect to mood disorders. Treatment focuses on symptom reduction, but there is limited evidence for efficacy in the ASD population (Siegel and Beaulieu 2011). Two recent case reports have shown that electroconvulsive shock therapy may hold promise for refractory bipolar disorder with severe challenging behavior (Siegel et al. 2012). Clearly, more work is needed in this area.

Considerations for Future Research

Study of co-occurring emotional psychopathology in children with ASD appears to be steadily increasing. Unfortunately, key barriers to expanding on what is known about psychopathology in this population must be addressed. Two major ones are intertwined: (a) the identification of appropriate diagnostic criteria for youth with ASD that are informed by theory and empirical data, and (b) the use of assessment measures that have been validated for children with ASD. Because theory influences the development of assessment measures, and research that utilizes such measures influences the ongoing refinement of theory, both issues need to be addressed simultaneously in order to advance our understanding of psychopathology in ASD.

The lack of an empirically established operational definition of anxiety and mood disorders in ASD represents a pivotal methodological issue in the study of these disorders in ASD (e.g., Gadow et al. 2012). Having a clear definition of anxiety and mood disorders in ASD including the extent to which specific disorders are similar to the general population with respect to phenomenology and how ASD and related developmental factors may moderate symptom presentation across gender, age, and functioning level are critical issues to be resolved. Such information will help inform both the development of new reliable and valid measures and the evaluation of currently used measures for the various purposes of assessment which include screening, diagnosis, progress monitoring, and outcome evaluation.

The conceptual and measurement issues that need to be resolved likely contribute to methodological differences across studies of anxiety and mood disorders in children with ASD. These include differences in participant characteristics, sampling methods used for participant selection, and assessment measures. Perhaps it is not surprising that we see mixed findings pertaining to prevalence estimates, correlates and risk factors, and the nature of psychopathology in this population. Much more work is needed to evaluate the effect of context on psychopathology and the longitudinal course of anxiety and mood disorders. Until more work is done to bridge gaps in the conceptualization and measurement of psychopathology, researchers and consumers of psychopathology research in ASD should consider the extent to which selected measures are appropriate in content given the authors' conceptualization of the disorder(s) in question. They should also evaluate the extent to which reliability and validity data are reported for the study sample.

Finally, more work is needed to evaluate the psychotherapeutic interventions for both anxiety and mood disorders. Efficacy should be evaluated across gender, age, and developmental levels and more consistent use of validated measures for subject characterization and outcome assessment are critical. The extent to which therapies such as CBT need to be modified for successfully addressing problematic cognitions, behavior, and physiological and emotional dysregulation awaits further study.

The research literature to date suggests that anxiety and mood disorders are relatively common in children with ASD. Although much more needs to be learned, the variables that have been studied to date that affect the risk and manifestation of psychopathology should be routinely assessed by clinicians and considered during treatment planning. A broadly focused approach to assessment and treatment is indicated until more specific data are available. Advances in research can greatly inform clinical practice, and perhaps more importantly, improve the lives of children with ASD and their families.

References

Albano, A. M., Chorpita, B. F., & Barlow, D. H. (2003). Childhood anxiety disorders. In E. J. Mash & R. A. Barkley (Eds.), *Child psychopathology*, 2nd ed (pp. 279–329). New York: Guilford.

American Academy of Child & Adolescent Psychiatry. (2007a). Practice parameter for the assessment and treatment of children and adolescents with anxiety disorders. *Journal of the American Academy of Child and Adolescent Psychiatry, 46*(2), 267–283.

American Academy of Child & Adolescent Psychiatry. (2007b). Practice parameter for the assessment and treatment of children and adolescents with depressive disorders. *Journal of the American Academy of Child and Adolescent Psychiatry, 46*(11), 1503–1526.

American Academy of Pediatrics. (2002). The medical home. *Pediatrics, 110,* 184–186.

American Psychiatric Association. (2013). *Diagnostic and statistical manual of mental disorders* (5th edn.). Washington, D.C.: Author.

Blumberg, S. J., Bramlett, M. D., Kogan, M. D., Schieve, L. A., Jones, J. R., & Lu, M. D. (2013). *Changes in prevalence of parent-reported autism spectrum disorder in school-aged U.S. children: 2007 to 2011–2012. National health statistics report, no 65*. Hyattsville: National Center for Health Statistics.

Bradley, E., & Bolton, P. (2006). Episodic psychiatric disorders in teenagers with learning disabilities with and without autism. *The British Journal of Psychiatry, 189,* 361–366. doi:10.1192/bip.bp.105.018127.

Cicchetti, D., & Toth, S. L. (2009). The past achievements and future promises of developmental psychopathology: The coming of age of a discipline. *Journal of Child Psychology and Psychiatry, 50*(1–2), 16–25.

Clarke, D., Baxter, M., Perry, D., & Prasher, V. (1999). The diagnosis of affective and psychotic disorders in adults with autism: Seven case reports. *Autism: The International Journal of Research and Practice, 3,* 149–164. doi:10.1177/1362361399003002005.

Cooray, S., Gabriel, S., & Gaus, V. (2007). Anxiety disorders. In R. Fletcher, E. Loschen, C. Stavrakaki, & M. First (Eds.), *Diagnostic manual- intellectual disability: A textbook of diagnosis of mental disorders in persons with intellectual disability* (pp. 317–348). Kingston: National Association for the Dually Diagnosed.

Deprey, L., & Ozonoff, S. (2009). Assessment of comorbid psychiatric conditions in autism spectrum disorders. In S. Goldstein, J. A. Naglieri, & S. Ozonoff (Eds.), *Assessment of autism spectrum disorders* (pp. 290–317). New York: Guilford.

Eussen, M. L. J. M., van Gool, A. R., Verheij, F., de Nijs, P. F. A., Verhulst, F. C., & Greaves-Lord, K. (2012). The association of quality of social relations, symptom severity and intelligence with anxiety in children with autism spectrum disorders. *Autism: the International Journal of Research and Practice, 17*(6), 723–735. doi:10.1177/1362361312453882.

Evans, D. W., Canavera, K., Kleinpeter, F. L., Maccubbin, E., & Taga, K. (2005). The fears, phobias and anxieties of children with autism spectrum disorders and down syndrome: Comparisons with developmentally and chronologically age matched children. *Child Psychiatry and Human Development, 36,* 3–26.

Foa, E. B., Costello, E. J., Franklin, M., Kagan, J., Kendall, P., Klein, R., & Spear, L. (2005). Defining anxiety disorders. In D. L. Evans, E. B. Foa, R. E. Gur, H. Hendin, C. P. O'Brien, M. E. P. Seligman, & B. T. Walsh (Eds.), *Treating and preventing adolescent mental health disorders: What we know and what we don't know. a research agenda for improving the mental health of our youth* (pp. 162–182). New York: Oxford University Press.

Gadow, K. D., DeVincent, C., & Schneider, J. (2008). Predictors of psychiatric symptoms in children with an autism spectrum disorder. *Journal of Autism and Developmental Disorders, 38,* 1710–1720. doi:10.1007/s10803-008-0556-8.

Gadow, K. D., Guttmann-Steinmetz, S., Rieffe, C., & DeVincent, C. J. (2012). Depression symptoms in boys with autism spectrum disorder and comparison samples. *Journal of Autism and Developmental Disorders, 42,* 1353–1363. doi:10.1007/s10803-011-1367x.

Ghaziuddin, M., & Greden, J. F. (1998). Depression in children with autism/pervasive developmental disorders: A case-control family history study. *Journal of Autism and Developmental Disorders, 28,* 111–115.

Hallett, V., Lecavalier, L., Sukhodolsky, D. G., Cipriano, N., Aman, M. G., McCracken, J. T., & Scahill, L. (2013). Exploring the manifestations of anxiety in children with autism spectrum disorders. *Journal of Autism and Developmental Disorders, 43,* 2341–2352. doi:10.1007/s10803-013-1775-1.

Hammen, C., & Rudolph, K. D. (2003). Childhood mood disorders. In E. J. Mash, & R. A. Barkley (Eds.), *Child psychopathology, 2nd Ed* (pp. 233–278). New York: Guilford.

Hess, J. A., Matson, J. L., & Dixon, D. R. (2010). Psychiatric symptom endorsement in children and adolescents diagnosed with autism spectrum disorders: A comparison to typically developing children and adolescents. *Journal of Developmental and Physical Disability, 22,* 485–496. doi:10.1007/s10882-009-9185-1.

Hurley, A. D., Levitas, A., Lecavalier, L., & Pary, R. J. (2007). Assessment and diagnostic procedures. In R. Fletcher, E. Loschen, C. Stavrakaki, & M. First (Eds.), *Diagnostic manual-intellectual disability: A textbook of diagnosis of mental disorders in persons with intellectual disability* (pp. 11–31). Kingston: National Association for the Dually Diagnosed.

Joshi, G., Biederman, J., Petty, C., Goldin, R., Furtak, S. L., & Wozniak, J. (2013). Examining the comorbidity of bipolar disorder and autism spectrum disorder: A large controlled analysis if phenotypic and familial correlates in a referred population of youth with bipolar I disorder with and without autism spectrum disorder. *Journal of Clinical Psychiatry, 74,* 578–586. doi:10.4088/JCP.12 m07392.

Kim, J. A., Szatmari, P., Bryson, S. E., Streiner, D. L., & Wilson, F. J. (2000). The prevalence of anxiety and mood problems among children with autism and Asperger syndrome. *Autism: The International Journal of Research and Practice, 4,* 117–132.

Klein, D. N., Dougherty, L. R., & Olino, T. M. (2005). Toward guidelines for evidence-based assessment of depression in children and adolescents. *Journal of Clinical Child and Adolescent Psychology, 34*(3), 412–432.

Lainhart, J. E. (1999). Psychiatric problems in individuals with autism, their parents and siblings. *International Review of Psychiatry, 11,* 278–298.

Lainhart, J. E., & Folstein, S. (1994). Affective disorders in people with autism: A review of published cases. *Journal of Autism and Developmental Disorders, 24,* 587–601.

Lidstone, J., Uljarevic, M., Sullivan, J., Rodgers, J., McConachie, H., Freeston, M., & Leekam, S. (2014). Relations among restricted and repetitive behaviors, anxiety, and sensory features in children with autism spectrum disorders. *Research in Autism Spectrum Disorders, 8,* 82–92. doi:10.1016/j.rasd.2013.10.001.

MacNeil, B. M., Lopes, V. A., Minnes, P. M. (2009). Anxiety in children and adolescents with autism spectrum disorders. *Research in Autism Spectrum Disorders, 3,* 1–21. doi:10.1016/j.rasd.2008.06.001.

Magnuson, K. M., & Constantino, J. N. (2011). Characterization of depression in children with autism spectrum disorders. *Journal of Developmental & Behavioral Pediatrics, 32,* 332–340.

Magyar, C. I., & Pandolfi, V. (2012). Considerations for establishing a multi-tiered problem-solving model for students with autism and emotional-behavioral disorders. *Psychology in the Schools, Special Edition, 49,* 975–987. doi:10.1002/pits.21645.

Mannion, A., & Leader, G. (2013). Comorbidity in autism spectrum disorder: A literature review. *Research in Autism Spectrum Disorders, 7,* 1595–1616. doi:10.1016/j.rasd.2013.09.006.

Matson, J. L., & Nebel-Schwalm, M. S. (2007). Comorbid psychopathology with autism spectrum disorder in children: An overview. *Research in Developmental Disabilities, 28,* 341–352.

Mayes, S. D., Calhoun, S.L., Murray, M.J., & Zahid, J. (2011a). Variables associated with anxiety and depression in children with autism. *Journal of Developmental and Physical Disabilities, 23,* 325–337. doi:10.1007/s10882-011-9231-7.

Mayes, S. D., Calhoun, S. L., Murray, M. J., Ahuja, M., & Smith, L. A. (2011b). Anxiety, depression, and irritability in children with autism relative to other neuropsychiatric disorders and typical development. *Research in Autism Spectrum Disorders, 5,* 474–485. doi:10.1016/j.rasd.2010.06.012.

Mazurek, M.O., & Kanne, S.M. (2010). Friendship and internalizing symptoms among children and adolescents with ASD, *Journal of Autism and Developmental Disorders,* 40, 1512-1520.

Mazzone, L., Postorino, V., DePeppo, L., Fatta, L., Lucarelli, V., Reale, L., & Vicari, S. (2013). Mood symptoms in children and adolescents with autism spectrum disorders. *Research in Developmental Disabilities, 34,* 3699–3708. doi:10.1016/j.ridd.2013.07.034.

McPheeters, M. L., Davis, A., Navarre, J. R., & Scott, T. A. (2011). Family report of ASD concomitant with depression or anxiety among US children. *Journal of Autism and Developmental Disorders, 41,* 646–653. doi:10.1007/s10803-010-1085-9.

Pandolfi, V., & Magyar, C.I. (2014). Assessment of co-occurring emotional and behavioral disorders in youth with ASD using the child behavior checklist 6–18. In V. B. Patel, V. R. Preedy, & C. R. Martin (Eds.), *The comprehensive guide to autism*. New York: Springer.

Reiss, S., Levitan, G. W., & Syzsko, J. (1982). Emotional disturbance and mental retardation: Diagnostic overshadowing. *American Journal of Mental Deficiency, 86,* 567–574.

Renno, P., & Wood, J. J. (2013). Discriminant and convergent validity of the anxiety construct in children with autism spectrum disorders. *Journal of Autism and Developmental Disorders, 43,* 2135–2146. doi:10.1007/s10803-013-1767-1.

Rodgers, J., Glod, M., Connolly, B., & McConachie, H. (2012). The relationship between anxiety and repetitive behaviours in autism spectrum disorder. *Journal of Autism and Developmental Disorders, 42,* 2404–2409. doi:10.1007/s10803-012-1531-y.

Selles, R. R., & Storch, E. A. (2013). Translation of anxiety treatment to youth with autism spectrum disorders. *Journal of Child and Family Studies, 22,* 405–413. doi:10.1007/s10826-012-9593-1.

Siegel, M., & Beaulieu, A. (2011). Psychotropic medications in children with autism spectrum disorders: A systematic review and synthesis for evidence-based practice. *Journal of Autism and Developmental Disorders, 42,* 1592–1605. doi:10.1007/s10803-011-1399-2.

Siegel, M., Milligan, B., Robbins, D., & Prentice, G. (2012). Electroconvulsive therapy in an adolescent with autism and bipolar I disorder. *Journal of Electroconvulsive Therapy, 28,* 252–255. doi:10.1097/YCT.0b013e31825cec86.

Simonoff, E., Pickles, A., Charman, T., Chandler, S., Loucas, T., & Baird, G. (2008). Psychiatric disorders in children with autism spectrum disorders: Prevalence, comorbidity, and associated factors in a population-derived sample. *Journal of the American Academy of Child and Adolescent Psychiatry, 47,* 921–929. doi:10.1097/CHI.0b013e3181799644f.

Spiker, M. A., Lin, C. E., van Dyke, M., Wood, J. J. (2012). Restricted interests and anxiety in children with autism. *Autism: The International Journal of Research and Practice, 16*(3), 306–320. doi:10.1177/1362361311401763.

Stavrakaki, C., & Lunsky, Y. (2007). Depression, anxiety, and adjustment disorders in people with intellectual disabilities. In N. Bouras, & G. Holt (Eds.), *Psychiatric and behavioural disorders in intellectual and developmental disabilities* (2nd edn., pp. 113–130). New York: Cambridge.

Stewart, M. E., Barnard, L., Pearson, J., Hasan, R., & O'Brien, G. (2006). Presentation of depression in autism and Asperger syndrome: A review. *Autism: The International Journal of Research and Practice, 10,* 103–116. doi:10.1177/1362361306062013.

Strang, J. F., Kenworthy, L., Daniolos, P., Case, L., Wills, M. C., Martin, A., et al. (2012). Depression and anxiety symptoms in children and adolescents with autism spectrum disorders without intellectual disability. *Research in Autism Spectrum Disorders, 6,* 406–412. doi:10.1016/j.rasd.2011.06.015.

Stratis, W. A., & Lecavalier, L. (2013). Restricted and repetitive behaviors and psychiatric symptoms in youth with autism spectrum disorders. *Research in Autism Spectrum Disorders, 7,* 757–766. doi:10.1016/j.rasd.2013.017.

Sukhodolsky, D. G., Bloch, M. H., Panza, K. E., & Reichow, B. (2013). Cognitive-behavioral therapy for anxiety in children with high-functioning autism: A meta-analysis. *Pediatrics, 132*(5), 1341–1350.

Tantam, D. (2003). The challenge of adolescents and adults with Asperger syndrome. *Child and Adolescent Psychiatric Clinics of North America, 12,* 143–163.

Tonge, B. (2007). The psychopathology of children with intellectual disabilities. In N. Bouras & G. Holt (Eds.), *Psychiatric and behavioural disorders in intellectual and developmental disabilities, 2nd Ed* (pp. 93–112). New York: Cambridge.

Ung, D., Wood, J. J., Ehrenreich-May, J., Arnold, E. B., Fujii, C., Renno, P., & Storch, E. A. (2013). *Neuropsychiatry, 3*(2), 147–157.

van der Gaag, R. J., Buitelaar, J., van den Ban, E., Bezemer, M., Njio, L., & van Engeland, H. (1995). A controlled multivariate chart review of multiple complex developmental disorder. *Journal of American Academy of Child and Adolescent Psychiatry, 34,* 1096–1106.

Vasa, R. A., Kalb, L., Mazurek, M., Kanne, S., Freedman, B., Keefer, A., & Murray, D. (2013). Age-related differences in the prevalence and correlates of anxiety in youth with autism spectrum disorders. *Research in Autism Spectrum Disorders, 7,* 1358–1369. doi:10.1016/j.rasd.2013.07.005.

van Steensel, F. J. A., Bogels, S. M., & Perrin, S. (2011). Anxiety disorders in children and adolescents with autism spectrum disorders: A meta-analysis. *Clinical Child and Family Psychology Review, 14,* 302–317. doi:10.1007/s10567-011-0097-0.

Vickerstaff, S., Heriot, S., Wong, M., Lopes, A., & Dossetor, D. (2007). Intellectual ability, self-perceived social competence and depressive symptomatology in children with high-functioning autistic spectrum disorders. *Journal of Autism and Developmental Disorders, 37,* 1647–1644. doi:10.1007/s10803-006-0292-x.

Volkmar, F. R., & Klin, A. (2005). Issues in the classification of autism and related conditions. In F. R. Volkmar, A. Klin, R. Paul, & D. J. Cohen (Eds.), *Handbook of autism and pervasive developmental disorders*, 3rd Ed (pp. 5–41). Hoboken, NJ: Wiley.

Weissman, A. S., & Bates, M. E. (2010). Increased clinical and neurocognitive impairment in children with autism spectrum disorders and comorbid bipolar disorder. *Research in Autism Spectrum Disorders, 4,* 670–680. doi:10.1016/j.rasd.2010.01.005.

White, S.W., Oswald, D., Ollendick, T., & Scahill, L. (2009). Anxiety in children and adolescents with autism spectrum disorders. *Clinical Psychology Review, 29,* 216–229. doi:10.1016/j.cpr.2009.01.003.

White, S. W., Schry, A. R., & Maddox, B. B. (2012). Brief report: The assessment of anxiety in high-functioning adolescents with autism spectrum disorder. *Journal of Autism and Developmental Disorders, 42,* 1138–1145. doi:10.1007/s10803-011-1353-3.

Witwer, A. N., & Lecavalier, L. (2010). Validity of comorbid psychiatric disorders in youngsters with autism spectrum disorders. *Journal of Developmental and Physical Disabilities, 22,* 367–380. doi:10.1007/s10882-010-9194-0.

Zablotsky, B., Bradshaw, C. P., Anderson, C., & Law, P. A. (2013). The association between bullying and the psychological functioning of children with autism spectrum disorders. *Journal of Developmental and Behavioral Pediatrics, 34,* 1–8.

Chapter 8
Feeding Disorders

Jill C. Fodstad, Sandra McCourt, Lisa R. Minor and Noha F. Minshawi

Introduction

Feeding (and relatively eating) is an essential and highly complex behavior. Feeding requires the integration of numerous aspects of developmental, environmental or setting-specific contexts, and physiology; all systems which need to work simultaneously in order to achieve a successful outcome. The act of feeding oneself or being fed by another (e.g., caregiver) is a noble social activity. This often requires a positive relationship between each other, whether that is with the feeder of a nonself feeder or with peers or others during mealtime for the self-feeder. When one or more of the prerequisites for successful feeding (e.g., swallowing reflex, gastrointestinal/gut motility, and appetite) are delayed, dysfunctional, disturbed, or absent, significant problems may occur. Medical conditions, feeder–child relationship or other social problems, and structural abnormalities of the mouth or tongue can lead separately or together to the final common pathway of problems in feeding. Given the wide range of associated variables and the heterogeneous nature of feeding problems, successful assessment and treatment of these conditions require an integrated, multidisciplinary approach.

In view of the complexity of feeding behavior, it is perhaps not surprising that feeding problems are relatively common in young children. Mealtime difficulties can occur in children, who are typically developing, those diagnosed with a developmental delay, and those who have a whole range of medical conditions. The term *feeding problems* typically refers to some pattern of oral or enteral consumption of nutrients that deviate from the norm enough to lead to negative social or health consequences. In general, feeding difficulties are typically considered to be problematic when they interfere with the individual's social integration or the family's

J. C. Fodstad (✉) · S. McCourt · L. R. Minor · N. F. Minshawi
Department of Psychiatry, Indiana University School of Medicine, 355 W. 16th Street, Indianapolis, IN, 46202 USA
e-mail: jfodstad@iupui.edu

Johnny L. Matson (ed.), *Comorbid Conditions Among Children with Autism Spectrum Disorders,* Autism and Child Psychopathology Series,
DOI 10.1007/978-3-319-19183-6_8

daily routine (Nadon et al. 2011). Feeding problems can vary by etiology, behavioral topography, and severity. Thus, germane to our discussion are severe feeding difficulties associated with an inadequate amount of nutrients consumed and/or extensive weight abnormalities (loss or gain) which are life-threatening and do not cede without intense intervention (Babbitt et al. 1994).

While feeding problems are most often associated with childhood, one population that appears to be at a high risk for feeding disorders and other mealtime difficulties throughout the lifespan are those with autism spectrum disorder (ASD). As detailed in previous chapters, ASD is a lifelong neurodevelopmental disorder with heterogeneous symptom presentation (Matson et al. 1996; Nicholson and Stzatmari 2003). ASD is characterized by clinically significant deficits in social and communication behavior, as well as the presence of repetitive behaviors, restricted interests, and/or sensory abnormalities (APA 2013). Researchers have noted that comorbid psychiatric conditions such as cognitive impairment, mood lability, anxiety, and behavioral disorders occur among individuals with ASD at higher rates than in the general population (Konst and Matson 2014; Matson and Nebel-Schwalm 2007). ASD and comorbid conditions often covary with each other, presenting an interactive effect which places individuals at even greater risk for additional difficulties (Holden and Gittlesen 2008; Matson et al. 2005a).

Feeding problems have long been reported as a common comorbid problem for individuals with ASD. In fact, Leo Kanner included feeding problems as a defining feature in the first modern description of ASD (Kanner 1943). Through his initial descriptions of 11 children, Kanner listed difficulties with food and dysfunctional mealtime behaviors occurring in over half (i.e., 6 out of 11) of those observed. Current conceptualization of ASD as per the *Diagnostic and Statistical Manual of Mental Disorders, 5th edition* (DSM-5; APA 2013) and *International Classification of Diseases, 10th edition* (ICD-10; World Health Organization (WHO; 2010) criteria do not include feeding difficulties as a necessary criterion for an ASD diagnosis, nor has previous diagnostic conceptualizations of the disorder (DSM-IV-TR; APA 2000) included this in their diagnostic conceptualizations. Despite the omission of these difficulties in diagnostic symptomatology, clinicians and caregivers have continued to suggest that aberrant feeding and mealtime problems are present in a substantial number of individuals with ASD. Among the most commonly described aberrant feeding and mealtime behavior issues described for those with an ASD include restricted food intake, selectivity or strong preferences for foods or textures, and ritualized eating patterns (Matson et al. 2009a; Schreck and Williams 2006; Sharp et al. 2013). These feeding difficulties could potentially be related to core symptoms of ASD such as circumscribed or restricted patterns of behaviors or interests, need for sameness, hyper- or hyposensitivities to sensory stimulation, or limited flexibility in routines (Johnson et al. 2014; Matson et al. 2009a; Nadon et al. 2011); however, environmental and medical/physiological factors may also contribute to the presence and maintenance of feeding dysfunctions (Piazza et al. 2003; Rommel et al. 2003). Regardless of the cause or potential interaction of all contributing variables, all of these issues require systematic evaluation and consideration if interventions are to be effective.

The purpose of the present chapter is to review the nature of feeding development and feeding problems. Development of feeding skills in typical development will be reviewed in order to highlight the complexity of this seemingly natural set of behaviors. Feeding disorders in the general population, as well as in those with ASD and other intellectual and developmental disabilities will then be presented. Various etiologies for feeding disorders, including physiological and behavioral etiologies are also reviewed.

Typical Development of Feeding Skills

Eating and ingesting liquids and solid foods involve a relatively complex repertoire of behavior and anatomy. The structures of the oral cavity (e.g., teeth, jaw, soft/soft palate, and tongue) must work in close coordination with the structures involved in swallowing (e.g., pharynx, larynx, and epiglottis) and eating (Matsuo and Palmer 2008). Food and liquids are processed in the mouth, swallowed, and transported to the esophagus for further processing in the gastrointestinal system. The appropriate development of feeding skills across the first few years of life (see Table 8.1) is highly dependent upon the proper integration and functioning of these anatomical structures, central nervous system development, and learning from one's environment.

In addition to the anatomy of feeding skill development, the individual's experience while eating also contributes to the development of feeding skills. Textures and types of food to which an individual is exposed, the reaction to foods consumed by the individuals, and the reaction of a caregiver or others present during meals can contribute to a successful outcome during mealtimes (Stevenson and Allaire 1991). At birth, infants are already prepared to find and be nourished by milk either

Table 8.1 Chronological development of appropriate eating/feeding behaviors

Age (months)	Oral-motor development	Feeding skills or abilities
Birth-12		Suck/swallow liquids by breast/bottle
3–6	four "innate" reflexes diminish Munching Upper lip closure at spoon removal	Pureed solids by spoon (fruits, vegetables, meats, and cereal)
8–9	Controls food position in mouth/jaw to chew curves lips around cup rim	Cup drinking Ground or junior foods by spoon Finger feeding (soft foods/dissolvable foods)
10–12	Rotary chewing uses jaw and tongue to mash food	Soft table foods
12–18		Finely chopped table foods
24		Self-feeding with utensils
36+		Advanced textures

The "innate" reflexes are suck/swallow, tongue thrust, rooting, and gag via breast or bottle feedings (de Costa et al. 2010). The four reflexive responses that enable infants to locate the source of nourishment and swallow liquids successfully include (1) the rooting reflex (i.e., moving the head toward the source of the stimulus that touches the cheek); (2) the suck/swallow reflex (i.e., suckling and swallowing precipitated by a stimulus touching the lips/mouth area); (3) the tongue thrust reflex (i.e., tongue protrusion precipitated by a stimulus touching the lips, can be used in combination with the gag reflex); and (4) the gag reflex (i.e., gagging when any object is placed deep in the mouth). These reflexes fade during an infant's first 3–5 months of life and are then replaced with more mature feeding behaviors that are shaped by the child's experience with food (Matsuo and Palmer 2008; Stevenson and Allaire 1991). Around 4–6 months of age, a child can take pureed food via spoon-feedings and with further experience is able to actively take food off the spoon with his/her upper lip. After this skill has developed, chewing patterns emerge and soft or dissolvable foods (e.g., crackers) can be mouthed. The successful development of chewing facilitates the eating of ground or mashed table food and the progression to more mature feeding skills. The eating of regular solids/table foods emerges with continued practice and the systematic exposure to a variety of food textures and types. Any interruption of this process can contribute to or directly cause problematic feeding patterns (Brisson et al. 2012; Manno et al. 2005).

The development of mature oral-motor skills is generally a byproduct of the systematic and gradual exposure to food textures (i.e., pureed before mashed, mashed before chopped pieces of table food, etc.) and the successful coordination and practice of oral-motor movements (i.e., tongue movements, sucking, munching, and chewing) across periods of neurological and anatomical development(Stevenson and Allaire 1991). Failure to experience textures during these early developmental periods results in anatomical and neurological maturation occurring without the accompanying skill acquisition (Lindberg et al. 1991). For example, children who require tube or other enteral (e.g., intravenous hydration) feedings prior to acquiring mature eating skills often take a longer period of time to reintroduce oral feedings. Often, attempts to initiate or reintroduce oral feedings are resisted by the child, and these children often continue to have persistent mealtime difficulties (e.g., food refusal, avoidant behaviors) once they have transitioned to predominantly oral feedings (Wright et al. 2011). Therefore, difficulties encountered in the development of appropriate feedings skills, particularly those that involve the failure to develop age-appropriate oral-motor skills, can certainly impact the success of mealtime and contribute to the development of feeding disorders.

Feeding Disorders Definition and Classification

An important setting event for the discussion of feeding problems in those with ASD is to define the problem adequately. However, there is much debate regarding the most appropriate method of classifying and subsequently identifying when aberrant feeding and eating patterns are present in those with a developmental delay such as ASD, as well as those who are typically developing (Bryant-Waugh and Piepenstock 2008; Burklow et al. 1998; Matson and Fodstad 2009). Certainly the easiest method for identifying if a feeding disorder exists is to note if a child is exhibiting a significant growth failure (height and/or weight) compared to same-aged peers. Commonly referred to as failure to thrive or more recently feeding disorder of infancy, and childhood as per the DSM-IV-TR (APA 2000), children were classified as having a feeding disorder if they displayed a "persistent failure to eat adequately with significant failure to gain weight or significant loss of weight over at least 1 month" with the onset of these difficulties occurring prior to the age of 6 years (p. 108). Furthermore, the feeding difficulties captured under this diagnosis had to occur without accompanying gastrointestinal, endocrinological, or neurological disorders or other general medical conditions, another mental disorder, or lack of available food. The most recent version of the ICD-10 (WHO 2010) provided further clarification to feeding disorder of infancy and childhood as "generally involv(ing) food refusal and extreme faddiness in the presence of an adequate food supply, a reasonably competent caregiver, and the absence of organic disease" with or without "associated rumination (repeated regurgitation without nausea or gastrointestinal illness)."

Unfortunately, these previous formal classifications have been found to be lacking in their ability to adequately capture many of the feeding and mealtime difficulties most often observed in the clinical setting for those diagnosed as having ASD or other developmental disabilities, but also those with a range of medical conditions. First, not all feeding problems observed in those with ASD occur exclusively in infancy or in childhood. Individuals with ASD are noted to have feeding and mealtime problems well into adulthood (Fodstad and Matson 2008). Second, many individuals with significant feeding problems do not have growth failure. For example, a child fed through a gastrostomy tube will gain weight adequately but consume nothing by mouth (Wright et al. 2011). Similarly, an individual with ASD who has severe food selectively (e.g., only eats junk food) may consume enough food/calories to gain weight adequately, although he/she might be at risk for nutritional deficiency (Johnson et al. 2014; Lane et al. 2014; Schmitt et al. 2008). Third, many feeding problems are associated or precipitated by a concomitant medical condition(s) (Rommel et al. 2003). Fourth, feeding disorders may not occur or may not be considered of a severe nature until well into adolescence or adulthood (Bryant-Waugh 2013a; Gravestock 2000).

One prospective longitudinal study following a sample of children from 2 to 11 years of age determined that 13–22 % of the children engaged in problematic "picky eating" at any given age and 39 % were described as picky eaters across the course of the study, with 47 % of the picky eaters experiencing chronic and severe feeding difficulties lasting more than 2 years (Mascola et al. 2011). Similarly, in a study by Fodstad and Matson (2009) adults diagnosed with ASD and intellectual disability (ID) ranging in age from 18 to 60 years old were found to have significant feeding difficulties including food selectivity, eating too rapidly, pica, rumination/vomiting, mealtime behavior problems, food refusal, and food stealing. Finally, individuals with ASD are often observed to engage in a wide variety of feeding problems that may not be specifically captured by these previous classification systems including unusual eating patterns, rituals regarding food preparation/presentation, rumination or vomiting, pica, food refusal, abnormal eating pace (eating too quickly or too slowly), overeating, polydipsia (i.e., consuming large amounts of liquids), mealtime problem behaviors (e.g., aggression, self-injury, batting at utensils, or other disruptive behaviors) and/or a strong emotional response elicited by the presentation of new foods, and food selectivity (by type, texture, and/or presentation) (Fodstad and Matson 2008; Ledford and Gast 2006; Schreck et al. 2004).

To address many of these concerns regarding the applicability of the formal classification of feeding disorders, the current version of the DSM-5 (APA 2013) replaced and expanded the diagnosis of feeding disorder of infancy or early childhood to include feeding dysfunction with onset after childhood. This new feeding disorder, named avoidant/restrictive food intake disorder (ARFID), was designed to encompass a broader range of feeding and eating disturbances, including lack of interest in food, sensory-based avoidance, and concerns about possible aversive consequences of eating (Bryant-Waugh 2013a, 2013b. Additionally, the diagnoses of pica and rumination disorder were retained in the DSM-5, but along with ARFID were acknowledged as occurring across the age range, including adulthood (Bryant-Waugh 2013a; Call et al. 2013).

Avoidant/Restrictive Food Intake Disorder

The DSM-5 Criteria Defined ARFID as a Feeding Disturbance Involving:

…persistent failure to meet appropriate nutritional and/or energy needs associated with one (or more) of the following: significant weight loss (or failure to achieve expected weight gain or faltering growth in children); significant nutritional deficiency; dependence on enteral feeding or oral nutritional supplements; marked interference with psychosocial functioning" (APA 2013, p. 334).

To address the expansion of the onset of feeding disorders beyond childhood, the DSM-5 diagnostic criteria included exclusions for other eating disorders such as anorexia nervosa, bulimia, and distorted body image. DSM-5 continued the exclusions adopted in DSM-IV for feeding disturbances that resulted from inadequate access to food or that were adequately accounted for by another mental disorder or medical condition and added a new exclusion for "an associated culturally sanctioned practice."

At this time, little research has been done incorporating the diagnosis of ARFID. It is likely that this broader definition will better capture the heterogeneity of feeding disorders seen across the range of persons diagnosed with ASD and other conditions. This could potentially lead to more accurate prevalence estimates which would assist with identifying those who have severe feeding issues who do not have significant weight loss. An additional advantage of the update and inclusion of ARFID is that it may provide some guidelines in establishing criteria for feeding disorders that may facilitate comparisons across studies for those with ASD (Seiverling et al. 2010). Certainly, accurately defining feeding disorders observed in those with ASD will assist in extending research in this area. This can lead to a better understanding of why individuals with ASD are at a high risk for having significant feeding and mealtime problems, as well as assisting with better assessment and intervention methodologies.

Pica

Pica is a feeding disorder characterized by the repeated consumption of inedible, nonnutritive items (APA 2013). Current DSM-5 criteria specify that the behavior must be part of a persistent pattern occurring for at least 1 month, is at a level developmentally inappropriate for the individual, and is not part of a cultural practice. Pica is a very serious and potentially life-threatening disorder associated with lead poisoning, intestinal perforation, intestinal parasites, encephalitis, failure to thrive/malnutrition, and even death in very severe cases (Paisey and Whitney 1989). Common examples of pica within the ASD/ID population include ingestion of cigarette butts, paint chips, fecal matter (i.e., coprophagia), paper, dirt/clay (i.e., geophagia), hair, and cloth (Matson and Bamburg 1995; Stiegler 2005). Although pica is generally associated with infancy or childhood, the disorder can occur at any age; often pica is not identified until well into adulthood (Bryant-Waugh et al. 2010).

Pica is generally subdivided into a few categories to account for the various aspects of the disorder (McLoughlin 1987). These subtypes include nonfood pica (e.g., eating items not meant to be eaten and with no nutritive value), food pica (e.g., consumption of rotten or frozen food), non-ingestion pica (e.g., mouthing, licking, or sucking on inedible objects), or a combination of these subtypes. Pica behavior can be limited to a single substance (i.e., specific pica) or may be exhibited across an array of substances (i.e., generalized pica). There is no single etiology for pica and, as such, the causes may range from cultural, medical, nutritional, environmental, sensory, and psychopathological factors. In those with ASD as well as those with severe ID, pica generally serves an automatic or sensory-seeking purpose (Matson and Bamburg 1995; Matson et al. 2005b); however, there are some reports of pica occurring to access attention for others, to escape/avoid a perceived aversive stimulus, or to access a preferred item (Piazza et al. 1998).

Prevalence data indicate that pica is relatively common in residential settings. In an extensive literature review, researchers have estimated that pica is observed in approximately 9.2–25.8 % of individuals in residential settings (Ashworth et al. 2008) and among those with more severe levels of ID (Matson and Bamburg 1999). However, anecdotal reports and an extensive literature review by Ali (2001) indicate that pica may occur at a higher rate, especially when less severe forms of the condition (e.g., non-ingestion pica, pagophagia, amylophagia, eating frozen/non-cooked foods, eating food scraps from trash bins) are present. Although more evidence is necessary, these rates may be even higher in ASD than in other developmental disabilities. For instance, Kinnell (1985) found that adults with ASD were more likely to engage in pica than those with Down's syndrome. Specifically 60 % of those with ASD exhibited in pica, whereas only 4 % of those with Down's syndrome exhibited the behavior. Despite some of these estimates, the incidence of pica continues to be under identified and undertreated (Ali 2001; Matson et al. 2011).

Rumination Disorder

Rumination refers to the voluntary, chronic regurgitation of stomach contents into the mouth and, typically, the chewing and re-swallowing of the rumitus in a repetitive cycle during mealtimes (APA 2013). Per current DSM-5 criteria, this pattern is recurrent for at least 1 month and is not associated to a gastrointestinal or general medical condition (pyloric stenosis, gastroesophageal reflux disease (GERD)). Similarly, the behavior must not be comorbid with an eating disorder such as anorexia nervosa or bulimia nervosa. For those with an ASD or ID, rumination must be of a severe enough level of behavior to merit a diagnosis. Rumination is a serious condition as it can lead to a multitude of life-threatening consequences such as weight loss, esophageal irritation, dental erosion, decreased immunity, aspiration, esophageal cancer, and death (Johnston 1993).

Initiation of ruminative behaviors by the individual may occur in different ways depending on physical capabilities, repertoire, and skill development. To ruminate, individuals may stimulate their gag reflexes manually; may rock forward sharply or arch their torso, tilt back their head, and/or create suction with their tongue on the roof of the mouth to initiate their gag reflex; and others may make no noticeable or consistent outward movements (Johnston 1993). The rate with which one ruminates is highly variable, and factors such as the texture, quantity, or type of food consumed as well as the taste or the rumitus and amount of oropharyngeal stimulation have been found to influence the likelihood that rumination will occur. As with pica, associated behavioral features vary among individuals with rumination disorder. Ruminative behaviors most often occur in those with ASD or severe ID as a self-soothing or self-stimulating behavior (Paclawskyj et al. 2004).

Rumination is noted to occur across a wide range of ages and developmental levels. The prevalence of rumination with respect to those with ASD is unknown. Most investigations regarding rumination focus on early infancy, or institutionalized adults with severe to profound ID (5–10% engage in rumination; Gravestock 2000). Out of the few investigations and single-case studies on this behavior in those with ASD, it does appear that rumination does occur and is treatable often with intensive and individualized interventions (Chial et al. 2003; Rhine and Tarbox, 2009; Luiselli et al. 1994). Part of the difficulties in ascertaining the frequency with which rumination occurs in those with ASD or other populations due to significant variability in terminology used and how it is defined across medical and psychological specialties (Hartmann et al. 2012). A further hindrance is the fact that regurgitation and rumination are often covert behaviors, and often go unreported by those engaging in the behavior or by caregivers.

Food Selectivity and Food Refusal

Food selectivity and food refusal have long been considered to be a common phenomenon among those with ASD. Food selectivity is most often subdivided into two forms: by type and by texture (Field et al. 2003). *Food selectivity by type* is defined as selected intake of only certain foods, severely limiting and appropriately varied, nutritional diet. *Food selectivity by texture* is defined as refusal to eat foods consisting of developmentally appropriate textures. *Food refusal* is often viewed as a consequence of food selectivity and is defined as the refusal or rejection of presented foods, resulting in insufficient dietary intake to meet caloric or nutritional requirements. The incidence of complete food refusal is less prevalent that either refusal occurring with food selectivity or than just food selectivity alone (Ledford and Gast 2006; Marí-Bauset et al. 2013).

What some have termed the "picky eater" syndrome, food selectivity in its milder form may impose very few serious consequences. Usually selective eating preferences do not affect the individual's ability to consume adequate calories throughout the day and often does not lead to significant weight loss or underweight status. However, an individual whose "picky" preference is deemed severe may lead to malnutrition, severe developmental delays, and social isolation (Nadon et al. 2011). Numerous case studies documenting food selectivity have shown a varied pattern of problematic eating behavior. In these studies, there have been reports of selectivity specific to food type or brand (e.g., only breadsticks; only McDonald's chicken nuggets), by the temperature of the food (e.g., eat only foods at room temperature), by foods of particular texture (e.g., eat only pureed foods), by the person who feeds them (e.g., will only eat if feed by their mother), by particular people present during the meal, by the location or "look" of the meal (e.g., will only eat alone; no foods must be touching), or a mixed combination of many of these variables (Ahearn et al. 2001; Hubbard et al. 2014; Kuhn and Matson 2002; Kozlowski et al. 2011; Schreck et al. 2004). Insufficient food intake may require the use of invasive feeding tubes, such as nasogastric or gastronomy tubes (Manno et al. 2005). This type of intervention does increase an individual's food intake. However, it can be associated with additional health risks, while failing to aid in the development of appropriate and effective eating behavior.

The development and maintenance of food selectivity may be linked to various organic and environmental factors (Schwarz et al. 2001). Organic factors most commonly associated with interference in food intake include physical obstructions and abnormalities. The environmental factors that are described at the onset of food selectivity include a lack of opportunities for skill development and aversive feeding experiences. Following the onset of food selectivity, reinforcement contingencies have been found to be responsible for the maintenance of the problem behavior (Piazza et al. 2003; Sharp et al. 2013).

Feeding Skills Problems

Feeding skill deficits are observed to occur among individuals with ASD. However, those with accompanying significant developmental delays or ID appear to be at the greatest risk for developing feeding difficulties associated by skill deficits (Fodstad and Matson 2008; Linscheid 1983; Schwarz 2003; Schwarz et al. 2001). When a person is unable to complete basic skills such as utensil use, neatness, table manners, proper pacing, and oral-motor skills, the ability to eat properly decreases and the risk for developing a feeding problems increases. The problems associated with poor feeding skills include difficulties swallowing, chewing, and accessing food. When an individual is unable, either from an inability or unwillingness to complete these tasks for a period of time, consequences may occur including malnutrition and starvation. Similarly, if a person is unable to eat at a regular pace (i.e., eating too fast), the risk of choking or aspirating increases dramatically and can cause a potentially life-threatening situation.

Overweight/Obesity

Obesity is often reported to be a significant problem for those with ASD. Unfortunately, research on this topic is sparse. Out of the scant amount of data that are present, it does appear that obesity and weight related issues do occur with regularity in those with ASD, and even more so for those who have a concomitant diagnosis of ID (Hinckson et al. 2013; Rimmer et al. 2010). Similar to those with ID, individuals with ASD demonstrate atypical cognitive, social, motor, and behavioral difficulties that may render them, more vulnerable to the development of obesity. Curtin et al. (2010) conducted a survey on obesity and weight-related concerns amongst children with ASD versus children without ASD. Outcomes indicated that children with ASD were 40 % more likely to be obese when compared with children without ASD. More recently, Zuckerman et al. (2014) found out that of 376 children and adolescents with ASD, 18.1 % of children met criteria for being overweight using current Center for Disease Control normative data and 17.0 % met criteria to be classified as being obese. Several studies have suggested that children with more severe ASD symptoms are at higher risk for overweight or obesity. For instance, Ho et al. (1997) found that obesity had a positive correlation with autism severity as measured by the childhood autism rating scale (CARS). Similarly, Egan et al. (2013) reported that children with autistic disorder are more likely to have obesity than children with Asperger's disorder or pervasive developmental disorder—not otherwise specified. In a study by Matson et al. (2009a), eating patterns that were observed significantly more often in children and adolescents with ASD than atypically or typically developing peers which could contribute to weight gain included eating too much (often of highly specific foods) and eating at a rapid pace. Adults with ASD are also noted to be at risk for being overweight or obese. Eaves and Ho (2008) conducted a follow-up assessment of 48 adults (age range 19–31 years of age) diagnosed with ASD in childhood and found that 42 % were considered to be in the overweight or obese range.

Obesity within the ASD community has been linked to not only behavioral or genetic reasons but also the environment in which the individual lives. Research, comparing various living arrangements of adults with similar levels of ID and ASD, has shown that those who live in less restrictive settings (i.e., at home with family or independently) are more likely to be obese than those who live in more supervised settings (i.e., residential group homes, developmental centers) (Lewis et al. 2002). A major issue with obesity is that being in the overweight (body mass index ≥ 25) or obese (body mass index ≥ 30) ranges of body composition places the individual at an increased risk for numerous health complications including diabetes, hypertension, dyslipidemia, orthopedic problems, sleep apnea, and premature death (Daniels 2009). It has also been suggested that nutritional imbalances which may accompany severe food selectivity and food refusal, may increase the likelihood of associated behaviors such as food stealing or overeating to compensate for the relative imbalances (Gravestock 2000). Independent of the reason, these behaviors can place the individual at risk for illness (e.g., if the individual steals food out of the trash) and potentially harmful environmental consequences (e.g., aggression from those from whom the food is stolen).

Research is needed to establish more firmly the prevalence of obesity and weight-related issues in those with ASD and to examine associated factors in this population. Findings from such lines of inquiry would have important implications for devising appropriate prevention and intervention strategies that take the unique needs of this population into account. Given that those with ASD with or without ID may be more likely to experience obesity and associated issues than the typical population, the study of weight related issues and associated risks appears all the more urgent.

Prevalence of Feeding Disorders

Prevalence figures of feeding disorders and mealtime difficulties vary considerably across studies. This finding is believed to be largely in part to an inability of previous formal classification systems to accurately represent the full range of feeding problems that can occur in those with ASD as well as other populations. Furthermore, there is a large variability in presentation and complications arising from feeding difficulties, including food selectivity, oral supplementation, and dependence on gastronomy or nasogastronomy tubes that have only been recently addressed with the current diagnosis of ARFID (APA 2013). Thus, the prevalence of severe feeding disturbances that meet previous diagnostic criteria (i.e., DSM-IV-TR; ICD-10) for a feeding disorder is believed to be significantly lower than reports of feeding problems. For example, a study by Williams et al. (2009) examined the proportion of children referred to a hospital-based feeding program who met full criteria for a feeding disorder of infancy or early childhood under the DSM-IV-TR. Only 8% of these children met the diagnostic criteria for a feeding disorder. The remaining 92% of the children failed to satisfy the criterion of failure to gain weight or significant weight loss despite demonstrating significant feeding difficulties. Despite the relative paucity of specific prevalence data on feeding disorders, feeding difficulties among children are commonly reported by parents, with estimates of feeding problems among typically developing children ranging from approximately 20–50% (Carruth et al. 2004; Lindberg et al. 1991; Manikam and Pernam 2000), and 33–90 % for children with developmental delays and disabilities (Bandini et al. 2010; Burklow et al. 1998; Ledford and Gast 2006).

Even with the variability of prevalence estimates, researchers have suggested that individuals with ASD experience higher rates of feeding problems than neurotypical peers, or even those diagnosed with other developmental disabilities (Field et al. 2003; Ledford and Gast 2006; Matson et al. 2009a; Schreck et al. 2004, Schmitt et al. 2008). For example, in a survey of the eating habits of children, Shreck et al. (2004) found that children with ASD experienced significantly more feeding problems than typically developing children. According to parent report, 72 % of the children with ASD were noted eating a limited variety of foods. Moreover, children with ASD were also significantly more likely to refuse foods, require specific utensils or food presentations, and consume only low texture foods than typically developing children.

Similar results were obtained by Matson et al. (2009). This study compared rates of feeding problems as reported on parent questionnaires for 279 children and adolescents with ASD (i.e., autistic disorder or PDD-NOS), other developmental disabilities, and typically developing children. Compared to typically developing children and children with other developmental disabilities, children with ASD were more likely to demonstrate feeding problems centered on food selectivity, preference for foods with a certain texture or smell, and consume nonnutritive items. These results were replicated by Kozlowski et al. (2012), who used psychometrically derived cutoff scores to which compared rates of feeding problems in children diagnosed with autistic disorder, PDD-NOS, or other developmental delays. Outcomes indicated that both ASD groups were reported to have higher rates of feeding difficulties than peers with other developmental delays, but rates of reported feeding problems were also significantly higher for the autistic disorder group than the PDD-NOS group. Thus, these results may indicate that overall symptom severity (e.g., higher level of symptoms) may be associated with increased rates of feeding and other problems. However, the relationship between severity of ASD symptoms and presence of feeding problems is mixed as other researchers have found no effect between these two variables (Johnson et al. 2014; Matson et al. 2009; Schreck and Williams 2006).

Martins et al. (2008) compared scores on questionnaires of feeding problems and family mealtime practices as completed by mothers of children with ASD or mothers of typically developing children who were matched for adaptive skill level. Results indicated that 54 % of children with ASD had ever experienced feeding difficulties, compared to 42 % reported for typically developing children. However, the rate of children currently experiencing a feeding problem was twice as high for children with ASD than typically developing children. Moreover, children with ASD were reported to demonstrate an average of three times as many simultaneous problems as compared to their typically developing peers. Overall, these studies suggest that feeding difficulties exhibited by children with ASD appear to be less transient, are more severe, and occur more frequently than feeding difficulties reported by parents of typically developing children. Finally, Sharp et al. (2013) conducted a meta analysis of 17 studies reporting the occurrence of feeding problems among children with ASD and typically developing children. All studies included in the analysis reported significant differences between groups, with standardized mean difference estimates ranging from 0.48 to 1.56. When collapsed across comparison groups, an odds ratio of 5– 1 was found, suggesting that children with ASD are five times more likely than typically developing children to exhibit feeding difficulties.

While most of the research on prevalence has been in relation to children, there have been a few studies conducted using adult populations. Across inpatient and community samples, prevalence rates for feeding and mealtime difficulties range from 1 to 64 % (Fodstad and Matson 2009; Gravestock 2000; Hove 2007; Matson et al. 1991). Overall, these studies have confirmed that feeding problems are a significant issue across the lifespan for those with ASD. Given the reclassification of feeding disorders per the DSM-5 to acknowledge that feeding dysfunction can occur across the lifespan as well as the new diagnosis of ARFID which encompasses food selectivity and other feeding difficulties without inadequate weight or growth, it is not yet clear how prevalence estimates may change.

Potential explanations for the discrepancies across studies where researchers looked at the prevalence in feeding disorders in those with ASD include differences in the methodology, instruments, and criteria used to assess for the presence of feeding problems. First, the majority of studies addressing feeding problems in this population have sample sizes of 150 or fewer participants, which limits the extrapolation of prevalence rates to the larger ASD population. Most studies use data from parent-completed questionnaires, which may be subject to response bias, as families of children with feeding difficulties may be more motivated to respond (Twachtman-Reilly et al. 2008). Finally, there are no established criteria for determining what level of difficulty constitutes a feeding problem. For example, Kerwin et al. (2005) found that 60 % of parents of children with ASD surveyed reported strong food preferences, but only 6.7 % reported that their child experienced feeding problems. Finally, many studies looking at feeding disorders or difficulties in those with ASD often focus on specific issues, such as food selectivity or food refusal, and fail to include the full range of issues (e.g., pica, meal time problems behaviors, rumination/vomiting, obesity and weight-related issues, feeding skill deficits, etc.) that are also noted to occur in this population.

Behavioral Versus Physiological Classifications of Feeding Disorders in ASD

A variety of feeding problems experienced by individuals with ASD have been reported in the literature. In describing feeding problems, several researchers distinguish between physiological and behavioral feeding disorders. Schwarz et al. (2001) described functional oral-motor disorders as difficulties with oral-motor coordination (e.g., sucking, chewing, etc.), swallowing disorders, pharyngoesophageal dyskinesia, and esophageal disorders. Similarly, Field et al. 2003 distinguished between behavioral problems exhibited by those who are safe oral feeders, and physiological problems demonstrated by those deemed to be unsafe oral feeders.

Schwarz (2003) categorized behavioral eating disorders as aversive feeding behaviors, which include food refusal, choking, gagging, and vomiting, expulsion without an identifiable medical cause, or sensory-based feeding disorders, typically selectivity by texture. Field et al. (2003) classified behavioral feeding problems into food refusal, food selectivity by type, and selectivity by texture. Other commonly reported behavioral feeding problems associated with ASD include neophobia, the refusal of novel food items; mealtime disruptive behaviors; and food selectivity by brand, color, temperature, or presentation (e.g., requiring the use of certain utensils, arrangement of food on the plate, pica, rumination or vomiting, refusing foods with visible blemishes, etc.) (Bandini et al. 2010; Mari-Bauset et al. 2013; Williams and Fox 2007).

The distinction between physiological and behavioral feeding problems is necessary for treatment planning purposes, as physiological problems tend to require more intensive medical intervention and careful supervision. Swallowing, dyskinesia, and esophageal disorders may require the services of a multidisciplinary feeding team, which may include pediatricians, nutritionists, speech and language pathologists, occupational therapists, and psychologists. In some cases, placement of a gastric feeding tube may be required to maintain adequate nutritive intake (Babbitt et al. 1994; Field et al 2003; Manikam and Perman 2000). Feeding skill problems, such as oral-motor disorders, difficulties with self-feeding using utensils, neatness, and inappropriate rates of eating, may also lead to serious consequences such as risk of aspiration and malnutrition over time (Fodstad and Matson 2008; Kuhn and Matson 2002, 2004; Schwarz 2003). Psychologists, speech and language pathologists, or occupational therapists with expertise in feeding disorders may treat these issues by teaching necessary motor skills and appropriate meal behaviors. Such strategies may include the use of direct instruction, prompting, rehearsal, and contingent reinforcement (Anglesea et al. 2008; Matson and Fodstad 2009). For behavioral feeding difficulties, parents may provide treatment at home or in an outpatient clinic under the guidance of a behavioral psychologist or board certified behavior analyst with expertise in feeding problems. Behavioral treatments include antecedent- and consequence-based strategies such as choice, simultaneous presentation, differential reinforcement, escape extinction (e.g., non-removal of spoon), physical guidance, repeated exposure (tasting sessions), shaping, and stimulus fading. (Laud et al. 2009; Ledford and Gast 2006; Piazza and Addison 2007).

While children with ASD have higher rates of both physiological and behavioral feeding difficulties in comparison to their typically developing peers, behavioral feeding problems appear to be much more common among children with ASD. Studies have generally found food selectivity to be most commonly experienced feeding problem reported in children with ASD (Ahearn et al. 2001; Collins et al. 2003; Schreck et al. 2004). In an audit of case reports from a feeding clinic, Field et al. (2003) reported that 62 % of children with a diagnosis of ASD exhibited selectivity by type, followed by 31 % with selectivity by texture. Of note, all three children who exhibited food refusal were also found to experience gastroesophageal reflux. Food refusal, oral-motor delay, and dysphagia were less common occurring at 12, 15, and 12 % respectively. In contrast, oral-motor delays were the most common presenting feeding problem among children with Down syndrome (85 %), and cerebral palsy (68 %), with dysphagia and food refusal also commonly reported. In a study of adults by Fodstad and Matson (2008), those with ASD and ID were found to engage in a higher level of behavioral feeding problems compared to those with ID. Individuals with ASD and ID were noted to engage in higher rates of mealtime problems behaviors (43 %), food selectivity issues (26 %), and food refusal (33 %) compared to those with ID only (13, 6, and 16 %, respectively). Comparatively, those with ID only were found to have more physiological feeding difficulties such as chewing difficulties (10 %), food choking/aspiration (22 %), and swallowing difficulties/dysphagia (20 %). Although those with ASD and ID also had difficulties with similar issues, they were noted to occur with less regularity (0, 3, 6, and 3 %, respectively).

Etiology of Feeding Dysfunction

The causes of feeding and mealtime problems are complex and interrelated. Rommel et al. (2003) conducted a thorough record review of 700 children under the age of 10 referred for a multidisciplinary assessment of feeding problems, 74 % of whom were diagnosed with a developmental disability. Outcomes indicated that out of these children 86 % had at least one associated medical condition, 61 % had some oropharyngeal dysfunction, and 18 % had behavioral difficulties or psychological disorder. Similarly, Burklow et al. (1998) examined the etiology of complex feeding disorders in children (64 % diagnosed with a developmental disability) by categorizing five non-mutually exclusive contributing categories: structural abnormalities, neurological conditions, behavioral and psychosocial issues, cardiorespiratory problems, and metabolic dysfunctions. Although, 85 % of the children in Burklow et al.'s sample had a behavioral component to their feeding disorder (e.g., dysfunctional parent–child interaction, negative feeding behaviors maintained by internal or social reinforcement, and phobias), only 12 % of the children were categorized as having only a behavioral etiology. Similar outcomes to those by Rommel et al. (2003) and Burklow et al (1998) have been reported by other researchers both in samples with typically developing children, children with general developmental delays, and those with an ASD (Carruth et al. 2004; Lindberg et al. 1991; Martins et al. 2008; Schmitt et al. 2008; Schreck et al. 2004). Thus, feeding difficulties, in general, appear to be a complex issue resulting from the combination of multiple variables. Due to this reason, there is generally not one "root cause" of an individual's difficulties surrounding eating food. Variables which should always been assessed and taken into account prior to the development and execution of an individualized feeding intervention should include medical conditions or anatomical abnormalities, the general developmental or ability level of the individual, behavioral and environmental factors, and specific variables related to the diagnosis of ASD.

Medical In order to diagnose a feeding disorder, the effects of general medical conditions that may contribute to or account for feeding difficulties typically should be ruled out first (see Table 8.2 for commonly associated medical conditions).

Those with ASD appear to be more likely to experience gastroenterological (GI) problems than typically developing peers. Estimates of comorbid gastroenterological issues among this population vary widely, with estimates ranging from 9% to as high as 70% (Buie et al. 2010). Commonly reported GI issues include chronic constipation, encopresis, GERD, abdominal pain, bloating, and diarrhea. GI disturbances may also be expressed as irritability, increased aggression or self-injurious

Table 8.2 Medical conditions commonly associated with dysfunctional feeding/eating patterns

Prematurity/low birth weight
Mitochondrial disease
Metabolic disorders
Niemann—Pick disease
Tay—Sachs disease
Muscular disorders
Cerebral palsy
Muscular dystrophy
Anatomical abnormalities of the mouth or oropharyngeal regions
Cleft palate
Cleft lip
Ankyloglossia (i.e., tongue-tied)
Oral-motor dysfunction
Dysphagia
Oral apraxia
Esophageal spasms
Aspiration
Gastrointestinal diseases
Gastroesophageal reflux disease (GERD)
Gastroparesis
Crohn's disease
Food allergies
Lactose intolerance
Celiac disease
Other medical diseases/conditions
Liver disease
Cancer/leukemia
Heart disease
GI inflammation (e.g., gastritis, duodenitis, and esophagitis)
Infections
Central nervous system infections
Adrenal hyperplasia
Constipation/impaction of bowels

GI gastrointestinal

behavior, and/or sleep disturbances (Erickson et al. 2005; Horvath and Perman 2002). Yet many GI disturbances may go unreported, as many children with ASD may have difficulty communicating their distress and most pediatricians and primary care doctors do not routinely assess these issues (Buie et al. 2010).

GI and feeding disorders may have interactive effects among individuals with ASD who experience these symptoms. For example, limited consumption of fiber may result in constipation and bloating, making eating uncomfortable. Similarly, experiencing GERD, an allergic reaction or GI distress after eating may make certain foods or eating in general an aversive event. Side effects of certain medications may also produce this effect. Individuals who experience these conditions should be treated medically first to reduce discomfort and eliminate the pairing of eating with GI pain (Marí-Bauset et al. 2013; Williams and Foxx 2007).

For individuals affected by GERD, eating may be associated with vomiting and the pain that occurs when excess acid is released into the stomach or esophagus. An individual with GERD might develop behavior problems surrounding mealtimes to avoid eating. The same may be true for those with food allergies, which are often difficult to detect until the food containing an allergen has been consumed. The individual may experience severe pain from an allergic reaction, which in turn could make eating unpleasant. Nausea has long been highly correlated to the development and maintenance of aversions to food (Bernstein 1999). That is when nausea and food consumption are paired, aversions to certain tastes may develop after only one or a limited number of trials, may generalize to other foods, and may be highly resistant to intervention (Birch 1999). Often, even if a painful medical condition (e.g., GERD, gastritis, esophagitis, etc.) or associated condition (e.g., nausea) is treated, the individual may continue to refuse food due to their prior experience of significant pain surrounding eating and limited or no experience of learning that eating is not painful.

Similarly, chronic medical problems may also indirectly contribute to the presence of feeding problems. Individuals with complex medical histories are often subjected to invasive diagnostic tests and procedures that may involve manipulation of the face and mouth (e.g., with a laryngoscope). The child may learn to associate the presentation of objects to the face and mouth (e.g., a spoon or cup) with these early negative experiences, and as such may develop aversion or avoidance to mealtimes. Parents of hospitalized and medically fragile children often report oral aversions and association conditions that affect feeding and other behaviors associated with the face and mouth (e.g., tooth brushing, face washing). For example, children with childhood cancer and cardiac problems have been noted to be two subgroups that often develop feeding problems (Davis 1998; Field et al. 2003; Rommel et al. 2003). These two subgroups of individuals often are subjected to extended periods of time not eating by mouth due to treatments and/or surgeries often necessitating lengthy hospitalizations. In these cases, it is likely that their internal motivation (i.e., hunger) to eat or drink by mouth wanes due to feeling nauseous or fatigued, or may dissipate due to side effects of medications (i.e., loss of appetite).

Oral-Motor Difficulties Oral-motor dysfunction may include problems such as difficulty swallowing, inability to lateralize food (i.e., move it from side to side), tongue thrust, and difficulty sucking. Individuals with anatomical abnormalities (e.g., cleft palate, enlarged tongue, misalignment of jaw, and esophageal stenosis), hypotonia/weak muscles of the oral-esophageal regions, oral-esophageal tumors, prematurity, neurological or genetic conditions (e.g., cerebral palsy, Down's syndrome, Rett syndrome, and traumatic brain injuries/strokes), and more may be more likely to have feeding problems due to difficulties with congenital or acquired defects to structures necessary for successful consumption of foods/drinks. Over and beyond the actual physiology and functional oral skills which contribute to successful eating, difficulties with motor coordination may impact a person's ability to grasp utensils or finger foods, to scoop or spear foods, bring the bolus to his or her mouth to consume, and eat at a regular pace (i.e., eat too quickly, chew insufficiently, and pack food in mouth). Without the basic skills (proper oral-motor reflexes or self-feeding skills), the natural eating process may be interrupted and become too effortful for the individual. This may cause more long-term disruptions during mealtime including continued difficulties with or delays in the development of oral-motor skills, refusal behaviors to avoid eating, severe aspiration/choking, malnutrition, and starvation (Kuhn and Matson 2002).

Intellectual Disability Symptoms of ASD and ID are noted to overlap considerably. This is no surprise given that the core symptoms of ID include deficits in adaptive functioning (i.e., social and communication skills, daily living skills) as well as a significant deficit of delay in cognitive functioning (APA 2013). Furthermore, those with severe to profound levels of ID often present with stereotypical and repetitive behaviors and limited/restricted interests. Thus, there are many areas where symptoms of ASD and ID covary (Matson et al. 2009b; Matson et al. 2009). Researchers have indicated that ASD and ID are often comorbid, with those individuals demonstrating more severe forms of ASD being the most likely to also have a comorbid diagnosis of ID (Matson and Shoemaker 2009; Vig and Jedrysek 1999).

Individuals diagnosed with ID are also noted to be a patient population at high risk for developing feeding disorders (Fodstad and Matson 2008; Hove 2007). Prevalence estimates indicate that approximately 30% of individuals with ID engage in eating or feeding problems; however, it has been noted that those with severe and profound ID are at an even greater risk for significant and severe feeding problems (Gravestock 2000; Matson et al. 2008). Children who are functioning within the severe to profound range of ID have been estimated to have a prevalence rate of mealtime problems as high as 80% (Field et al. 2003). Similar rates have also been estimated in adult populations across both inpatient and community samples (Gravestock 2000; Hove 2007; Matson et al. 2008). Linscheid (1983) described ten mealtime problems that were likely to occur within this population, including tantrums; bizarre food habits; multiple food dislikes/food refusal; food selectivity (type and texture); delay or difficulty in chewing, swallowing, or sucking; delay in self-feeding skills; pica; excessive overeating; malnutrition through eating very little; and rumination. Subsequent work suggested that feeding problems for those with

ID could be parceled into four distinct categories: (1) lack of independent skills; (2) disruptive behavior; (3) eating too much or too little; and (4) selectivity by type or texture (Sisson and Van Hasselt 1989).

Despite the increased prevalence of feeding difficulties among those with severe deficits in cognitive and adaptive functioning, it has proven to be rather difficult to accurately identify and assess these problems within such a handicapped group. Individuals who have limited functional language or are nonverbal might be unable to describe their symptoms (e.g., ruminating due to exacerbation of GERD/discomfort) or indicate their preference or tastes with respect to foods. Other issues within the ID population that may contribute to the high prevalence rate of feeding problems are deficits in motor skills/abilities, physical abnormalities, nutritional imbalances, and a higher rate of medical complications (Gravestock 2000). It is unclear how the overlapping symptoms and increased comorbidity of ASD and ID might be related to feeding disorders in those diagnosed with both conditions. What is known is that individuals with ASD only or ASD and ID are more likely to have behavioral feeding disorders (e.g., food selectivity, food refusal) compared to those with ID only, who are more likely to have feeding difficulties due to organic/physiological reasons (e.g., medical conditions, anatomical abnormalities, and feeding skill deficits) (Field et al. 2003; Fodstad and Matson 2009; Schwarz 2003). More research is needed to deduce if there are distinct features of ASD, as opposed to ID, that may place individuals with ASD at risk for developing feeding disorders. However, at this time research in this area has been restricted to investigating these feeding/eating patterns among individuals with ID only or among individuals with both ASD and ID versus ID only; there is no known research to date that has investigated patterns of feeding difficulties across all the three groups (i.e., ASD only, ID only, and both ASD and ID) taking into account the respective severity of these diagnoses.

Biological/Disorder-Specific Issues It is logical to assume that the feeding and mealtime behaviors observed in those with ASD likely interact with and may be exacerbated by the behavioral symptoms and features of the disorder. Several researchers have proposed that high rates of feeding problems in individuals with ASD may be related to core diagnostic criteria including perseveration, rigidity or difficulties with change, sensory impairments, ritualistic patterns of behavior, deficiencies in social skills/reciprocity, sensory abnormalities, and communication difficulties (Ahearn et al. 2001; Ledford and Gast 2006; Rastam 2008). As mentioned previously, those with ASD are also known to have presentations complicated by other medical conditions that can affect feeding behaviors, such as constipation. Children with ASD are more likely to eat a selective and low-fiber diet (Bandini et al. 2010). A low-fiber diet can cause constipation, producing stomach discomfort, pain, and lack of appetite, which can lead to further food refusal. Finally, although there are some reports that individuals with more severe symptoms of ASD are more likely to have more severe feeding disturbances (Kozlowski et al. 2012), data is mixed regarding whether the severity of ASD symptoms contributes to the presence or severity of feeding and mealtime difficulties (Matson et al. 2009; Schreck and Williams 2006).

Eating is generally regarded as a social activity, involving interactions with others (e.g., feeder, peers or family members present, etc.). For those with ASD who already have difficulties with social reciprocity and communication, the social expectations during mealtimes can be especially challenging, as success requires an integration and understanding of several complex social features, including social approach, table etiquette, and social norms. Additionally, co-occurring cognitive deficits or ID could impede an individual's ability to learn mealtime expectations and rules. Those with ASD may not be socially motivated to participate in mealtimes either with a feeder or in a group format, may not be able to model the eating habits and behaviors of others, may not be responsive to their caregivers' verbal praise for appropriate feeding behavior, or may not have the necessary communication abilities to effectively influence their mealtime environment. Further, the ritualistic and repetitive behaviors exhibited by those with ASD, as well as the "need for sameness" and behavioral inflexibility are likely to contribute to rigid mealtime routines. Thus, problematic feeding behaviors may be, at least in part, secondary to the repetitive and ritualistic behaviors ubiquitous in ASD. In the context of feeding and mealtime difficulties, repetitive behaviors and ritualistic routines might include demanding specific utensils and dishware, requiring that food be presented in a specific order, insisting on food not touching, having only certain people present, and sitting in specific places at the table (Schrek and Williams 2006; Sieverling et al. 2010; Williams and Foxx 2007). Rigid and routine-based mealtime behaviors in a more social context (e.g., at school, in restaurants, and with peers) may further impact the individual's ability to develop relationships, as their strong preferences may cause them to be more socially isolated. Acceptable behavior when eating with others is something that, to a certain extent, can be learned. Skills training, increasing flexibility in routines with the use of positive reinforcement and shaping, video modeling, and social stories have all been used in single-case studies to teach individuals with ASD mealtime etiquette, conversational skills to use during meal times, and basic meal preparation behaviors (Bledsoe et al. 2003; Pierce and Schreibman 1994; Rehfeldt et al. 2003).

Feeding and mealtime behaviors in ASD may be further impacted by sensory difficulties.

Sensory sensitivity (also known as sensory under- or over-reactivity) relates to difficulties in the detection of, and reaction to, sensory information, including information from the taste, touch, vision, and smell senses (Dunn 1997). In a study by Bennetto et al. (2007), children and adolescents with high-functioning ASD were significantly less accurate in identifying basic tastes and odors than 27 typically developing, same-aged peers. These results have also been replicated with adults. That is, high-functioning adults with ASD compared to adults without ASD were more likely to misidentify basic tastes using chemical taste strips, especially those related to bitter, sour, and sweet tastes (Tavassoli and Baron-Cohen 2012). While sensory sensitivities (e.g., tactile and oral defensiveness; hyper- or hyposensitivity) are seen in typically developing children and adults, they are much more common in those with ASD (Tomchek and Dunn 2007). Children with sensory issues who are not diagnosed with ASD are significantly more likely to engage in food refusal when presented with a specific food category (e.g., vegetables, fruit), smell, or temperature, and are less likely to try new foods (Farrow and Coulthard 2012). Furthermore, researchers have suggested that sensory abnormalities may play a role in feeding issues (e.g., food selectivity) in those with ASD (Cermak et al. 2010; Martins et al. 2008; Nadon et al. 2011). In a recent study of children with ASD, Johnson et al. (2014) found that sensory impairment was highly correlated with feeding and mealtime behaviors, suggesting that those with more significant sensory impairment were more likely to have more pervasive feeding difficulties.

Apart from physiological or sensory processing factors, food selectivity and neophobia are thought to be manifestations of the restricted, repetitive patterns of behaviors or interests observed in those with ASD (Kozlowski et al. 2012; Ledford and Gast 2006; Matson et al. 2009; Rastam 2008). In a parent survey on food preferences, children with ASD were reported to eat fewer foods within each food group category compared to same-aged peers (Schreck et al. 2004). In general, children with ASD ate about half the number of foods in each food group except starches, where they ate about two-thirds the number of foods as typically developing children. Children with ASD also were considerably more likely to accept only low-texture foods (e.g., pureed). Similarly, Schreck and Williams (2006) observed that those with ASD often made their food choices based upon texture (70 %) than did same-aged peers without ASD (11 %). It is important to note that neophobia, which refers to the resistance to trying novel foods, is also common in young, typically developing children. For example, children who have had choking or vomiting experiences with certain foods, may also develop an avoidance or neophobia to certain foods if they associate these behaviors/reactions/experience with these, or certain, foods (Nicholls and Bryant-Waugh 2009).

Research has suggested that the establishment of new food preferences is linked to repeated exposure to novel foods (Birch 1982). Therefore, avoidance of new foods limits the development of new food preferences. In other words, if children refuse to taste new foods, they are not likely to expand their preferences (Williams and Foxx 2007). Similar to methods used for treating phobias, gradual exposure to novel food items is central to treating food selectivity (Seiverling et al. 2012; Williams et al. 2008). This is often accomplished by the use of tasting sessions in order to repeatedly expose children to small amounts of novel foods. Shaping may also be necessary in order for children to consume the novel food initially. Tasting sessions may be conducted during regular meals, or during separate sessions and later generalized into meals. In our clinical experience, we have observed previously-refused novel foods become frequently-requested foods. Similarly, in a recent study by Beighley et al. (2013), food selectivity was observed to decline across age groups, which ranged from 2 years to 18 years of age for all ASD groups (Autistic Disorder, PDD-NOS, and Asperger's Disorder), and over time approached similar levels of food selectivity as that displayed by peers with ID or general cognitive delays as well as by typically developing peers. This data suggests that over time and with repeated exposures, food selectivity may decrease in those with ASD; however, to date, there are no data investigating the course and longevity of food selectivity across the lifespan in those with ASD.

Behavioral/Environmental With respect to behavioral or social-environmental influences on complex feeding disorders, caregiver responses to behavior during meals also contribute to the maintenance of feeding problems. That is, feeding problems are also maintained by the events, settings, or people present at the beginning of meals (i.e., antecedents) as well as how other individuals (e.g., caregiver/feeder, others present during meals) react and respond when a feeding difficulty or mealtime misbehavior occurs (i.e., consequences). On the antecedent end, factors such as free access to snacks throughout the day, providing meals in a highly stimulating environment, and transitions to meals from a preferred activity may also produce problem behaviors at mealtime (Nadon et al. 2011; Williams and Foxx 2007). Additionally, there is some evidence that a family's food preference may be related to the child's food preferences. Specifically, in a study by Schreck et al. (2004), families who ate more restrictive diets were more likely to also have children with ASD with engaged in more restrictive or selective eating behavior. However, it is unclear which came first—the food selectivity of the child or the restrictive family diet. It is also possible that the eating habits of the whole family adapt to the more "picky" eater over time. Unfortunately, there is limited data in this area.

In terms of consequence-based variables, problematic feeding behavior may be maintained by a variety of reinforcement contingencies such as escape from eating the presented food (i.e., negative reinforcement) and caregiver attention to problematic behaviors or access to preferred foods (i.e., positive reinforcement) (Piazza et al. 2003). That is, when confronted with significant refusal behavior, caregivers will often provide attention to the refusal or remove food items and/or terminate a meal of novel foods. Caregivers may resort to using coercive tactics (e.g., threats, reprimands, and negative physical contact) or use other techniques (e.g., bribing/pleading, repeating prompts, time out/"calm down," provide a soothing activity, and remove nonpreferred food) in an attempt to reduce or stop the individual's behavior, get them to eat at least some portion of their meal, and reduce caregiver stress. Unfortunately, this pattern of caregiver response to the food refusal may increase the probability of an extreme emotional response of the individual (e.g., temper tantrums, self-injury, and aggression) to the point that problem behaviors and food refusal occurs at the majority, if not all, mealtimes. That is, what may start out as an occasional rigid pattern of behavior is often inadvertently negatively and/or positively reinforced due to caregivers' attempts to reduce the amount of conflict and problem behavior that may arise during mealtime. A functional analysis may be necessary to identify maintaining contingencies and assist the development of a function-based intervention (Najdowdki et al. 2008; Piazza et al. 2003).

Piazza et al. (2003) conducted an observational assessment of child and caregiver behaviors during mealtimes. Outcomes of the observations indicated that caregivers responded to child inappropriate behaviors with one of the following consequences: allowing escape from bites of food or the entire meal; coaxing or reprimanding; or providing the child with a toy or preferred food. That is, how the caregiver responds either with positive reinforcement (i.e., attention or provide preferred item) and/or negative reinforcement (i.e., remove the unwanted food item) may increase problem behaviors (e.g., physical aggression, whining/tantrums, vomiting/expulsion of bite, swiping at the utensils/tableware, disruptive/destructive behavior, self-injury, and food stealing) during mealtimes and may cause food refusal and selectivity issues to persist (Girolami and Scotti 2001; Matson et al. 2005; Piazza et al. 2003). Multiple functions were identified for 80% of the children, suggesting that many feeding problems can often be maintained by concurrent negative reinforcement (e.g., escape or avoidance) and positive reinforcement (e.g., access to attention or preferred food/tangible).

Matson et al. (2005) identified 125 adults with developmental disabilities (ID with or without ASD) who displayed one or more feeding problems categorized as problem behaviors (e.g., aggression, self-injury, and temper tantrums) during a meal, pica, rumination, food stealing, or food refusal. The behavioral function of these behaviors was assessed across the group using an indirect functional assessment measure, the *Questions About Behavioral Function* (QABF; Matson and Vollmer 1995). Results were consistent with the findings of other researchers, in that, mealtime problem behavior and food refusal behavior were found to be primarily maintained by negative reinforcement (Girolami and Scotti 2001; Najdowski et al., 2008; Piazza et al. 2003). Positive reinforcement contingencies in the form of access to attention or preferred foods were most commonly associated with food stealing and food refusal behaviors. Behaviors most commonly found to be maintained independent of social consequences (i.e., had an automatic or sensory function) included pica and rumination.

Consequences of Feeding Dysfunction

Extended feeding difficulties can lead to a failure to gain weight or even weight loss. Symptoms of constipation, vomiting, irritability, lethargy, and behavior problems are common. Inadequate food intake or food selectivity issues can cause nutritional deficiencies, including anemia (Bandini et al. 2010). Feeding disorders can interrupt children's physical and mental growth and development (Frank and Drotar 1994). Feeding disorders in infancy and childhood also place children at risk of developing eating disorders as adolescents or adults or continuing to have feeding/eating difficulties during mealtimes (Kotler et al. 2001; Marchi and Cohen 1990). Feeding dysfunction can lead to social isolation from peer groups, increase stress on families significantly (Ledford and Gast 2006; Sanders et al. 1993; Singer et al. 1990), and increase the likelihood of obesity and weight-related complications (Curtin et al. 2010; Zuckerman et al. 2014). Feeding disorders may require surgeries, use of feeding tubes, or hospitalization to ensure adequate nutrition. In the most severe circumstances, malnutrition and dehydration from feeding disorders can be life-threatening.

Conclusions

Feeding disorders in individuals diagnosed with ASD occur frequently and have the potential to cause serious outcomes. Therefore, a better understanding of the nature of the problem is warranted. Until recently, investigations into the interrelationship between ASD and feeding, and mealtime difficulties have been somewhat stymied by appropriate terminology and classification methods. With the recent inclusion of ARFID into the DSM-5 (APA 2013) and an acknowledgement that feeding disorders can and do occur across the lifespan in individuals with ASD and other developmental disabilities (e.g., ID), it would appear that being able to better understand that nature of these difficulties in this population could be more easily obtainable. However, there is still much to investigate to be able to fully understand the complex biological and environmental factors which likely contribute to the condition. Areas related to the topic of feeding disorders in those with ASD that are of extreme importance to continue to focus on better understanding the contribution of core features of ASD to the presentation or emergence of feeding difficulties, how environmental variables contribute to the maintenance of problematic eating patterns, investigating underlying medical or biological factors related to the presentation of feeding disorders, and how associated issues (e.g., mealtime behavior problems, sensory sensitivity, adaptive skill deficits, and cognitive deficits) impact the individual's ability to achieve mealtime independence. It would also be beneficial for clinicians to broaden their own definitions of what is an ASD-specific feeding difficulty, as most research in this area focuses primarily on food selectivity or food refusal. With researchers indicating that there are other feeding disorders that also occur across the lifespan of those with ASD (e.g., pica, rumination, obesity, and neophobia), it seems intuitive that to best address and remediate feeding and mealtime problems clinicians and researchers need to focus on the entire range of conditions that can occur and likely exacerbate or precipitate other feeding difficulties. Further elucidating these issues will assist in developing better assessment methodologies and informing appropriate and effective interventions to address feeding and mealtime difficulties in those diagnosed as having ASD. Thus, the end result of these efforts will increase the quality of life for the individual and for their family/caregivers, which appears to be the most important outcome.

References

Ahearn, W. H., Castine, T., Nault, K., & Green, G. (2001). An assessment of food acceptance in children with autism or pervasive developmental disorder-not otherwise specified. *Journal of Autism and Developmental Disorders, 31,* 505–511.

Ali, Z. (2001). Pica in people with intellectual disability: A literature review of aetiology, epidemiology and complications. *Journal of Intellectual and Developmental Disability, 26,* 205–215.

American Psychiatric Association. (2000). *Diagnostic and statistical manual of mental disorders* (5th ed., text rev.). Washington, DC: American Psychiatric Association.

American Psychiatric Association. (2013). *Diagnostic and statistical manual of mental disorders* (5th ed.). Arlington: American Psychiatric Association.

Anglesea, M. M., Hoch, H., & Taylor, B. A. (2008). Reducing rapid eating in teenagers with autism: Use of a pager prompt. *Journal of Applied Behavior Analysis, 41,* 107–111.

Ashworth, M., Martin, L., & Hirdes, J. P. (2008). Prevalence and correlates of pica among adults with intellectual disability in institutions. *Journal of Mental Health Research in Intellectual Disabilities, 1,* 176–190.

Babbitt, R. L., Hoch, T. A., Coe, D. A., Cataldo, M. F., Kelly, K. J., Stackhouse, C., et al. (1994). Behavioral assessment and treatment of pediatric feeding disorders. *Journal of Developmental and Behavioral Pediatrics, 15,* 278–291.

Bandini, L. G., Anderson, S. E., Curtin, C., Cermak, S., Evans, E. W., Scampini, R., et al. (2010). Food selectivity in children with autism spectrum disorders and typically developing children. *Journal of Pediatrics, 157,* 259–264.

Beighley, J. S., Matson, J. L., Rieske, R. D., & Adams, H. L. (2013). Food selectivity in children with and without an autism spectrum disorder: Investigation of diagnosis and age. *Research in Developmental Disabilities, 34,* 3497–3503.

Bennetto, L., Kuschner, E. S., & Hyman, S. L. (2007). Olfaction and taste processing in autism. *Biological Psychiatry, 62,* 1015–1021.

Bernstein, I. L. (1999). Taste aversion learning: A contemporary perspective. Nutrition, *15,* 229–234.

Birch, L. L. (1999). Development of food preferences. *Annual review of nutrition, 19,* 41–62.

Birch, L. L., & Marlin, D. W. (1982). I don't like it. I've never tried it: Effects of exposure on two-year-old children's food preferences. *Appetite, 3,* 353–360.

Bledsoe, R., Smith, B., & Simpson, R. L. (2003). Use of a social story intervention to improve mealtime skills of an adolescent with Asperger syndrome. *Autism: the international journal of research and practice, 7,* 289–295.

Brisson, J., Warreyn, P., Serres, J., Foussier, S., & Adrien-Louis, J. (2012). Motor anticipation failure in infants with autism: A retrospective analysis of feeding situations. *Autism: The International Journal of Research and Practice, 16,* 420–429.

Bryant-Waugh, R. (2013a). Feeding and eating disorders in children. *Current Opinion in Psychiatry, 26,* 537–542.

Bryant-Waugh, R. (2013b). Avoidant restrictive food intake disorder: An illustrative case example. *International Journal of Eating Disorders, 46,* 420–423.

Bryant-Waugh, R. J., & Piepenstock, E. H. (2008). Childhood disorders: Feeding and related disorders of infancy or early childhood. In A. Tasman, J. Kay, J. A. Lieberman, M. B. First & M. Maj (Eds.), *Psychiatry, Third Edition* (pp. 830–846.). Chichester: Wiley.

Bryant-Waugh, R., Markham, L., Kreipe, R. E., & Walsh, B. T. (2010). Feeding and eating disorders in childhood. *International Journal of Eating Disorders, 43,* 98–111.

Buie, T., Campbell, D. B., Fuchs, G. J., Furuta, G. T., Levy, J., VandeWater, J., Whitaker, A.H., Atkins, D., Bauman, M.L., Beaudet, A.L., Carr, E.G., Gershon, M.D., Hyman, S.L., Jirapinyo, P., Jyonouchi, H., Kooros, K., Kushak, R., Levitt, P., Levy, S.E., Lewis, J.D., Murray, K.F., Natowicz, M.R., Sabra, A., Wershil, B.K., Weston, S.C., Zeltzer, L., & Winter, H. (2010). Evaluation, diagnosis, and treatment of gastrointestinal disorders in individuals with ASDs: A consensus report. *Pediatrics, 125*(Suppl. 1), S1–S18.

Burklow, K. A., Phelps, A. N., Schultz, J. R., McConnell, K., & Rudolph, C. (1998). Classifying complex pediatric feeding disorders. *Journal of Pediatric Gastroenterology and Nutrition, 27,* 143–147.

Call, C., Walsh, B. T., & Attia, E. (2013). From DSM-IV to DSM-5: Changes to eating disorder diagnoses. *Current opinion in psychiatry, 26,* 532–536.

Carruth, B. R., Ziegler, P. J., Gordon, A., & Barr, S. I. (2004). Prevalence of picky eaters among infants and toddlers and their caregivers' decisions about offering a new food. *Journal of the American Dietetic Association, 104,* S57–S64.

Cermak, S. A., Curtin, C., & Bandini, L. G. (2010). Food selectivity and sensory sensitivity in children with autism spectrum disorders. *Journal of the American Dietetic Association, 110,* 238–246.

Chial, H. J., Camilleri, M., Williams, D. E., Litzinger, K., & Perrault, J. (2003). Rumination syndrome in children and adolescents: Diagnosis, treatment, and prognosis. *Pediatrics, 111,* 158–162.

Collins, M. S., Kyle, R., Smith, S., Laverty, A., Roberts, S., & Eaton-Evans, J. (2003). Coping with the usual family diet eating behaviour and food choices of children with down's syndrome, autistic spectrum disorders, or cri du chat syndrome and comparison groups of siblings. *Journal of Learning Disabilities, 7,* 137–155.

Curtin, C., Anderson, S. E., Must, A., & Bandini, L. (2010). The prevalence of obesity in children with autism: A secondary data analysis using nationally representative data from the National Survey of Children's Health. *BMC pediatrics, 10,* 11.

da Costa, S. P., van der Schans, C. P., Boelema, S. R., van der Meij, E., Boerman, M. A., & Bos, A. F. (2010). Sucking patterns in fullterm infants between birth and 10 weeks of age. *Infant Behavior and Development, 33,* 61–67.

Daniels, S. R. (2009). Complications of obesity in children and adolescents. *International Journal of Obesity, 33,* S60–S65.

Davis, M. K. (1998). Review of the evidence for an association between infant feeding and childhood cancer. *International Journal of Cancer, 78*(S11), 29–33.

Dunn, W. (1997). The impact of sensory processing abilities on the daily lives of young children and their families: A conceptual model. *Infants and Young Children, 9,* 23–35.

Eaves, L. C., & Ho, H. H. (2008). Young adult outcome of autism spectrum disorders. *Journal of Autism and Developmental Disorders, 38,* 739–747.

Egan, A. M., Dreyer, M. L., Odar, C. C., Beckwith, M., & Garrison, C. B. (2013). Obesity in young children with autism spectrum disorders: Prevalence and associated factors. *Childhood Obesity, 9,* 125–131.

Erickson, C. A., Stigler, K. A., Corkins, M. R., Posey, D. J., Fitzgerald, J. F., & McDougle, C. J. (2005). Gastrointestinal factors in autistic disorder: A critical review. *Journal of Autism and Developmental Disorders, 35,* 713–727.

Farrow, C. V., & Coulthard, H. (2012). Relationships between sensory sensitivity, anxiety and selective eating in children. *Appetite, 58,* 842–846.

Field, D., Garland, M., & Williams, K. (2003). Correlates of specific childhood feeding problems. *Journal of Paediatrics and Child Health, 39,* 299–304.

Fodstad, J. C., & Matson, J. L. (2008). A comparison of feeding and mealtime problems in adults with intellectual disabilities with and without autism. *Journal of Developmental and Physical Disabilities, 20,* 541–550.

Frank, D. A., & Drotar, D. (1994). Failure to thrive. In R. M. Reece (Ed.), *Child abuse: Medical diagnosis, treatment and management* (pp. 298–324). Philadelphia: Lea & Febiger.

Girolami, P. A., & Scotti, J. R. (2001). Use of analog functional analysis in assessing the function of mealtime behavior problems. *Education and Training in Mental Retardation and Developmental Disabilities, 26,* 207–223.

Gravestock, S. (2000). Eating disorders in adults with intellectual disability. *Journal of Intellectual Disability Research, 44,* 625–637.

Hartmann, A. S., Becker, A. E., Hampton, C., & Bryant-Waugh, R. (2012). Pica and rumination disorder in DSM-5. *Psychiatric Annals, 42,* 426–430.

Hinckson, E. A., Dickinson, A., Water, T., Sands, M., & Penman, L. (2013). Physical activity, dietary habits and overall health in overweight and obese children and youth with intellectual disability or autism. *Research in Developmental Disabilities, 34,* 1170–1178.

Ho, H. H., Eaves, L. C., & Peabody, D. (1997). Nutrient intake and obesity in children with autism. *Focus on Autism and Other Developmental Disabilities, 12,* 187–192.

Holden, B., & Gitlesen, J. P. (2008). The relationship between psychiatric symptomatology and motivation of challenging behaviour: A preliminary study. *Research in Developmental Disabilities, 29,* 408–413.

Horvath, K., & Perman, J. A. (2002). Autistic disorder and gastrointestinal disease. *Current Opinion in Pediatrics, 14,* 583–587.

Hove, O. (2007). Survey on dysfunctional eating behavior in adult persons with intellectual disability living in the community. *Research in Developmental Disabilities, 28,* 1–8.
Hubbard, K. L., Anderson, S. E., Curtin, C., Must, A., & Bandini, L. G. (2014). A comparison of food refusal related to characteristics of food in children with Autism Spectrum Disorder and typically developing children. *Journal of the Academy of Nutrition and Dietetics.* doi:10.1016/j.jand.2014.04.017.
Johnson, C. R., Turner, K., Stewart, P. A., Schmidt, B., Shui, A., Macklin, E., et al. (2014). Relationships between feeding problems, behavioral characteristics and nutritional quality in children with ASD. *Journal of Autism and Developmental Disorders, 44,* 2175–2184.
Johnston, J. M. (1993). Phenomenology and treatment of rumination. *Eating and Growth Disorders, 2,* 93–107.
Kanner, L. (1943). Autistic disturbances of affective contact. *Nervous child, 2,* 217–250.
Kerwin, M. E., Eicher, P. S., & Gelsinger, J. (2005). Parental report of eating problems and gastrointestinal symptoms in children with pervasive developmental disorders. *Children's Health Care, 34,* 217–234.
Kinnell, H. G. (1985). Pica as a feature of autism. *The British Journal of Psychiatry, 147,* 80–82.
Konst, M. J., & Matson, J. L. (2014). Comorbid psychopathology symptom rates in infants and toddlers with autism spectrum disorders. *Research in Autism Spectrum Disorders, 8,* 147–155.
Kotler, L. A., Cohen, P., Davies, M., Pine, D. S., & Walsh, B. T. (2001). Longitudinal relationships between childhood, adolescent, and adult eating disorders. *Journal of the American Academy of Child and Adolescent Psychiatry, 40,* 1434–1440.
Kozlowski, A. M., Matson, J. L., Fodstad, J. C., & Moree, B. N. (2011). Feeding therapy in a child with autistic disorder: Sequential food presentation. *Clinical Case Studies, 10,* 236–246.
Kozlowski, A. M., Matson, J. L., Belva, B., & Rieske, R. (2012). Feeding and sleep difficulties in toddlers with autism spectrum disorders. *Research in Autism Spectrum Disorders, 6,* 385–390.
Kuhn, D. E., & Matson, J. L. (2002). A validity study of the screening tool of feeding problems (STEP). *Journal of Intellectual and Developmental Disability, 27,* 161–167.
Kuhn, D. E., & Matson, J. L. (2004). Assessment of feeding and mealtime behavior problems in persons with mental retardation. *Behavior Modification, 28,* 638–648.
Lane, A. E., Geraghty, M. E., Young, G. S., & Rostorfer, J. L. (2014). Problem eating behaviors in autism spectrum disorder are associated with suboptimal daily nutrient intake and taste/smell sensitivity. *ICAN: Infant, Child, and Adolescent Nutrition.* doi:1941406414523981.
Laud, R. B., Girolami, P. A., Boscoe, J. H., & Gulotta, C. S. (2009). Treatment outcomes for severe feeding problems in children with autism spectrum disorder. *Behavior Modification, 33,* 520–536.
Ledford, J. R., & Gast, D. L. (2006). Feeding problems in children with autism spectrum disorders: A review. *Focus on Autism and Other Developmental Disabilities, 21,* 153–166.
Lewis, M. A., Lewis, C. E., Leake, B., King, B. H., & Lindemann, R. (2002). The quality of health care for adults with developmental disabilities. *Public Health Reports, 117,* 174.
Lindberg, L., Bahlin, G., & Hagekull, S. (1991). Early feeding problems in a normal population. *International Journal of Eating Disorders, 10,* 395–405.
Linscheid, T. R. (1983). Eating problems in children. In C. E. Walker & M. C. Roberts (Eds.), *Handbook of clinical child psychology* (pp. 616–639). New York: Wiley.
Luiselli, J. K., Medeiros, J., Jasinowski, C., Smith, A., & Cameron, M. J. (1994). Behavioral medicine treatment of ruminative vomiting and associated weight loss in an adolescent with autism. *Journal of Autism and Developmental Disorders, 24,* 619–629.
Manikam, R., & Perman, J. (2000). Pediatric feeding disorders. *Journal of Clinical Gastroenterology, 30,* 34–46.
Manno, C. J., Fox, C., Eicher, P. S., & Kerwin, M. E. (2005). Early oral-motor interventions for pediatric feeding problems: What, when and how. *Journal of Early and Intensive Behavior Intervention, 2,* 145–159.
Marchi, M., & Cohen, P. (1990). Early childhood eating behaviors and adolescent eating disorders. *Journal of the American Academy of Child and Adolescent Psychiatry, 29,* 112–117.

Marí-Bauset, S., Zazpe, I., Mari-Sanchis, A., Llopis-González, A., & Morales-Suárez-Varela, M. (2013). Food selectivity in Autism Spectrum Disorders: A systematic review. *Journal of Child Neurology*. doi:10.1177/0883073813498821.

Martins, Y., Young, R. L., & Robson, D. C. (2008). Feeding and eating behaviors in children with autism and typically developing children. *Journal of Autism and Developmental Disorders, 38,* 1878–1887.

Mascola, A., Bryson, S. W., & Agras, W. S. (2011). Picky eating during childhood: A longitudinal study to age 11-years. *Eating Behaviors, 11,* 253–257.

Matson, J. L., & Bamburg, J. W. (1999). A descriptive study of pica behavior in persons with mental retardation. *Journal of Developmental and Physical Disabilities, 11,* 353–361.

Matson, J. L., & Fodstad, J. C. (2009). The treatment of food selectivity and other feeding problems in children with autism spectrum disorders. *Research in Autism Spectrum Disorders, 3,* 455–461.

Matson, J. L., & Nebel-Schwalm, M. S. (2007). Comorbid psychopathology with autism spectrum disorder in children: An overview. *Research in Developmental Disabilities, 28,* 341–352.

Matson, J. L., & Shoemaker, M. (2009). Intellectual disability and its relationship to autism spectrum disorders. *Research in developmental disabilities, 30,* 1107–1114.

Matson, J. L., & Vollmer, T. R. (1995). *User's guide: Questions about behavioral function (QABF).* Baton Rouge: Disability Consultants, LLC.

Matson, J. L., Gardner, W. I., Coe, D. A., & Sovner, R. (1991). A scale for evaluating emotional disorders in severely and profoundly mentally retarded persons. development of the diagnostic assessment for the severely handicapped (DASH) scale. *The British Journal of Psychiatry, 159,* 404–409.

Matson, J. L., Baglio, C. S., Smiroldo, B. B., Hamilton, M., Packlowskyj, T., Williams, D., et al. (1996). Characteristics of autism as assessed by the diagnostic assessment for the severely handicapped—II (DASH-II). *Research in Developmental Disabilities, 17,* 135–143.

Matson, J. L., Dixon, D. R., & Matson, M. L. (2005a). Assessing and treating aggression in children and adolescents with developmental disabilities: A 20—year overview. *Educational Psychology, 25,* 151–181.

Matson, J. L., Mayville, S. B., Kuhn, D. E., Sturmey, P., Laud, R., & Cooper, C. (2005b). The behavioral function of feeding problems as assessed by the questions about behavioral function (QABF). *Research in Developmental Disabilities, 26,* 399–408.

Matson, J. L., Fodstad, J. C., & Boisjoli, J. A. (2008). Cutoff scores, norms and patterns of feeding problems for the Screening Tool of feeding Problems (STEP) for adults with intellectual disabilities. *Research in Developmental Disabilities, 29,* 363–372.

Matson, J. L., Fodstad, J. C., & Dempsey, T. (2009a). The relationship of children's feeding problems to core symptoms of autism and PDD-NOS. *Research in Autism Spectrum Disorders, 3,* 759–766.

Matson, J. L., Fodstad, J. C., & Rivet, T. T. (2009b). The relationship of social skills and problem behaviors in adults with intellectual disability and autism or PDD-NOS. *Research in Autism Spectrum Disorders, 3,* 258–268.

Matson, J. L., Rivet, T. T., Fodstad, J. C., Dempsey, T., & Boisjoli, J. A. (2009c). Examination of adaptive behavior differences in adults with autism spectrum disorders and intellectual disability. *Research in Developmental Disabilities, 30,* 1317–1325.

Matson, J. L., Belva, B., Hattier, M. A., & Matson, M. L. (2011). Pica in persons with developmental disabilities: Characteristics, diagnosis, and assessment. *Research in Autism Spectrum Disorders, 5,* 1459–1464.

Matsuo, K., & Palmer, J. B. (2008). Anatomy and physiology of feeding and swallowing: Normal and abnormal. *Physical Medicine and Rehabilitation Clinics of North America, 19,* 691–707.

McLoughlin, I. J. (1987). The picas. *British journal of hospital medicine, 37,* 286–290.

Nadon, G., Feldman, D. E., Dunn, W., & Gisel, E. (2011). Association of sensory processing and eating problems in children with autism spectrum disorders. *Autism Research and Treatment.* doi:10.1155/2011/541926.

Najdowski, A. C., Wallace, M. D., Penrod, B., Tarbox, J., Reagon, K., & Higbee, T. S. (2008). Caregiver-conducted experimental functional analyses of inappropriate mealtime behavior. *Journal of Applied Behavior Analysis, 41,* 459–465.

Nicholls, D., & Bryant-Waugh, R. (2009). Eating disorders of infancy and childhood: Definition, symptomatology, epidemiology, and comorbidity. *Child and Adolescent Psychiatric Clinics of North America, 18,* 17–30.

Paclawskyj, T. R., Kurtz, P. F., & O'Connor, J. T. (2004). Functional assessment of problem behaviors in adults with mental retardation. *Behavior Modification, 28,* 649–667.

Paisey, T. J., & Whitney, R. B. (1989). A long-term case study of analysis, response suppression, and treatment maintenance involving life-threatening pica. *Behavioral Interventions, 4,* 191–211.

Piazza, C. C., & Addison, L. R. (2007). Function-based assessment and treatment of pediatric feeding disorders. In P. Sturmey (Ed) *Functional analysis in clinical treatment* (pp. 129–150). New York: Academic Press.

Piazza, C. C., Fisher, W. W., Hanley, G. P., LeBlanc, L. A., Worsdell, A. S., Lindauer, S. E., et al. (1998). Treatment of pica through multiple analyses of its reinforcing functions. *Journal of Applied Behavior Analysis, 31,* 165–189.

Piazza, C. C., Fisher, W. W., Brown, K. A., Shore, B. A., Patel, M. R., Katz, R. M., Sevin, B. M., Gulotta, C. S., & Blakely-Smith, A. (2003). Functional analysis of inappropriate mealtime behaviors. *Journal of Applied Behavior Analysis, 36,* 187–204.

Pierce, K. L., & Schreibman, L. (1994). Teaching daily living skills to children with autism in unsupervised settings through pictorial self-management. *Journal of Applied Behavior Analysis, 27,* 471–481.

Rastam, M. (2008). Eating disturbances in autism spectrum disorders with focus on adolescent and adult years. *Clinical Neuropsychiatry, 5,* 31–42.

Rehfeldt, R. A., Dahman, D., Young, A., Cherry, H., & Davis, P. (2003). Teaching a simple meal preparation skill to adults with moderate and severe mental retardation using video modeling. *Behavioral Interventions, 18,* 209–218.

Rhine, D., & Tarbox, J. (2009). Chewing gum as a treatment for rumination in a child with autism. *Journal of Applied Behavior Analysis, 42,* 381–385.

Rimmer, J. H., Yamaki, K., Lowry, B. M., Wang, E., & Vogel, L. C. (2010). Obesity and obesity-related secondary conditions in adolescents with intellectual/developmental disabilities. *Journal of Intellectual Disability Research, 54,* 787–794.

Rommel, N., De Meyer, A. M., Feenstra, L., & Veereman-Wauters, G. (2003). The complexity of feeding problems in 700 infants and young children presenting to a tertiary care institution. *Journal of Pediatric Gastroenterology and Nutrition, 37,* 75–84.

Sanders, M. R., Patel, R. K., Le Grice, B., & Shepherd, R. W. (1993). Children with persistent feeding difficulties: An observational analysis of the feeding interactions of problem and non-problem eaters. *Health Psychology, 12,* 64–73.

Schmitt, L., Heiss, C. J., & Campbell, E. E. (2008). A comparison of nutrient intake and eating behaviors of boys with and without autism. *Topics in Clinical Nutrition, 23,* 23–31.

Schreck, K. A., & Williams, K. (2006). Food preferences and factors influencing food selectivity for children with autism spectrum disorders. *Research in Developmental Disabilities, 27,* 353–363.

Schreck, K. A., Williams, K., & Smith, A. F. (2004). A comparison of eating behaviors between children with and without autism. *Journal of Autism and Developmental Disorders, 34,* 433–438.

Schwarz, S. M. (2003). Feeding disorders in children with developmental disabilities. *Infants and Young Children, 16,* 317–330.

Schwarz, S. M., Corredor, J., Fisher-Medina, J., Cohen, J., & Rabinowitz, S. (2001). Diagnosis and treatment of feeding disorders in children with developmental disabilities. *Pediatrics, 108,* 671–676.

Seiverling, L., Williams, K., & Sturmey, P. (2010). Assessment of feeding problems in children with autism spectrum disorders. *Journal of Developmental and Physical Disabilities, 22,* 401–413.

Seiverling, L., Williams, K., Sturmey, P., & Hart, S. (2012). Effects of behavioral skills training on parental treatment of children's food selectivity. *Journal of Applied Behavior Analysis, 45,* 197–203.

Sharp, W. G., Berry, R. C., McCracken, C., Nuhu, N. N., Marvel, E., Saulnier, C. A., Klin, A., Jones, W., & Jaquess, D. L. (2013). Feeding problems and nutrient intake in children with autism spectrum disorders: A meta-analysis and comprehensive review of the literature. *Journal of Autism and Developmental Disorders, 43,* 2159–2173.

Singer, L. T., Song, L., Hill, B. P., & Jaffe, A. C. (1990). Stress and depression in mothers of failure-to-thrive children. *Journal of Pediatric Psychology, 15,* 711–720.

Sisson, L. A., & Van Hasselt, V. B. (1989). Feeding disorders. In J. K. Luiselli (Ed.), *Behavioral medicine and developmental disabilities* (pp. 45–73). New York: Springer.

Stevenson, R. D., & Allaire, J. H. (1991). The development of normal feeding and swallowing. *Pediatric Clinics of North America, 38,* 1439–1453.

Stiegler, L. N. (2005). Understanding pica behavior a review for clinical and education professionals. *Focus on Autism and Other Developmental Disabilities, 20,* 27–38.

Tavassoli, T., & Baron-Cohen, S. (2012). Taste identification in adults with autism spectrum conditions. *Journal of Autism and Developmental Disorders, 42,* 1419–1424.

Tomchek, S. D., & Dunn, W. (2007). Sensory processing in children with and without autism: A comparative study using the short sensory profile. *American Journal of Occupational Therapy, 61,* 190–200.

Twachtman-Reilly, J., Amaral, S. C., & Zebrowski, P. P. (2008). Addressing feeding disorders in children on the autism spectrum in school-based settings: Physiological and behavioral issues. *Language, Speech, and Hearing Services in Schools, 39,* 261–272.

Vig, S., & Jedrysek, E. (1999). Autistic features in young children with significant cognitive impairment: Autism or mental retardation? *Journal of Autism and Developmental Disorders, 29,* 235–248.

Williams, K. E., & Foxx, R. M. (2007). *Treating eating problems of children with autism spectrum disorders and developmental disabilities: Interventions for professionals and parents*. Austin: Pro-Ed.

Williams, K. E., Paul, C., Pizzo, B., & Riegel, K. (2008). Practice does make perfect. A longitudinal look at repeated taste exposure. *Appetite, 51,* 739–742.

Williams, K. E., Riegel, K., & Kerwin, M. L. (2009). Feeding disorder of infancy or early childhood: How often is it seen in feeding programs? *Children's Health Care, 38,* 123–136.

World Health Organization. (2010). International statistical classification of diseases and related health problems (10th ed.). http://apps.who.int/classifications/icd10/browse/2010/en. Accessed 10 Feb 2014.

Wright, C. M., Smith, K. H., & Morrison, J. (2011). Withdrawing feeds from children on long term enteral feeding: Factors associated with success and failure. *Archives of Disease in Childhood, 96,* 433–439.

Zuckerman, K. E., Hill, A. P., Guion, K., Voltolina, L., & Fombonne, E. (2014). Overweight and obesity: Prevalence and correlates in a large clinical sample of children with autism spectrum disorder. *Journal of Autism and Developmental Disorders, 44,* 1708–1719.

Chapter 9
Sleep Disorders

Karen McKenzie, Halina Rzepecka and Iain McClure

Introduction

Prevalence of ASD in Children

Autism spectrum disorder (ASD) is a relatively common developmental disorder (Yates and Le Couteur 2012). Whilst there are recognised difficulties in estimating prevalence rates due to differing diagnostic criteria and inclusion/exclusion criteria in studies (Volkmar et al. 2004), there is some consensus that it affects approximately one person in 100 (Allison et al. 2012; Baron-Cohen et al. 2009). Individuals with ASD are part of a heterogeneous group, with representation across a range of intelligence quotient (IQ) levels. Intellectual disability (ID) is the most common co-morbid condition with ASD, with estimates suggesting that up to 70% of those with ASD also meet the criteria for ID (see Matson and Goldin 2013, for an overview). This co-morbidity has implications for sleep difficulties, as sleep problems have been found to be common in children with ASD, ID and ASD and ID (Rzepecka et al. 2011) and many studies which research sleep difficulties including those with both ASD and ID (Cortesi et al. 2010).

K. McKenzie (✉)
Northumbria University, Department of Psychology, Northumberland Building,
Newcastle-upon-Tyne, Edinburgh, NE1 8ST, UK
e-mail: k.mckenzie@northumbria.ac.uk

Northumbria University, NE1 8ST Newcastle upon Tyne, UK

H. Rzepecka
NHS Tayside, Centre for Child Health, 19 Dudhope Terrace, Dundee, DD3 6HH, UK

I. McClure
NHS Lothian, The Esk Centre, Ladywell way, Musselburgh, EH21 6AB, UK

Johnny L. Matson (ed.), *Comorbid Conditions Among Children with Autism Spectrum Disorders,* Autism and Child Psychopathology Series,
DOI 10.1007/978-3-319-19183-6_9

Introduction to Sleep Problems

Sleep is thought to serve many important functions including facilitating brain as well as physical and psychological functioning (Czeisler 2011). Sleep deprivation, can, therefore, have a number of negative consequences, including extreme tiredness and sleepiness, reduced cognitive performance, such as memory, learning and attentional difficulties, increased risk of accidents and poorer cardiovascular, immune and metabolic functioning (Czeisler 2011; Fallone et al. 2005; Gozal 1998). The detrimental impact on cognitive performance is likely to be particularly concerning for children with ASD/ID who, by definition, already have significant cognitive difficulties. It is also widely acknowledged that caring for a child with ID and/or ASD is generally more stressful than caring for a typically developing child (Eisenhower et al. 2005), and this can be exacerbated by the child's sleep problems (e.g. Hoffman et al. 2008).

Measuring sleep problems can be difficult, particularly in children where self-report may not be possible. Richdale and Schreck (2009) outline a number of factors which may impact on estimated prevalence rates including: the population being studied (including age and level of IQ), how sleep problems are defined and measured and who is reporting on the sleep problem. These difficulties need to be borne in mind when considering the research outlined in the chapter.

This chapter provides an overview of the sleep problems experienced by children with ASD, beginning with a definition of sleep problems and sleep architecture, followed by a discussion of relevant developmental/biological, psychological and social factors and ending with an overview of potential interventions.

Definition of Sleep Disorders and Problems

It is important to distinguish between sleep disorders and sleep problems. Whilst mainly of adult orientation, there are over 80 different sleep disorders included in the International Classification of Sleep Disorders-Revised, (American Sleep Disorders Association 1997). Stores and Wiggs (2001) identify three main categories of sleep problems: difficulty falling asleep or remaining asleep, too much sleep and disturbed sleep. Within these broader categories, common sleep problems include refusal to go to bed and distress around going to bed, refusal to sleep in own bed, co-sleeping, delayed sleep onset, frequent waking during the night, nightmares, sleep walking, snoring, early morning waking and excessive daytime sleepiness (Espie 2000).

There are also three main types of sleep disorders. Dysomnias are disorders which result in difficulty falling asleep, remaining asleep or excessive sleepiness during the day. Many of the difficulties reported by parents of children with ASD and confirmed by objective measures, fall within this category (Richdale and Schreck 2009). Parasomnias are disorders whereby the sleep process is disrupted. The third category covers sleep disorders which are related to neurological or medical conditions.

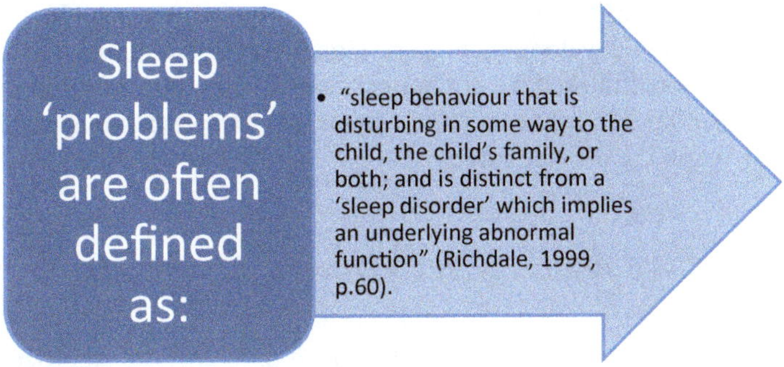

Sleep Architecture and Normal Sleep Development

The circadian clock (the suprachiasmatic nucleus of the hypothalamus) regulates endogenous circadian rhythms which are aligned with social and environmental cues (Brandon and Zee 2006). Essentially, this clock programs humans to be awake during the day and to sleep at night. As we move from awake to asleep, there is a progressive slowing of electrical activity in the brain (Stores 2001a), which can be monitored by an electroencephalogram (EEG). There are four stages of non-rapid eye movement (NREM) sleep, with EEG activity slowing as the stage number increases. Rapid eye movement (REM) sleep is a separate stage of sleep, characterised by high rates of brain activity (Stores 2001a). There is a high frequency of REM sleep in early life, which decreases with age (Brandon and Zee 2006).

Newborn babies and infants do not differentiate between night and day. However, this distinction is established quite quickly as sleep develops to be mainly at night and naps are shortened during the day (Richdale and Prior 1995). Many young typically developing children will be sleeping through the night by 1 year of age, daytime naps will be extinguished by around age 3–5 years, and an adult pattern of sleep will gradually develop and be established by adolescence (Robinson and Waters 2008). However, difficulties with settling, night-time waking and early morning waking are common in up to 25% of typically developing school age children, but will generally improve with age (Scher et al. 1995).

Sleep Problems in Children with ASD

There is a wealth of literature regarding sleep problems in children with ASD. Studies examining prevalence rates have estimated that sleep problems in children with ASD range from 53 to 81% (Couturier et al. 2005; Mannion Leader and Healy 2013; Paavonen et al. 2008; Polimeni et al. 2005; Rzepecka et al. 2011). Significantly more sleep problems have been identified in children with ASD when compared with typically developing children (Allik et al. 2006; Honomichl et al. 2002; Patzold et al. 1998; Richdale and Prior 1995) or with other groups such as children with epilepsy (Tsai et al. 2012). In contrast to these findings, Hering et al. (1999) did not report significant differences between the sleep patterns of children with ASD compared to typically developing children. However, these authors note that a very small sample size and limited ASD diagnosis information may have contributed to these results. Similar difficulties are likely to have contributed to the varying prevalence rates noted in the previous studies.

Aetiology of Sleep Problems in Children with ASD/ID

The research presented above indicates that sleep problems are significantly more prevalent in those with ASD/ID compared to the typically developing population. Whilst there is no single definitive theory to explain this, there are several developmental/biological, psychological and social factors which indicate why this may be the case. Indeed, Richdale and Schreck (2009) suggest that sleep difficulties in people with ASD may be the outcome of complex interactions between many of these factors (see Fig. 9.1).

Developmental/Biological Factors

Syndromes and Medical Conditions There is some evidence to suggest that there is a higher prevalence of sleep disorders and problems in some syndromes and medical conditions associated with ID. Children with Down syndrome (DS) are vulnerable

Fig. 9.1 Some of the factors which are thought to influence sleep difficulties in children with ASD

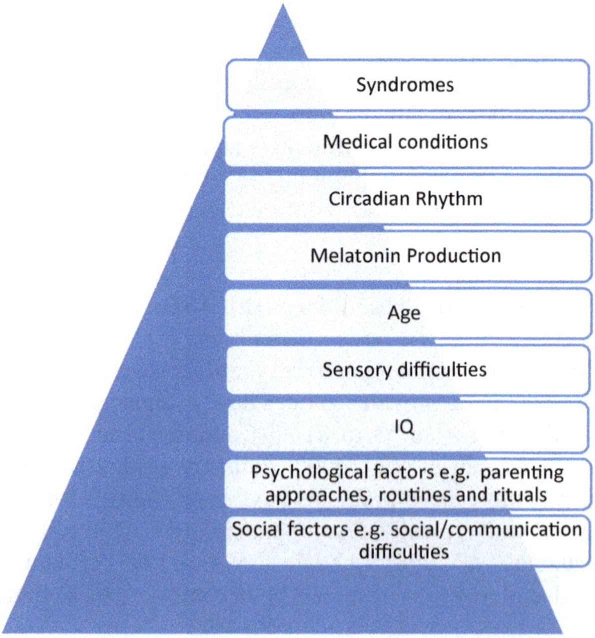

to upper airway obstructions, unusual tongue position and enlarged tonsils and adenoids, which can lead to breathing difficulties and disruption of REM sleep, thereby increasing the likelihood of sleep problems (Levanon et al. 1999; Miano et al. 2008; Stores 2001b). Many studies have found sleep problems in children with DS to be more common than in typically developing children (e.g. Fields et al. 1995). Stores et al. (1996) examined sleep problems in children with DS, non-specific ID and typically developing children. The authors found that both the children with DS and ID had significantly more sleep problems than the typically developing children. Children with Prader-Willi Syndrome (PWS) have been reported to show excessive daytime sleepiness (Richdale et al. 1999). In a study by Cotton and Richdale (2006), children with ASD, DS, PWS and ID were all found to have up to four times more sleep problems than typically developing children, and these were most common in the ASD group.

Epilepsy is one of the most common medical conditions associated with ID and sleep problems, and has also been found to impact negatively on the sleep of typically developing children (e.g. Stores et al. 1998) as well as individuals with ID (Giannotti et al. 2008).

In terms of other physical conditions, Mannion et al. (2013) found that sleep anxiety, parasomnias and daytime sleepiness in children with ASD were predicted by gastrointestinal symptoms as well as the Autism Spectrum Disorders Comorbidity-Child Version (ASD-CC: Matson and Gonzalez 2007) subscales of under-eating and avoidant behaviour.

Circadian Rhythm/Melatonin Production It has been proposed that individuals with ASD/ID may have circadian rhythm dysfunction or disorders, and abnormalities in melatonin production which can impact on normal sleep patterns (e.g. Richdale and Schreck 2009). Individuals with ASD and/or ID have been found to have increased stage one sleep and less REM sleep (Brandon and Zee 2006; Levanon et al. 1999). Melatonin is an endogenous hormone, produced by the pineal gland during darkness, and appears to be involved in the phase setting of the circadian clock (Wehr et al. 2001). Melatonin should be produced during daylight and activated at night, but this cycle has been found to be disrupted in individuals with ASD/ID, leading to a deficiency in melatonin production (Hare et al. 2006; Sajith and Clarke 2007).

IQ Sleep problems occur at all levels of IQ within ASD and ID, but there is some debate in the literature as to how IQ impacts on the severity of the sleep problem, if at all. Richdale and Prior (1995) found more sleep problems in children with ASD with a higher IQ when compared to children with ASD with a lower IQ. Richdale (1999) reports that some studies suggest that sleep problems increase as IQ decreases. Other studies, however, have found no impact of IQ level on sleep problems (e.g. Mayes and Calhoun 2009; Patzold et al. 1998; Williams et al. 2004).

Age There has been mixed evidence in the literature to suggest that sleep problems in children with ASD and/or ID might improve with age, as is seen in typically developing children. For example, in a study of children (aged 3–19 years) with ASD, Richdale and Prior (1995) found that sleep problems did improve with age, with the most severe problems occurring when the children were under 8 years of age. Goldman and colleagues (2011) also found age differences, with younger children with ASD who slept poorly having an increased likelihood of also having language difficulties, hyperactivity, aggression and eating problems compared with the older children who were also poor sleepers. However, Quine (2001) found that most sleep problems in children attending mainstream school improved with age, but only night waking and sleeping in the parental bed improved with age in children attending special school. Likewise, Mayes and Calhoun (2009) found no relationship between sleep problems and age. Instead they found that the severity of ASD symptoms was the strongest predictor of sleep problems. Therefore, it is unclear if sleep problems in children with ASD and/or ID will improve with age, as is expected in typically developing children.

Sensory Problems Children with ASD/ID are particularly prone to sensory impairments and these, in turn, have been associated with sleep problems. Hodapp (1998) reports that 17% of children with ID have hearing impairments and 30% have visual impairments. It seems reasonable that, given the impact of the environment, daylight and darkness on the circadian clock, individuals with severe visual impairments may have difficulties sleeping. Children with ID and a visual impairment have been found to have significantly more sleep problems than healthy controls (e.g. Carvil 2001), and it has been reported that a visual impairment impacts negatively on sleep, out with the possible influence of the ID.

Psychological Factors

Parental Factors It has been noted that some parents of children with ASD/ID may believe that sleep problems are inherently associated with the condition and, therefore, not amenable to change (Honomichl et al. 2002; Robinson and Richdale 2003). Additionally, it has been shown that sleep problems in children with ASD/ID result in greater levels of parental stress (e.g. Hoffman et al. 2008). Parental stress has also been shown to impact on quality of care, possibly resulting in ineffective and inconsistent parenting strategies being implemented around the child's sleep problems (Quine 2001).

Routines and Rituals One of the core features of ASD is the need for routine and consistency. It has been speculated that some children with ASD may have established a poor bedtime routine. As children with ASD have a strong need for routine and become distressed when routines are changed, parents may find it particularly difficult to set new boundaries and structure around bedtime behaviour (Patzold et al. 1998).

Social Factors

Social/Communication Difficulties Children with ASD are likely to be affected by social and communication difficulties, which can potentially impact on the sleep/wake

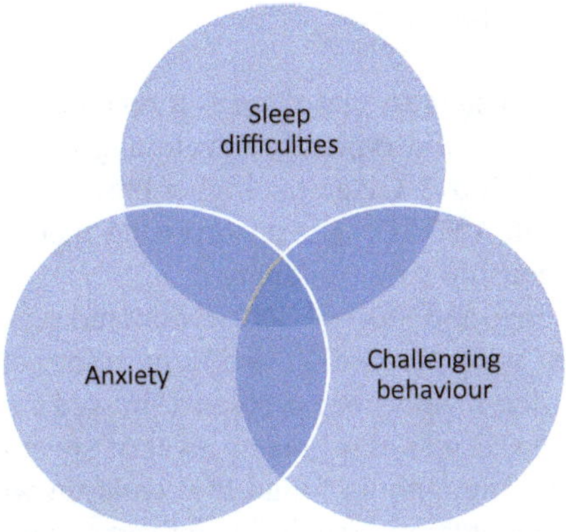

Fig. 9.2 Conditions that have been found to coexist in children with ASD

cycle. Humans are thought to use social cues (such as the family getting ready for bed) as well as environmental cues (such as light and dark) to help maintain their circadian rhythm (Brandon and Zee 2006). If a child is unable to identify social and environmental cues, this could lead to problems in the sleep/wake cycle (Richdale 1999).

Sleep Difficulties and Co-occurring Conditions

There is a body of research that states that sleep difficulties often co-occur with other clinical difficulties, such as anxiety and challenging behaviour (CB) in both typically developing children and those with ASD/ID (see Fig. 9.2).

Sleep and Anxiety

There is a substantial literature which has found a relationship between sleep problems and anxiety in typically developing children (e.g. Alfano et al. 2006; Alfano et al. 2007), but far less is known about this relationship in children with ASD. Patzold et al. (1998) suggested that psychological factors such as anxiety may be impacting on sleep problems in this latter group, but this is not directly addressed. Allik et al. (2006) reported a positive correlation between the emotional subscale of the Strength and Difficulties Questionnaire (Goodman 1997) and insomnia in children with ASD. Whilst this suggests a relationship between emotional difficulties and sleep problems in children with ASD, it does not address anxiety specifically. Rzepecka et al. (2011) examined the relationship between sleep difficulties, anxiety and CB in children with ASD/ID and found significant correlations between the three, with medication, sleep problems and anxiety significantly predicting CB. Sleep problems were found to be the strongest of the three predictive factors.

Sleep and Challenging Behaviour

There is some evidence to suggest that there is a relationship between sleep problems and behaviour problems in typically developing children (e.g. Blunden and Chervin 2008; Stein et al. 2001). Given the higher prevalence of both CB and sleep problems in children with ASD/ID, it is unsurprising that there is substantial evidence to suggest a relationship between the two.

An early study by Wiggs and Stores (1996) examined severe sleep problems and daytime CB in children with severe ID, 16.5 % of whom also had a diagnosis of ASD, and found that children with sleep problems showed a greater number of types of CB. Furthermore, the CB was at a greater level of severity than in the children without sleep problems. The authors found that children who showed poor sleep were more likely to show daytime irritability, lethargy, stereotyped behaviour and hyperactivity. They suggested that the disrupted sleep had a direct impact on daytime functioning. A similar study was conducted with adults with ID by Brylewski and Wiggs (1999). The authors divided the sample into good sleepers and poor sleepers and found that the poor sleepers showed significantly more CB, including daytime irritability, stereotyped behaviours and hyperactivity. This suggests that the difficulties seen in childhood are likely to continue into adulthood.

Richdale et al. (2000) explored stress, behaviour and sleep problems in 52 children with ASD/ID compared to children without these diagnoses. The results suggested that the presence of sleep problems was significantly associated with intensity and frequency of parental hassles and the presence of CB. The level of ID was not found to impact on the findings. The authors noted that whilst a relationship was found between sleep and CB, no direction could be predicted. Didden et al. (2002) also examined sleep problems and daytime behaviour in children with a range of levels of ID. Just over one fifth of this sample also had ASD. The results suggested that the children with severe sleep problems also showed higher scores on aggression, screaming, temper tantrums, non-compliance and impulsivity compared to the children without a sleep disorder.

A more recent study by DeVincent et al. (2007) compared preschool children with and without a pervasive developmental disability (PDD) on measures of sleep and behaviour. A relationship was found between sleep and behaviour in both groups and the authors highlighted the fact that this relationship was similar between the two groups. However, significantly more sleep problems were evident in those with PDD and these were associated with inattentiveness, hyperactivity and oppositional behaviour. Children in the sleep disturbance group also showed more elevated scores on scales of separation anxiety, generalised anxiety disorder and major depressive disorder.

Rzepecka et al. (2011) found significant relationships between sleep problems, anxiety and CB, with sleep problems, anxiety and medication being found to account for 42% of the variance in CB. Goldman et al. (2011) conducted a comparison of good and poor sleepers and found the latter group of children with ASD had increased CB, including self-injury. The authors also found the poorer sleepers had increased anxiety amongst other difficulties.

Wiggs and Stores (1996) and Brylewski and Wiggs (1999) suggest three possible associations for the relationship found between sleep and CB. First, they suggest that sleep problems are a form of CB. They speculate that refusal to go to bed or a delay in going to sleep could be seen in itself as CB, and not as a separate sleep problem. Second, they suggest that sleep problems cause daytime behaviour problems and/or contribute to their maintenance. The loss of REM sleep found in children with ASD/ID is thought to impair the learning process which is already challenging for these children (Brandon and Zee 2006). This could not only impact on the child's ability to learn academically but also on their ability to learn adaptive and appropriate coping strategies. Lack of sleep at night has also been shown to lead to either daytime sleepiness or hyperactivity in children (Hoban 2000), neither of which provide a suitable environment for a child to learn or for a parent to teach appropriate behaviour. Parents may unknowingly reinforce both sleep and CB problems, and high stress levels make it difficult to be consistent in setting boundaries. Third, they suggest that both are connected to the underlying pathology of ASD and ID. This could include communication difficulties, as CB has been suggested to be a maladaptive way of communicating. The authors suggest that there is no definitive explanation as to the relationship as yet, and further research is required.

Summary

The evidence suggests that children with ASD/ID show significantly more sleep problems than typically developing children. There are several developmental/biological, psychological and social factors which may contribute to the high prevalence of sleep problems in children with ASD/ID. There is a substantial amount of literature that suggests that sleep problems, anxiety and CB are significantly more common in children with ASD and/or ID than in typically developing children. Whilst there have been some conflicting results from studies, overall it appears that having ASD as well as ID may lead to increased difficulty in these three areas.

The research to date, looking at the relationship between sleep problems and anxiety, is predominantly with typically developing children and this shows a positive relationship between sleep problems and anxiety. Whilst a minority of studies have suggested that this relationship may be present in a child ASD/ID population, this relationship was only recently examined directly by Rzepecka et al. (2011). This study found a significant positive correlation between sleep problems and anxiety. The relationship between sleep problems and CB is fairly well established in the child ASD/ID literature. The picture is, however, complicated somewhat by the co-occurring relationships between sleep problems, anxiety and CB (Rzepecka et al. 2011). This suggests that clinicians need to be mindful of the need to take account of potential co-morbid conditions when assessing and treating any one of these difficulties.

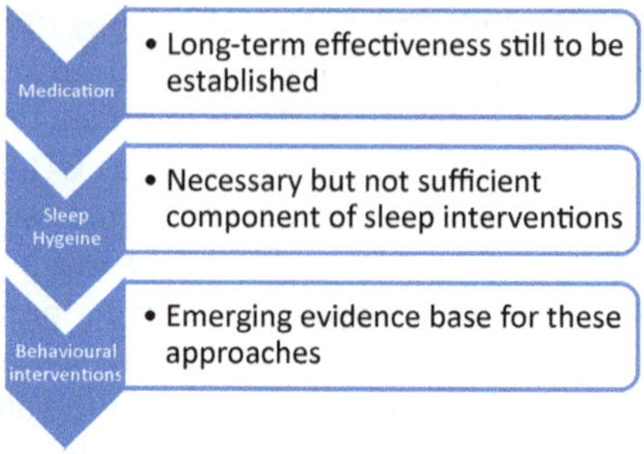

Fig. 9.3 Interventions for sleep difficulties

Interventions for Sleep Difficulties

There are a range of interventions available to address sleep difficulties in children with ASD, although the number of published evaluations of their effectiveness is relatively small and not always of the highest methodological quality (see Fig. 9.3 for a summary). The range of interventions is discussed in more detail below.

Medication

Melatonin is often used to help sleep problems in children with ID/ASD (Bramble and Feehan 2005; Keenan et al. 2007) and this has been found to be effective in the short term at least (Sajith and Clarke 2007). A recent review by Guénolé et al. (2011), however, concluded that the long term impact of melatonin has yet to be established. In addition, due to the small number of studies in this area and their associated methodological limitations, the authors note that it cannot yet be concluded that there is an evidence base for the use of melatonin for sleep disorders in children with ASD. There are also disadvantages to the use of medication in terms of parental perceptions; parents prefer behavioural interventions to medication as a solution to their childrens' sleep problems (Williams et al. 2006).

Sleep Hygiene

There is a body of literature testifying to the effectiveness of sleep hygiene and behavioural approaches with sleep difficulties in typically developing children (e.g. Mindell et al. 2006). There is, however, much less literature relating to children with ASD/ID and there is limited research that is methodologically robust (Vriend et al. 2011).

Components of good sleep hygiene include choosing a bedtime appropriate to the age and needs of the child; implementing a consistent and positive bedtime and waking routine; minimising stimulation and distractions before bedtime and ensuring the sleeping environment is comfortable. Which elements comprise a comfortable environment is likely to vary from child to child and the parents are likely to have to take account of factors such as sensory sensitivities (Cortesi et al. 2010). Parents will also need to be mindful that a sleep routine does not become a ritual for the child that results in distress when it changes in some way. To avoid this, Kodak and Piazza (2008) suggest ensuring that small changes are regularly made to different parts of the routine. Vriend et al. (2011) review the limited literature on sleep hygiene approaches with children with ASD and conclude that it is not sufficient on its own to tackle sleep problems, but is included as a necessary component of broader sleep interventions.

Behavioural Interventions

Behavioural interventions comprise those which focus on antecedents that is, occurring prior to the sleep problem and consequences that is, occurring in response to the sleep problem.

Antecedent-based Approaches Turner and Johnson (2012) and Vriend et al. (2011) provide an overview of antecedent-based approaches to sleep problems. These have mainly consisted of interventions designed to establish an appropriate bedtime routine. These often have a bedtime fading component, whereby the child's bedtime is initially set at just before the point the child would normally fall asleep. This is gradually adjusted until the child falls asleep within a few minutes of going to bed.

Sleep restriction approaches involve giving the child 90% less sleep time he/she would usually have, to reduce the time that the child is awake in bed. This period is gradually reduced until the child returns to a recommended level once a better sleep pattern is established. In contrast to this, Vriend et al. (2011) describe chronotherapy. This involves systematically making bed and waking time later until it has progressed right around the clock and reset at an appropriate time. One case study by Piazza et al. (1998) effectively utilised this approach, but Vriend et al. (2011) note that more research is needed to establish if its effectiveness can be generalised.

Another approach is scheduled night-time wakening. The child is woken a short period (approximately 15 minutes) before he/she would spontaneously wake during the night. These time intervals are systematically reduced until they take place after longer periods of uninterrupted sleep. Turner and Johnson (2012) conclude that the literature on these approaches fit the category of emerging evidence.

For children who are unable to sleep alone (co-sleeping) stimulus fading has been used to gradually reduce the time the parent spends in the child's room. In practice this may mean the gradual change over a series of nights from the parent sleeping on a mattress next to the child to moving further away from the child's bed until the parent ends up outside the child's room. Vriend et al. (2011) note the very limited research into this approach and conclude that its effectiveness is still to be established.

Consequence-based Procedures Turner and Johnson (2012) and Vriend et al. (2011) also review the evidence for consequence based approaches. Standard extinction, that is, withholding reinforcement, such as attention, following unwanted behaviour such as the child shouting out rather than going to sleep has been used. In practice, this can mean not interacting with the child between bedtime and morning, which can result in parental discomfort because of feeling they are ignoring their child when he/she is distressed (Vriend et al. 2011). In addition, a resultant extinction burst may occur, whereby the child increases the unwanted behaviour in an attempt to get the previous reinforcement. If a parent responds to this sudden increase, the unwanted behaviour may be reinforced at an increased rate or severity. Graduated extinction attempts to address these limitations. Here, the parent periodically checks on the child at night, but this is not related to the child's behaviour. This checking interval is gradually increased. Turner and Johnson (2012) conclude that the literature in this area also falls within the emerging evidence category.

Since the reviews conducted by Turner and Johnson (2012) and Vriend et al. (2011), two studies have evaluated the impact of behavioural parental training on the sleep problems of children with ASD. Malow et al. (2013) conducted a randomised trial of parental education, comparing individualised and group based education for parents of 80 children with ASD. The sleep-based educational package covered reasons why children with ASD sleep poorly, components of successful sleep, bedtime routines and behavioural strategies. Participants were also given homework to complete and were contacted by phone to review progress. The authors found no difference in the effectiveness of, or parental satisfaction with, group versus individual training. Both modes of delivery resulted in improvements in sleep difficulties. Whilst the study did not include a control group, it does provide some evidence that parental behavioural training can be helpful for sleep problems.

Johnson et al. (2013) used a small randomised control trial to evaluate a multicomponent parental training package which covered: behavioural principles, bedtime routines, reinforcement and extinction procedures, delayed sleep onset and sleep association procedures. They compared this with a group who received parental education which was unrelated to sleep. The authors found that the sleep difficulties of those children who had parents in the behavioural training group improved significantly more than those in the control group based on parental report, but not on objective measures of sleep. Both Johnson et al. and Malow et al. (2013) suggest that the results of their studies indicate that further research into the effectiveness of parental behavioural training for sleep difficulties is warranted.

Multicomponent Interventions

The research on the association of sleep difficulties with other conditions such as anxiety and CB in children with ASD/ID suggests that interventions may need to comprised of more than one component in order to address these multiple difficulties. Despite an increasing call for such approaches (e.g. Cortesi et al. 2010; Rzepecka et al. 2011), many interventions continue to only focus on the presenting difficulty.

Interventions for Sleep Difficulties, CB and Anxiety Treatment of CB has developed greatly over the past 40 years, with a move from 'behaviour modification' to positive approaches including functional analysis and creating an enabling environment (Halliday and Mackrell 1998). The British Psychological Society guidelines (2004) for CB indicate that treatment should be both proactive (preventative) and reactive (when the behaviour is occurring). Interventions may include behavioural approaches, adapting the environment, general skills training, staff training, relaxation and functional communication training (Baker et al. 1998; Lindsay and Walker 1999). Whilst positive outcomes for these interventions are reported in relation to CB (e.g. Braithwaite and Richdale 2000), a few interventions also assess or target co-morbid difficulties such as sleep difficulties.

One exception is a treatment study by Wiggs and Stores (1999) who examined a behavioural intervention for sleep problems and also monitored the impact on daytime CB. This study found an improvement in sleep following intervention, but the authors note that an observed reduction in CB was not related specifically to the sleep intervention. This was not the expected finding and the authors suggest that it is possible that the participants had such extreme behaviour that change was not easily detected. Alternatively, confounding variables such as medical conditions, genetic factors or family dynamics may have contributed to the CB to such an extent that the sleep intervention did not lessen these behaviours. Additionally, they note that a small sample size and low statistical power may have contributed to this outcome.

The present authors are unaware of any intervention studies that have assessed and/or treated both anxiety and sleep problems in children with ASD/ID. Most studies only focus on the specific factor identified for treatment, whether sleep problems, anxiety or CB, and do not assess or monitor additional factors. The significant relationships that researchers have found between sleep, CB, anxiety and other conditions suggest that assessing, monitoring and developing interventions that take account of co-occurring difficulties would be beneficial.

Overall Summary

ASD is a complex, heterogeneous condition, with a high overlap with ID. Likewise, sleep difficulties in children with ASD are often complex, coexisting with a range of other clinical difficulties. The research in this area suggests the need for further, high quality research into interventions for sleep difficulties and further, the need to develop assessment, monitoring and intervention processes that take account of the fact that children with sleep difficulties may also present with anxiety, CB or other clinical difficulties. Dosen (2007) suggests that assessment and treatment should be carried out by a multidisciplinary team in order to take account of biological, developmental, psychological and social factors. Health professionals involved in the care of children with ASD/ID should be aware of the potential relationships between the different conditions and how they may interact to provide the most effective interventions.

References

Alfano, C. A., Beidel, D. C., Tuner, S. M., & Lewin, D. S. (2006). Preliminary evidence for sleep complaints among children referred for anxiety. *Sleep Medicine, 7,* 467–473.

Alfano, C. A., Ginsburg, G. S., & Kingery, J. N. (2007). Sleep-related problems among children and adolescents with anxiety disorders. *Journal of American Academy of Child and Adolescent Psychiatry, 46*(2), 224–232.

Allik, H., Larsson, J-O., & Smedje, H. (2006). Insomnia in school-age children with Asperger syndrome or high-functioning autism. *BMC Psychiatry, 6,* 18–29.

Allison, C., Auyeung, B., & Baron-Cohen, S. (2012). Toward brief "Red Flags" for autism screening: The Short Autism Spectrum Quotient and the Short Quantitative Checklist for autism in toddlers in 1000 cases and 3000 controls. *Journal of the American Academy of Child and Adolescent Psychiatry, 51*(2), 202–212.e7.

American Sleep Disorders Association [ASDA]. (1997). *International classification of sleep disorders (revised): Diagnostic and coding manual.* Rochester: ASDA.

Baker, P. A., LaVigna, G. W., & Willis, T. J. (1998). Managing behaviours: Understanding and responding to challenging behaviour: A multi-element approach. In W. Fraser, D. Sines, & M. Kerr (Eds.), *Hallas' The care of people with intellectual disabilities.* Ninth Edition. UK: Butterworth-Heinemann.

Baron-Cohen, S., Scott, F. J., Allison, C., Williams, J., Bolton, P., Matthews, F. E., et al. (2009). Prevalence of autism-spectrum conditions: UK school-based population study. *The British Journal of Psychiatry, 194*(6), 500–509.

Blunden, S. L., & Chervin, R. D. (2008). Sleep problems are associated with poor outcomes in remedial teaching programmes: A preliminary study. *Journal of Paediatrics and Child Health, 44,* 237–242.

Braithwaite, K. L., & Richdale, A. L. (2000). Functional communication training to replace challenging behaviour across two behaviour outcomes. *Behavioural Interventions, 15,* 21–36.

Bramble, D., & Feehan, C. (2005). Psychiatrists' use of melatonin with children. *Child and Adolescent Mental Health, 10*(3), 145–149.

Brandon, S. L., & Zee, P. C. (2006). Circadian rhythm sleep disorders. *Chest, 130,* 1915–1923.

British Psychological Society [BPS]. (2004). *Clinical practice guidelines: Psychological interventions for severely challenging behaviours shown by people with learning disabilities.* Leicester: BPS.

Brylewski, J., & Wiggs, L. (1999). Sleep problems and daytime challenging behaviour in a community based sample of adults with intellectual disability. *Journal of Intellectual Disability Research, 43*(6), 504–512.

Carvil, S. (2001). Sensory impairments, intellectual disability and psychiatry. *Journal of Intellectual Disability Research, 45*(6), 467–483.

Cortesi, F., Giannotti, F., Ivanenko, A., & Johnson, K. (2010). Sleep in children with autistic spectrum disorder. *Sleep Medicine, 11,* 659–664.

Cotton, S., & Richdale, A. (2006). Brief report: Parental descriptions of sleep problems in children with autism, down syndrome, and Prader–Willi syndrome. *Research in Developmental Disabilities, 27,* 151–161.

Couturier, J. L., Speechley, K. N., Steele, M., Norman, R., Stinger, B., & Nicolson, R. (2005). Parental perception of sleep problems in children of normal intelligence with pervasive developmental disorders: Prevalence, severity, and pattern. *Journal of American Academy of Child and Adolescent Psychiatry, 44*(8), 815–822.

Czeisler, C. A. (2011). Impact of sleepiness and sleep deficiency on public health—utility of biomarkers. *Journal of Clinical Sleep Medicine, S7*(5), s6–s8.

DeVincent, C. J., Gadow, K. D., Delosh, D., & Geller, L. (2007). Sleep disturbance and its relation to DSM-IV psychiatric symptoms in preschool-age children with pervasive developmental disorder and community controls. *Journal of Child Neurology, 22,* 161–169.

Didden, R., Korzilius, H., van Aperlo, B., van Overloop, C., & de Vries, M. (2002). Sleep problems and daytime problem behaviours in children with intellectual disability. *Journal of Intellectual Disability Research, 46*(7), 537–547.

Dosen, A. (2007). Integrative treatment in persons with mental health problems. *Journal of Intellectual Disability Research, 51*(1), 66–74.

Eisenhower, A. A., Baker, B. L., & Blacher, J. (2005). Preschool children with intellectual disability: Syndrome specificity, behaviour problems, and maternal wellbeing. *Journal of Intellectual Disability Research, 49,* 657–671.

Espie, C. (2000). Sleep and disorder of sleep in people with mental retardation. *Current Opinion in Psychiatry, 13,* 507–511.

Fallone, G., Acebo, C., Seifer, R., & Carskadon, M. A. (2005). Experimental restriction of sleep opportunity in children: Effects on teacher ratings. *Sleep, 28,* 1561–1567.

Fields, D., Egers, J., & Griffin, I. (1995). Patterns of sleep behaviour in children with Down syndrome. *Sleep Research, 24,* 95–99.

Giannotti, F., Cortesi, F., Cerquiglini, A., Miraglia, D., Vagnoni, C., Sebastiani, T., & Bernabei, P. (2008). An investigation of sleep characteristics, EEG abnormalities and epilepsy in developmentally regressed and non-regressed children with autism. *Journal of Autism in Developmental Disorders, 38,* 1888–1897.

Goldman, S. E., McGrew, S., Johnson, K. P., Richdale, A. L., Clemons, T., & Malow, B. A. (2011). Sleep is associated with problem behaviors in children and adolescents with autism spectrum disorders. *Research in Autism Spectrum Disorders, 5,* 1223–1229.

Goodman, R. (1997). The strengths and difficulties questionnaire. *Journal of Child Psychology and Psychiatry, 38,* 581–586.

Gozal, D. (1998). Sleep disordered breathing and school performance in children. *Pediatrics, 102,* 616–620.

Guénolé, F., Godbout, R., Nicolasc, A., Franco, P., Claustrat, B., & Baleyte, J. (2011). Melatonin for disordered sleep in individuals with autism spectrum disorders: Systematic review and discussion. *Sleep Medicine Reviews, 15,* 379–387.

Halliday, S., & Mackrell, K. (1998). Psychological interventions in self-injurious behaviour. Working with people with a learning disability. *British Journal of Psychiatry, 172*(5), 395–400.

Hare, D. J., Jones, S., & Evershed, K. (2006). Objective investigation of the sleep-wake cycle in adults with intellectual disabilities and autism spectrum disorders. *Journal of Intellectual Disability Research, 50*(10), 701–710.

Hering, E., Epstein, R., Elroy, S., Iancu, D. R., & Zelnik, N. (1999). Sleep patterns in autistic children. *Journal of Autism and Developmental Disabilities, 29*(2), 143–147.

Hoban, T. F. (2000). Sleeplessness in children with neurodevelopmental disorders: Epidemiology and management. *CNS Drugs, 14*(1), 11–22.

Hodapp, R. M. (1998). *Development and disabilities: Intellectual, sensory and motor impairments.* New York: Cambridge University Press.

Hoffman, C. D., Sweeny, D. P., Lopez-Wagner, M. C., Hodge, D., Nam, C. Y., & Botts, B. H. (2008). Children with autism: Sleep problems and mothers' stress. *Focus on Autism and Other Developmental Disabilities, 23*(3), 155–165.

Honomichl, R. D., Goodlin-Jones, B. L., Burnham, M., Gaylor, E., & Anders, T. F. (2002). Sleep patterns of children with pervasive developmental disorders. *Journal of Autism and Developmental Disorders, 32*(6), 553–561.

Johnson, C. R., Turner, K. S., Foldes, E., Brooks, M. M., Kronk, R., & Wiggs, L. (2013). Behavioral parent training to address sleep disturbances in young children with autism spectrum disorder: a pilot trial. *Sleep Medicine, 14,* 995–1004.

Keenan, R. A., Wild, M. R., McArthur, I., & Espie, C. (2007). Children with developmental disabilities and sleep problems: Parental beliefs and treatment acceptability. *Journal of Applied Research in Intellectual Disabilities, 20,* 455–465.

Kodak, T., & Piazza, C. C. (2008). Assessment and behavioral treatment of feeding and sleeping disorders in children with autism spectrum disorders. *Child and Adolescent Psychiatric Clinics of North America, 17*(4), 887–905.

Levanon, A., Tarasiuk, A., & Tal, A. (1999). Sleep characteristics in children with Down syndrome. *Journal of Pediatrics, 134,* 755–760.

Lindsay, W. R., & Walker, B. (1999). Advances in behaviour methods in intellectual disability. *Current Opinion in Psychiatry, 12*(5), 561–565.

Malow, B. A., Adkins, K. W., Reynolds, A., Weiss, S. K., Loh, A., Fawkes, D., et al. (2013). Parent-based sleep education for children with Autism Spectrum Disorders. *Journal of Autism and Developmental Disorders. Early view*. doi:10.1007/s10803-013-1866-z.

Mannion, A., Leader, G., & Healy, O. (2013). An investigation of comorbid psychological disorders, sleep problems, gastrointestinal symptoms and epilepsy in children and adolescents with autism spectrum disorder. *Research in Autism Spectrum Disorders, 7,* 35–42.

Matson, J. L., & Goldin, R. L. (2013). Comorbidity and autism: Trends, topics and future directions. *Research in Autism Spectrum Disorders, 7,* 1228–1233.

Matson, J. L., & Gonzalez, M. L. (2007). *Autism spectrum disorders—comorbidity—child version.* Baton Rouge: Disability Consultants.

Mayes, S. D., & Calhoun, S. L. (2009). Variable related to sleep problems in children with autism. *Research in Autism Spectrum Disorders, 3,* 931–941.

Miano, S., Bruni, O., Elia, M., Scifo, L., Smerieri, A., Trovato, A., et al. (2008). Sleep phenotypes of intellectual disability: A polysomnographic evaluation in subjects with Down syndrome and Fragile-X syndrome. *Clinical Neuropsychology, 119,* 1242–1247.

Mindell, J. A., Kuhn, B., Lewin, D. S., Meltzer, L. J., & Sadeh, A. (2006). Behavioral treatment of bedtime problems and night wakings in infants and young children. *Sleep, 29,* 1263–1276.

Paavonen, E. J., Vehkalahti, K., Vanhala, R., von Wendt, L., Nieminen-von Wendt, T., & Aronen, E. T. (2008). Sleep in children with Asperger Syndrome. *Journal of Autism and Developmental Disorders, 38,* 41–51.

Patzold, L. M., Richdale, A. L., & Tonge, B. J. (1998). An investigation into sleep characteristics of children with autism and Asperger's disorder. *Journal of Paediatrics and Child Health, 34*(6), 528–533.

Piazza, C. C., Hagopian, L. P., Hughes, C. R., & Fisher, W. W. (1998). Using chronotherapy to treat severe sleep problems: A case study. *American Journal on Mental Retardation, 102*(4), 358–366.

Polimeni, M. A., Richdale, A. L., & Francis, A. J. P. (2005). A survey of sleep problems in autism, Asperger's disorder and typically developing children. *Journal of Intellectual Disability Research, 49*(4), 260–268.

Quine, L. (2001). Sleep problems in primary school children: Comparison between mainstream and special school children. *Child: Care, Health, and Development, 27*(3), 201–221.

Richdale, A. L. (1999). Sleep problems in autism: Prevalence, cause and intervention. *Developmental Medicine and Child Neurology, 41,* 60–66.

Richdale, A., & Prior, M. R. (1995). The sleep/wake rhythm in children with autism. *European Child and Adolescent Psychiatry, 4*(3), 175–186.

Richdale, A. L., & Schreck, K. A. (2009). Sleep problems in autism spectrum disorders: Prevalence, nature, & possible biopsychosocial aetiologies. *Sleep Medicine Reviews, 13,* 403–411.

Richdale, A., Cotton, S., & Hibbit, K. (1999). Sleep and behaviour disturbance in Prader–Willi syndrome: A questionnaire study. *Journal of Intellectual Disability Research, 43,* 380–392.

Richdale, A., Frances, A., Gavidia-Payne, S., & Cotton, S. (2000). Stress, behaviour, and sleep problems in children with an intellectual disability. *Journal of Intellectual and Developmental Disability, 25*(2), 147–161.

Robinson, A. M., & Richdale, A. L. (2003). Sleep problems in children with an intellectual disability: parental perceptions of sleep problems, and views of treatment effectiveness. *Child: Care, Health and Development, 30*(2), 139–150.

Robinson, P. D., & Waters, K. (2008). Are children just small adults? The differences between paediatric and adult sleep medicine. *Internal Medicine Journal, 38,* 719–731.

Rzepecka, H., McKenzie, K., McClure, I., & Murphy, S. (2011). Sleep, anxiety and challenging behaviour in children with intellectual disability and/or autism spectrum disorder. *Research in Developmental Disabilities, 32,* 2758–2766.

Sajith, S. G., & Clarke, D. (2007). Melatonin and sleep disorders associated with intellectual disability: A clinical review. *Journal of Intellectual Disability Research, 51*(1), 2–13.

Scher, A., Tirosh, E., Jaffe, M., Rubin, L., Sadeh, A., & Lavie, P. (1995). Sleep patterns of infants and young children in Israel. *International Journal of Behaviour Development, 18,* 701–711.

Stein, M. A., Mendelsohn, J., Obermeyer, W. H., Amromin, J., & Benca, R. (2001). Sleep and behaviour problems in school age children. *Pediatrics, 107*(4), 86–75.

Stores, G. (2001a). Sleep and down syndrome. In: G. Stores & L. Wiggs (Eds.), *Sleep disturbance in children and adolescents with disorders of development: Its significance and management* (pp. 10–14). Mac Keith Press: London.

Stores, R. (2001b). Normal sleeping including developmental aspects. In: G. Stores & L. Wiggs (Eds.), *Sleep disturbance in children and adolescents with disorders of development: Its significance and management* (pp. 53–59). UK: Cambridge University Press.

Stores, G., & Wiggs, L. (2001). Sleep problems and sleep disorders: General. In: G. Stores & L. Wiggs (Eds.), *Sleep disturbance in children and adolescents with disorders of development: Its significance and management* (pp. 15–23). UK: Cambridge University Press.

Stores, R., Stores, G., & Buckley, S. J. (1996). The patterns of sleep problems in children with Down's syndrome and other learning disabilities. *Journal of Applied Research in Intellectual Disabilities, 9,* 145–159.

Stores, G., Wiggs, L., & Campling, G. (1998). Sleep disorders and their relationship to psychological disturbance in children with epilepsy. *Child: Care, Health, and Development, 24*(1), 5–19.

Tsai, F., Chiang, H., Lee, C., Gau, S. S., Lee, W., Fan, P., et al. (2012). Sleep problems in children with autism, attention-deficit hyperactivity disorder, and epilepsy. *Research in Autism Spectrum Disorders, 6,* 413–421.

Turner, K. S., & Johnson, C. R. (2012). Behavioral interventions to address sleep disturbances in children with autism spectrum disorders: A review. *Topics in Early Childhood Special Education, 33*(3) 144–152.

Volkmar, F. R., Lord, C., Bailey, A., Schultz, R. T., & Klin, A. (2004). Autism and pervasive developmental disorders. *Journal of Child Psychology and Psychiatry, 45*(1), 135–170.

Vriend, J. L., Corkum, P. V., Moon, E. C., & Smith, I. M. (2011). Behavioral interventions for sleep problems in children with autism spectrum disorders: Current findings and future directions. *Journal of Pediatric Psychology, 36*(9), 1017–1029.

Wehr, T. A., Aeschbach, D., & Duncan, W. C. (2001). Evidence for a biological dawn and dusk in the human circadian timing system. *Journal of Physiology, 535,* 937–951.

Wiggs, L., & Stores, G. (1996). Severe sleep disturbance and daytime challenging behaviour in children with severe learning disabilities. *Journal of Intellectual Disability Research, 40*(6), 518–528.

Wiggs, L., & Stores, G. (1999). Behavioural treatment for sleep problems in children with severe learning disabilities and challenging daytime behaviour: Effect on daytime behaviour. *Journal of Child Psychology and Psychiatry, 40*(4), 627–635.

Williams, P. G., Sears, L. L., & Allard, A. (2004). Sleep problems in children with autism. *Journal of Sleep Research, 13,* 265–268.

Williams, P. G., Sears, L. L., & Allard, A. (2006). Parent perceptions of efficacy for strategies used to facilitate sleep in children with autism. *Journal of Developmental and Physical Disabilities, 18*(1), 25–33.

Yates, K., & Le Couteur, A. (2012) Diagnosing autism. *Paediatrics and Child Health, 23*(1), 5–10.

Chapter 10
Epilepsy

Colin Reilly and Christopher Gillberg

Introduction

Epilepsy occurs much more often in autism than expected by chance. The reverse is also true (Steffenburg et al. 1996; Russ et al. 2012; Reilly et al. 2014). This chapter looks specifically at epilepsy in classic autism and in the broader category of autism spectrum disorder (ASD), and does not address the issue of autism in epilepsy. However, there are an increasing number of studies focussing on ASD in those who have epilepsy and recent studies suggest that the rate of ASD in active/current childhood epilepsy is 16–21 % (Russ et al. 2012; Reilly et al. 2014).

In the chapter, we discuss the prevalence of epilepsy and epileptiform abnormalities in ASD. We describe the diagnosis of epilepsy in ASD with respect to possible challenges and the overlap between symptoms of ASD and behavioural manifestations of seizures. The manifestation of epilepsy in ASD has been the subject of a number of studies with respect to both seizure types and also epilepsy syndromes, and we outline the research in this area. We also examine co-morbid epilepsy in ASD with respect to gender, age of onset, intellectual functioning, psychopathology and motor impairment with a particular emphasis on possible differences between those with ASD and epilepsy, and ASD alone. We subsequently describe the relationship between epilepsy and ASD with respect to possible shared pathophysiology including reference to possible shared genetic factors. We describe research which has focussed on the outcome of epilepsy in ASD and discuss the treatment of epilepsy in ASD. We conclude the chapter with a summary of what is a known and possible future direction for research and clinical practice.

C. Reilly (✉) · C. Gillberg
Research Department, National Center for Young People with Epilepsy,
Lingfield, Surrey RH7 6PW, UK
e-mail: colin.reilly@ucdconnect.ie

Gillberg Neuropsychiatry Centre, University of Gothenburg, Kungsgatan 12,
Gothenburg, Sweden

Johnny L. Matson (ed.), *Comorbid Conditions Among Children with Autism Spectrum Disorders,* Autism and Child Psychopathology Series,
DOI 10.1007/978-3-319-19183-6_10

Autism

Autism spectrum disorder (ASD) has complex and variable symptoms along with multiple aetiologies and phenotypic outcomes (Delorme et al. 2013). It involves persistent deficits in social communication across multiple environments, and restricted repetitive patterns of behaviours, interest and activities (American Psychiatric Association (APA) 2013). ASD is a neurodevelopmental disorder in that symptoms must be present early in life although the symptoms may not become manifest until social demands exceed limited capacities or may be masked by learned strategies in later life (APA 2013). Individuals with a previous DSM-IV-TR (APA 2000) diagnosis of autistic disorder, Asperger's disorder or pervasive developmental disorder-not otherwise specified should now be given the diagnosis of ASD. The prevalence of ASD is estimated at approximately 1 % (Posserud et al. 2010; Baird et al. 2006a). Classic autism (a subcategory of the DSM-IV construct of autistic disorder)—with extremes of autistic aloneness and elaborate repetitive routines from an early age—is probably as rare today as it was 40 years ago, that is, affecting fewer than 0.1 % of all individuals in the population (Gillberg 2010). The male:female ratio in ASD is 3.3:1 (Baird et al. 2006a). Half or more of all individuals with ASD have intellectual developmental disorder (IDD) (Baird et al. 2006a; Fernell et al. 2011), and the vast majority have at least one more diagnosable DSM-IV disorder other than ASD (Gillberg 2010). Epilepsy is also commonly encountered in ASD (see prevalence section). It is possible to find a genetic and/or medical cause for ASD in at least 20 % cases (Delorme et al. 2013).

Epilepsy

Epilepsy may be characterised by recurrent (two or more) epileptic seizures unprovoked by any immediate cause (Commission on Classification & Terminology of the International League against Epilepsy 1981). Epilepsy comprises a heterogeneous group of disorders including a variety of epilepsy syndromes that range in severity from relatively benign to progressive and catastrophic (Cross et al. 2013). There is an increased risk for a wide spectrum of cognitive, behavioural and psychiatric disorders in epilepsy (Jensen 2011). It is one of the most common neurological disorders that affects people of all ages and the most common serious neurological disorder in childhood with prevalence estimates of 0.5–1 % of all children from birth to 16 years (Camfield et al. 1996) with a roughly equal male:female ratio. It is estimated that 1 in 26 individuals will develop epilepsy at some point in their lives (Hesdorffer et al. 2011). Epileptic seizures can be classified into 'generalised' or 'focal'. 'Generalised' epileptic seizures originate at some point within, and rapidly engage, bilaterally distributed networks involving both cerebral hemispheres (Berg et al. 2010). Generalised seizures include tonic–clonic, absence, myclonic, clonic, tonic and atonic (Berg et al. 2010). 'Focal' indicates that the seizure begins primarily within networks limited to one cerebral hemisphere (Berg et al. 2010). Previously terms like 'simple partial', 'complex partial' and 'partial seizures secondarily generalised' were used as descriptors of focal seizures (Commission on Classification & Terminology of the International League against Epilepsy 1981). Epilepsy has increasingly been recognised as a disorder that reaches well beyond seizures. In an UK study, 60% of school-aged children with 'active epilepsy' (had a seizure in last year or currently on anti-epilepsy drugs or AEDs) met criteria for one or more DSM-IV-TR behavioural or motor disorder, and 40% were functioning in the IDD range (Reilly et al. 2014). One in five of the children with epilepsy who were assessed met DSM-IV-TR criteria for ASD (Reilly et al. 2014). In another US study, 16% of children with current epilepsy were reported to have ASD (Russ et al. 2012).

Given the neurodevelopmental nature of ASD, it is unsurprising that epilepsy often co-exists in individuals with ASD (Matson and Neal 2009), and children with ASD are at greater risk of epilepsy than children with other types of developmental problems (Gillberg and Neville 2010). The association between autism and childhood epilepsy was noted by Kanner (1943) in his original descriptions of autism. One of the 11 children with autism in Kanner's group had epilepsy, and in a follow-up of the patients, two had epilepsy (Kanner 1971). Early reports of the association between autism and epilepsy contributed to the understanding that ASD is a developmental disorder (Lotter 1966). The high prevalence of epilepsy in autism supports a neurobiological aetiology for ASD (Levisohn 2007). Epilepsy and ASD are both heterogeneous disorders with variable aetiologies and pathophysiologies (Brooks-Kayal 2010). It is likely that there is a more than coincidental association between ASD and epilepsy (Canitano 2007).

As a result of the increased prevalence of epilepsy in ASD, there has been interest in understanding what role epilepsy/seizures may play in the aetiology and development of ASD and how epilepsy in ASD should be treated. The association of autism with clinical or sub-clinical epilepsy might indicate common genetic factors in at least some cases (Tuchman and Rapin 2002), which may have implications for understanding the neurobiology of ASD and also the treatment of ASD and related disorders.

Prevalence of Epilepsy in ASD

The prevalence of epilepsy is greatly increased in individuals with ASD as compared with the general population (Woolfenden et al. 2012). Reported rates have varied significantly depending on how ASD and epilepsy have been defined or diagnosed and on the populations that have been sampled (Spence and Schneider 2009). There is a lack of truly systematic studies and much of the research has focussed on the prevalence of participants who have narrowly defined classic autism as opposed to the range of presentations within ASD (Matson and Neal 2009). With regard to methods of ascertainment in studies reporting prevalence of epilepsy in ASD, referral bias is likely to lead to clinic-based samples reporting higher rates of epilepsy or electroencephalogram (EEG) abnormalities (Spence and Schneider 2009) and those with milder presentation/higher cognitive functioning may not be included in such studies.

One of the first-ever population studies of epilepsy in autism found a rate of 20 % (Olsson et al. 1988). Woolfenden et al. (2012) reported a pooled prevalence of epilepsy of 1.8 % in studies in which the majority of individuals with ASD did not have intellectual disability (ID) and the mean age was < 12 years at follow-up, and 23.7 % in studies in which the majority did have an ID and the mean age at follow-up was more than 12 years. Based on a study of a nationwide register of children in Norway aged between 0 and 11 years, Surén et al. (2012) reported that 11.2 % of children with ASD had epilepsy. Spence and Schneider (2009) examined studies published since 2000 and reported rates between 7 % (for a group of individuals with idiopathic autism) to 46 %. The highest rates reported tended to be for studies that included older children or adults and most of the studies reported on were clinic-based studies.

A number of studies have included adults with ASD and/or looked at lifetime prevalence of epilepsy. This is important given that, while diagnostic criteria for ASD indicate that abnormalities must have been present from the first years of life, epilepsy can develop at any age. Therefore, studies that focus on lifetime prevalence or include adults are likely to have a higher prevalence than studies focussing exclusively on children with ASD. Danielsson et al. (2005) reported on 108 of 120 individuals initially diagnosed with autism in childhood in a population-based study. They were followed for a period of 13–22 years and revaluated at ages 17–40 years. Thirty eight percent of individuals with autistic disorder or an autistic-like condition had epilepsy at some point in their lives in this community-based cohort. Bolton et al. (2011) reported on 150 individuals diagnosed with autism in childhood who were followed up at 21+ years of age and reported that 22 % of cases had epilepsy. The overall prevalence of epilepsy in a Danish cohort with ASD was 24.6 % at middle adulthood (Mouridsen et al. 2011). Viscidi et al. (2013a) reported on a cross-sectional study of four samples of 5815 children with ASD. The average prevalence of epilepsy in children with ASD 2–17 years was 12.5 % and among children 13 years and older, 26 % had epilepsy. In relation to Asperger's syndrome, Cedurland and Gillberg (2004) looked at the medical files of 100 individuals with Asperger's syndrome diagnosed using Gillberg's (Gillberg and Gillberg 1989) criteria. In this study, routine EEGs had been performed on at least 56 patients, 20 of whom had shown abnormal results. However, clear epileptogenic discharges were seen in only 13 % of those examined and only 4 % of the individuals had a diagnosis of epilepsy. Gillberg and Neville (2010) have concluded that a reasonable minimum estimate for the prevalence of epilepsy across the 'autisms' would be in the range of 10–20 %.

Epileptiform Abnormalities in ASD

Epileptic EEG abnormalities are frequently observed in individuals with ASD (even in the absence of overt seizures) suggesting a low seizure threshold (e.g. Amiet et al. 2008). These EEG abnormalities should not by themselves be considered evidence of epilepsy (Spence and Schneider 2009). Much like prevalence rates of epilepsy, reports of epileptiform or EEG abnormalities in individuals with ASD have varied and there have been no population-based studies of these discharges among individuals with ASD (Spence and Schneider 2009). The lack of population-based data is likely to mean that children with ASD without cognitive impairment are less likely to have been included in previous studies. Definitions of EEG abnormality or epileptiform abnormalities and type of EEG monitoring are also likely to influence findings. One study noted that prolonged sleep EEGs significantly increased the yield of EEG abnormalities (Hrdlicka et al. 2004). Requesting EEG studies for children with ASD without a suspicion of epilepsy is not routine practice and there is considerable variability between paediatric neurologists, paediatricians and psychiatrists with respect to EEG investigation (Gabis et al 2005). Spence and Schneider (2009) reported on 12 studies which have focussed on EEG abnormalities in ASD published since 2000; the lowest reported rate in those without epilepsy was 4 % (Gabis et al. 2005) and the highest was 60.7 % (Chez et al. 2006). The Chez et al. study was the largest study, based on a sample of 889 children with ASD without overt seizures. Several studies in the review reported rates of epileptiform abnormalities of approximately 30 % in ASD populations without seizures (Hrdlicka et al. 2004; Akshomoff et al. 2007; Baird et al. 2006b). In a study which included individuals with ASD with and without epilepsy, Parmeggianai et al. (2010) reported that 24.9 % of 345 individuals with ASD had epilepsy/febrile convulsions and 45.5 % had abnormal EEG paroxysmal abnormality (including those with seizures/febrile convulsions). The treatment of EEG abnormalities in the absence of clinical seizures has proved controversial (see section on treatment).

The possible role of EEG epileptiform abnormalities in the development of regressive autism has been the subject of some discussion. Some clinicians have been concerned that the EEG abnormalities may indicate untreated epilepsy which could be a contributory factor to the development of ASD. Some authors, including Fong et al. (2008) have concluded that in the absence of clinical seizures, EEG investigation in children with regressive autism is not justified based on currently available evidence. Furthermore, Malow (2006) has concluded that while epileptiform discharges in the absence of clinical seizures are common in ASD, this may not be causative of cognitive and behavioural changes but may reflect underlying cortical dysfunction. Tuchman and Rapin (1997) noted that epileptiform abnormalities appear to occur more often in regressive as opposed to non-regressive autism. However, the majority of studies have not noted this relationship. Chez et al. (2006) noted that there was no difference between those with reported regressive and non-regressive autism in terms of the prevalence of epileptiform abnormalities. Baird et al. (2006b) and Canitano et al. (2005) also found no difference between the regressive and non-regressive groups.

Diagnosing Epilepsy in ASD

Epilepsy can be difficult to recognise and diagnose correctly since there is no definitive diagnostic test (Cross et al. 2013). Unusual mannerisms, movements and behaviours in infants, children and adults are common and may have a variety of causes, only some of which result from epileptic seizures (Hindley et al. 2006). Paroxysmal non-epileptic events present in both psychiatric and non-psychiatric conditions and can be difficult to distinguish from epileptic seizures (Reilly et al. 2013a).The non-psychiatric conditions can consist of physiologic and organic disorders including inattention/daydreaming, staring, sleep myoclonus, stereotyped movements, hypnic jerks, tonic posturing, parasomnias and movement disorders (Kotagal et al. 2002; Kim et al. 2012). Of those with a psychiatric basis, psychogenic non-epileptic seizures (PNES) are some of the most common non-epileptic events (Kotagal et al. 2002). Misdiagnosis of epilepsy is common, and one Danish study reported that 39 % of children referred to a tertiary centre due to suspected epilepsy did not have the condition (Udall et al. 2006).There have been reports that children with epilepsy and ASD are likely to be diagnosed with ASD at an older age than children with ASD alone (e.g. Turk et al. 2009), suggesting a possible difficulty with differential diagnosis for young children with epilepsy.

With respect to epileptic seizures in ASD, it is not clear if the time taken to diagnose epilepsy in those with ASD is different than the time taken to diagnose epilepsy in those without ASD. It is possible that seizure behaviours may mimic or overlap with behaviours commonly associated with the dyad of social communication and restricted repetitive patterns of behaviours associated with ASD, thus making diagnosis of ASD or identification of seizures more difficult. For example, the unusual repetitive and stereotyped behaviours common in children with ASD can be difficult to distinguish from clinical seizures (Tuchman and Rapin 2002). Absence seizures could be wrongly thought of as failure to respond to one's name, which is a common finding in young children with ASD (Tuchman and Rapin 2002). Complex partial seizures (now known as focal seizures) or absence seizures may be difficult to detect in children with ASD, especially in those who are non-verbal (Gillberg and Neville 2010). Typical absence seizures are staring spells—usually under 20 s duration—often accompanied by a slight flickering of the eyes (Gillberg and Neville 2010). A complex partial seizure usually lasts between 30 s and 3 min and is often accompanied by lip smacking, hand wringing, plucking at clothes or a temporary dreamy state (Gillberg and Neville 2010).

Epilepsy should be suspected in children on the autism spectrum who have paroxysmal events. Review of home or school videos in addition to routine EEGs may help in clarifying the diagnosis (Gabis et al. 2005). The clinical suspicion of epilepsy should always be high among the ASD population particularly if there is a history of convulsion and staring episodes (Gabis et al. 2005). Episodic events that are considered potentially symptomatic (e.g. breath holding spells, rage) rarely relate to epilepsy, especially if they occur in children who have a milder form of ASD (Gabis et al. 2005).

Autistic regression early in life is a real phenomenon. The prevalence of children who displayed 'regression' was 22 % (half of whom had lost skills, the other half plateauing) in a study of 208 preschoolers with ASD in Sweden (Fernell et al. 2010). Another group of individuals with ASD, a small minority, appear to deteriorate in adolescence (Gillberg and Neville 2010). Although epilepsy is likely to play only a minor role in autistic regression (Rapin 1995), children with ASD who display regression of normal development should be considered at risk for epilepsy (Gabis et al. 2005). A prolonged sleep EEG that includes study of stage III and IV of sleep is recommended for children without overt clinical seizures who have regressed or are suspected of regression or developmental stagnation (Gillberg and Neville 2010).

Seizure Types and Epilepsy Syndromes in ASD

All epileptic seizure types can be associated with ASD (Tuchman et al. 1991; Canitano 2007). Generalised tonic–clonic seizures are the most frequent form of epilepsy in the general population (Gillberg and Neville 2010). Based on published studies, it is not clear whether particular seizure types are more likely to be found in individuals with ASD and epilepsy compared with ASD alone and there is no consensus on this. It can be difficult to compare studies as seizure classification and description have varied considerably across studies. Bolton et al. (2011) reported that generalised tonic–clonic seizures predominated in a group of 29 individuals with ASD and epilepsy although they further commented that it is possible that this seizure type represented secondary generalised seizures arising from initial focal seizures. Hara (2007) reported that in 33 individuals with ASD and epilepsy, partial seizures with secondary generalised and generalised seizures were predominant while Danielsson et al. (2005) reported that of 45 individuals with ASD and epilepsy, partial seizures with or without secondarily generalised seizures were the dominant seizure type. Gillberg and Neville (2010) have suggested that infantile spasms and complex partial seizures are relatively more common in ASD. The differences between studies reflect both the heterogeneity of samples and also seizure classification systems employed.

There are several epilepsy syndromes in which regression/stagnation of language, cognition and behaviour may lead to clinical manifestations that overlap with the behavioural phenotype of ASD (Tuchman 2006; Deonna and Roulet-Perez 2005). Important in this overlap is the concept of epileptic 'encephalopathy'. Epileptic encephalopathies can be defined as conditions in which the epileptic activity itself is postulated to contribute to severe cognitive and behavioural impairments above and beyond what might be expected from the underlying pathology alone (Speechio et al. 2012). However, the term is often used to describe epilepsies with severe cognitive and behavioural outcomes regardless of whether the difficulties arise from the underlying aetiology or the epileptic activity, and teasing out the cause of difficulties in such conditions can be difficult. Disorders such as early myoclonic encephalopathy, Otahara syndrome, West syndrome (infantile spasms), Dravet syndrome, Myoclonic status in non-progressive encephalopathies, Lennox–Gastuat Syndrome, Landau-Kleffner syndrome (LKS) and epilepsy with continuous spike waves during slow wave sleep (CSWS) are often included in the epileptic encephalopathies (Engel 2001). As a group, the epileptic encephalopathies are associated with regression or slowing of cognitive, language or behavioural development and the supposition is that the seizures or the interictal epileptiform activity are responsible for the deterioration (Nabbout and Dulac 2003). Approximately 40% of all epilepsies occurring during the first 3 years of life fit the definition of epileptic encephalopathy (Guerrini 2006). Among the epileptic encephalopathies, West syndrome, LKS and CSWS are most commonly associated with an ASD phenotype (Ballaban-Gil and Tuchman 2000).

LKS usually affects children between 2 and 6 years of age who have developed speech and there are usually, but not always, clinical seizures and a bilateral paroxysmal centro-sylvian EEG pattern (Gillberg and Neville 2010). LKS is not a developmental disorder but an acquired aphasia associated with clinical seizures or an epileptiform EEG (Tuchman and Rapin 2002). Loss of language in LKS can be confused with regression noted by parents of children with ASD. In comparison to children with LKS, patients with 'autistic regression' have regression of both language and behaviour in association with significant social deficits (Tuchman 2006). The regression in language seen with LKS is more dramatic and other higher cortical functions may not deteriorate (Gillberg and Neville 2010). The social deficits in LKS are usually less severe than those associated with autistic regression, although the distinction may be very difficult to make in younger children (Tuchman 2006). Children with ASD are also more likely to regress earlier, usually prior to 2 years, in contrast to those with LKS.

CSWS or electrical status epilepticus (ESES) is an EEG diagnosis in which the epileptiform EEG is often, but not invariably, associated with severe behavioural disorder and developmental regression (Ballaban-Gil and Tuchman 2000). CSWS is sometimes regarded as a variation of LKS and may be a variation of the same syndrome in older children (Hirsch et al. 1990). It is usually diagnosed after 6 years of age (Gillberg and Neville 2010). Onset of CSWS may be associated with intellectual regression that is often global, including behaviour and cognition (Ballaban-Gil and Tuchman 2000). Behavioural changes can include decreased attention span, hyperactivity, aggressiveness, difficulty in interpersonal interactions and 'psychotic behaviour' with some of the behaviours similar to ASD (Ballaban-Gil and Tuchman 2000). Depression, psychosis, autism and substance use disorder are often the 'primary' diagnoses made, and it is common for the EEG changes not to be diagnosed for some time in the initial presentation of symptoms.

West syndrome (infantile spasms) is an early onset epilepsy syndrome with an associated severely abnormal background EEG pattern (hypsarrhythimia) and often poor developmental outcome (Spence and Schneider 2009). In West syndrome, regression occurs after some basic social and emotional competencies have developed and regression and recovery or evolution of ASD symptoms can be documented. The syndrome appears to increase the risk of developing ASD, and Riikonen and Amnell (1981) noted that 12.5% of 192 individuals with infantile spasms had 'infantile autism' but also noted that in 14 cases this was 'transient'. A prevalence of ASD as high as 35% depending on the severity of ID has been reported in West Syndrome (Saemundsen et al. 2007a) while Millichap (1997) estimated that approximately 10% with the syndrome will meet criteria for autism. The combination of infantile spasms and ASD may be found in a variety of syndromes such as Down syndrome, tuberous sclerosis complex, neurofibromatosis 1, minor hydrocephalus and phenylketonuria (Gillberg and Neville 2010).

Although there is a high risk for the development of ASD in children with epileptic encephalopathies, especially those with seizures in the first year of life, there is controversy around the notion that epileptiform activity can trigger autistic regression (Tuchman and Rapin 1997; Tuchman 2006; Humphrey et al. 2006). It would appear that epilepsy is not a causal factor in the majority of children with autism, even in those who undergo a developmental regression typically at 18–24 months. There are some situations where the role of epilepsy may arise with regard to the development of autism or display of autistic behaviours (Deonna and Roulet 2006). However, epilpetiform activity is more likely to be associated with language regression than with autistic regression (Tuchman 2006), and there is no evidence that autism is an epileptic encephalopathy (Tuchman and Rapin 2002). In the epileptic encephalopathies, symptoms of ASD may reduce as the child develops or when effective anti-epileptic therapy is given (Gillberg and Schaumann 1983; Deonna and Roulet 2006). However, for some with these epilepsy syndromes, significant features of ASD may persist, and for the practical issue of management they have ASD, albeit via a different route to that of developmental autism (Reilly et al. 2013b).

Intellectual Functioning in those with ASD and Epilepsy

Research suggests that a clear relationship exists between levels of intellectual functioning and rates of epilepsy in individuals with ASD with those with IDD and ASD being at a significantly higher risk. Amiet et al. (2008) reported on a meta-analysis of studies involving individuals with ASD and epilepsy and concluded that there was a strong and significant reduction in relative risk with increasing intellectual ability. Specifically, more individuals with ASD and IDD compared to individuals with ASD without IDD had epilepsy. The pooled prevalence of epilepsy in 1485 individuals with autism and IDD was 21.4% compared with 8% in 627 individuals with autism without IDD. Amiet et al. (2008) also reported that there was an increase in the prevalence of epilepsy in participants with an IQ less than 50 compared with individuals with autism with an IQ greater than or equal to 70. However, no difference was noted between those with an IQ between 50 and 70 and those with an IQ greater than or equal to 70. Therefore, the greater part of the association between epilepsy and IDD in autism related to moderate and severe IDD (IQ<50).

Mouridsen et al. (2011) reported that rates of epilepsy in individuals with ASD were 34.0% in those with IQ below 50, 26.7% in those with IQ between 50 and 69 and 8.8% in those with an IQ above 70 and thus low intelligence was a risk factor for epilepsy. Overall, the prevalence of epilepsy in the ASD population for those with an IQ below 70 was 33.7% and it was 8.8% in those without IDD (Mouridsen et al. 2011). Bolton et al. (2011) reported that those with ASD and epilepsy had significantly lower non-verbal IQ and lower verbal ability than those with ASD alone. Viscidi et al. (2013a) reported that for a one standard deviation increase in

IQ the odds of having epilepsy fell by 47 %. Hara (2007) reported that those with ASD and epilepsy had a lower IQ and adaptive level compared with those with ASD alone. In a population-based study, adults with ASD and epilepsy had more severe cognitive impairment (IQ < 50) and adaptive functioning than did adults with ASD and no epilepsy (Danielsson et al. 2005). Van Eeghen et al. (2012) reported that the level of autistic features in patients with epilepsy and tuberous sclerosis complex was strongly associated with intelligence outcomes with lower levels of cognition associated with a greater degree of ASD symptomatology. Therefore, epilepsy in ASD is associated with a lower level of intellectual functioning than ASD alone, highlighting the significant support needs of those with both epilepsy and ASD.

Gender of Individuals with ASD and Epilepsy

It has been reported in a number of studies that females with ASD are more likely to have epilepsy than males with ASD. In their meta-analysis, Amiet et al. (2008) reported a pooled prevalence of epilepsy in females with ASD of 34.5 % versus 18.5 % in males with ASD. In a population-based sample, Danielsson et al. (2005) reported that 58 % of women with ASD had epilepsy compared with only 32 % of men and this difference was statistically significant. Viscidi et al. (2013a) reported that females were significantly more likely to have epilepsy in one of two large samples of individuals with ASD, but significant differences between the genders were not noted in the other sample. The increased risk for ASD in females did not hold after controlling for IQ (Viscidi et al. 2013a). This suggests that the increased risk of epilepsy in ASD in females is due to the lower level of cognitive functioning in females with ASD and it has previously been reported that the female gender has been associated with lower cognitive ability in ASD (Newschaffer et al. 2007). However, Bolton et al. (2011) reported that female gender was independently associated with an increased risk of ASD even after controlling for IQ, indicting the possibility that the increased risk is not just due to the lower IQ often found in females with ASD.

It must be noted that some studies have not found a significant gender difference between males and females with respect to prevalence of epilepsy in ASD. Hara (2007) and Parmeggianai et al. (2010) did not find that gender was a predictor of prevalence of epilepsy in ASD. Mouridsen et al. (2011) reported that the female gender was not a statistically significant predictor of epilepsy in ASD, although the prevalence of epilepsy among females with ASD was slightly higher than males (30.3 versus 22.4 %). The possibility that females with ASD are underdiagnosed (Kopp and Gillberg 2011) may have implications with respect to the gender of those with ASD and epilepsy. It may be that females with ASD, particularly those with a higher level of cognitive functioning, are more likely to remain undiagnosed resulting in females with lower IQs being over-represented in the ASD population included in clinical studies, and that this will impact upon the gender balance of those with epilepsy and ASD.

Age of Onset of Epilepsy in ASD

Rates of epilepsy increase with age in ASD, so higher rates of lifetime epilepsy will be noted in adults compared with children. With regard to age of onset, there appears to be a bimodal age distribution of seizures in autism with one peak occurring before 5 years and the other in adolescence or later. Parmeggianai et al. (2010) reported a peak age of 20–25 years in 345 individuals with ASD, although the peak for EEG paroxysmal abnormalities was from 5 to 10 years. A study of 80 cases of idiopathic autism with epilepsy indicated two peaks at 3.2 years and 16.7 years (Nomura et al. 2010). Bolton et al. (2011) reported that for the majority of participants in their study, seizures began after 10 years.

Nomura et al. (2010) suggest that while the first peak of the age of onset of epilepsy is similar to epilepsy in the general population, the second peak is unique to ASD. Regarding the first peak of epilepsy before 5 years, the highest risk for children with epilepsy who develop ASD is in the first year of life (Saemundsen et al. 2007b) and this peak onset may be for syndromic/complex autism (autism and a genetic medical condition) in infancy, whereas the second peak onset of epilepsy may be in adolescence (Hara 2007) for those with idiopathic ASD. However, the only longitudinal prospective study of epilepsy in autism from early childhood well into adult age did not find a peak of onset of cases in adolescence (Danielsson et al. 2005) and more longitudinal work with larger samples is needed.

Psychopathology and Motor Problems in those with ASD and Epilepsy

Epilepsy is associated with significant behavioural and psychiatric co-morbidity in both childhood (Reilly et al. 2013b) and adulthood (O'Donoghue et al. 1999). A key question regarding the presence of epilepsy in those with ASD concerns whether those with epilepsy and ASD are more at risk for other (non-ASD) psychopathology than those with ASD alone. Turk and co-workers found significantly more challenging behaviour overall in a group with ASD and epilepsy than in those with ASD 'only' (Turk et al. 2009). Smith and Matson (2010a) reported that among a group of adults functioning in the IDD range, individuals with ASD and epilepsy were significantly more impaired than a group of adults with ASD alone or epilepsy alone in the area of disruptive behaviour. The presence of epilepsy contributed more to disruptive behaviour ratings than the presence of ASD. Smith and Matson (2010b) reported that adults with IDD who had both ASD and epilepsy had significantly more impaired social skills than those with IDD alone, or groups containing only IDD and ASD, or IDD and epilepsy even when IQ was controlled for. Viscidi et al. (2013b) reported on the association between epilepsy and ASD with respect to maladaptive behaviours in a sample of 2645 children with ASD of whom 139 had epilepsy. Children with ASD and epilepsy had more ASD symptoms and maladaptive behaviours than those with ASD without epilepsy. However, after adjusting for IQ, only hyperactivity symptoms remained significantly increased in those with ASD and epilepsy.It is possible that the use of AEDs with their mood-stabilizing and other psychotropic effects could reduce behavioural and psychiatric symptoms in those with epilepsy as has been suggested by Arshad et al. (2011). However, there are no studies in which the role of AEDs on psychopathology has been explored in those with both ASD and epilepsy.

Epilepsy is associated with a high risk for motor difficulties. Reilly et al. (2014) reported that of 85 school-aged children with active epilepsy, 15 (18 %) had cerebral palsy and a further 16 (19 %) had Developmental Coordination Disorder (DCD). Motor impairments are also common in children with ASD (Green et al. 2009; Kopp et al. 2010) and systematic assessment of motor functioning in ASD should be part of routine assessment in ASD (Green et al. 2009). There have been reports that those with epilepsy and ASD have increased difficulties with motor skills compared with ASD alone. Turk et al. (2009) attempted to compare a group of children with ASD and ASD and epilepsy. Although exact matching was not possible, the group with ASD and epilepsy displayed a greater number and severity of gross and fine motor problems. Nomura et al. (2010) reported that there was a higher rate of 'no crawling' in children with ASD and epilepsy compared with ASD alone. The authors suggested that the higher rate of 'no crawling' in the epilepsy group in contrast to the non-epilepsy group indicated that the neuronal system related to crawling is involved in the pathophysiology of epilepsy in autism. Tuchman et al. (1991) suggest that the cumulative risk for epilepsy in ASD rose with both age and presumed diffuseness of the underlying brain dysfunction as shown by the severity of the cognitive deficit and the presence of cerebral palsy or other overt motor deficit. There is a need for further studies investigating whether or not epilepsy in ASD increases the risk for motor impairments.

Pathophysiology of Epilepsy in ASD

ASD and epilepsy are both heterogeneous disorders with a variety of possible aetiologies. The relatively high rates of epilepsy in ASD and the fact that the onset of seizures can result in autistic features suggests the possibility of common underlying pathphysiological mechanisms in at least some cases. An increasing number of genetic causes have been identified as contributing to ASD and to epilepsy. Often patients with genetic mutations associated with ASD will also have epilepsy and vice versa, suggesting an underlying common aetiology for both disorders. Children with ASD and epilepsy have been reported more likely to have a genetic condition than children with ASD alone (Turk et al. 2009). Many of the medical/genetic conditions with a high rate of ASD such as Rett syndrome, fragile X syndrome and tuberous sclerosis complex frequently have epilepsy as well, suggesting a role for common genetic contributors in some cases.

Genetic studies of children with epilepsy syndromes also suggest shared molecular mechanisms between the two conditions. In children with LKS and CSWS, several copy number variant (CNV) alternations have been found in genomic regions or genes associated with ASD (Lesca et al. 2012). In tuberous sclerosis complex, the MTOR pathway has been identified as important in altered social behaviour and epileptogenesis, and work with animal models suggest that treatment using a MTORC inhibitor, Rapamycin, reduces seizure susceptibility but also attenuates autistic behaviour (Talos et al. 2012). Brooks-Kayal (2010) has suggested that ASD and epilepsy be understood as disorders of synaptic plasticity that result in imbalances of excitation and inhibition in the developing brain. The abnormal plasticity may result in both ASD and epilepsy with the possibility of seizures further contributing to maladaptive plasticity and further imbalances in excitation and inhibition that contribute to learning and behavioural difficulties (Brooks-Kayal 2010). However, all children with ASD do not develop epilepsy and vice versa. The higher association between epilepsy and ASD in those with ASD and IDD is suggestive that IDD may account for at least some of the co-occurrence, and thus understanding relationships between cognitive impairments and the process of development of epilepsy may also shed light on the pathophysiology of ASD.

Treatment of Epilepsy in ASD

Epilepsy is known to be associated with increased mortality and therefore, in individuals with ASD, the diagnosis of epilepsy and careful treatment of seizure disorders is important (Mouridsen et al. 2011). However, in the treatment of epilepsy, it is important to weigh seizure control with possible side effects of anti-epileptic treatments. It is also important that resources are available to treat the often associated cognitive and behavioural impairments as well as the seizures, as these impairments often have the greatest impact on quality of life (Baca et al. 2011). In terms of treatments, AEDs are usually the first choice. If AEDs are not deemed to be efficacious with respect to seizure control, the possibility of surgery may arise, particularly in cases where it is possible to identify where seizures initiate. Approximately 25 % of children with intractable epilepsy have surgically remediable epilepsy syndromes (Hemb et al. 2010). Other possible treatments include the ketogenic diet and vagus nerve stimulation (VNS). The ketogenic diet is a high fat, adequate protein, low carbohydrate diet used to treat AED-resistant epilepsy and has been shown to be an effective and well tolerated alternative for both paediatric and adult epilepsy (Neal et al. 2008; Payne et al. 2011). VNS is a treatment for patients with focal epilepsy which involves electrical stimulation of the left vagus nerve using a subcutaneously implanted pulse generator (Ben-Menachem 2002).

The treatment of seizures in ASD will not differ from that of epileptic seizures in individuals without ASD (Gillberg 1991) and in most instances, this will mean the use of AEDs. Given the possibility that prompt AED treatment in a small number of cases may limit or prevent cognitive and behavioural regression, clinicians must strive to identify children in whom deterioration might be prevented/lessened by appropriate AED treatment (Besag 2009). AEDs may be administered to children with ASD with and without epilepsy (Aman et al. 2003). There have been reports of improvements in ASD symptoms via the use of lamotrigine in some children with epilepsy and ASD (Uvebrant and Bauziene 1994), although in children with ASD without epilepsy, positive results have not been found on standardised measures of behaviour and ASD symptoms (Belsito et al. 2001). It appears that while current pharmacological and surgical treatments for epilepsy in children with ASD may be effective in treating seizures, they are rarely effective in treating the cognitive, language and social functioning defecits (Tuchman et al. 2010). Approximately 20–40 % of epilepsy surgery candidates have an ASD phenotype (McLellan et al. 2005; Taylor et al. 1999; Danielsson et al. 2009) and a small number of studies of children with epilepsy and autistic-like regression have suggested that aggressive treatment of seizures (including surgery) is associated with a decrease of autistic behaviours (e.g. Neville et al. 1997). Szabo et al. (1999) found that surgical intervention in a small group of children with autism and intractable seizures improved the seizures but not the ASD symptoms. Danielsson et al. (2009) reported that post-epilepsy surgery, all parents of children with epilepsy and ASD reported positive behavioural effects, but of the seven children diagnosed with ASD all kept this diagnosis based on results of standardised diagnostic instruments and with respect to DSM-IV criteria. Other potential interventions that been used in epilepsy such as VNS and the ketogenic diet have been tried in children with both epilepsy and ASD with mixed results (Warwick et al. 2007; Park 2003; Danielsson et al. 2008; Evaneliou et al. 2003).

The treatment of EEG paroxysmal abnormalities is frequently reported in children with ASD despite the absence of seizures (Chez et al. 2006) and whether or not these abnormalities should be treated in a manner similar to actual seizures is controversial (Spence and Schneider 2009; Parmeggianai et al. 2010). There is also controversy with regard to the treatment of autistic regression and epileptiform abnormalities without clinical epilepsy (Canitano 2007). Several clinical reports note improvement in children with either ASD with seizures or ASD without clinical seizures but with EEG epileptiform abnormalities (Childs and Blair 1997; Plioplys 1994). Pharmacotherapy seems to be a reasonable approach when regression of language and behaviour associated with an abnormal EEG is ongoing, but current evidence on efficacy of treatment of these conditions is limited (Canitano 2007). The mere presence of EEG abnormalities in these cases may not be an indication for the use of anti-epileptic therapy, as the EEG abnormalities may reflect an underlying brain disorder responsible for ASD (Deonna and Roulet 2006). In the case of LKS, there exists the possibility of benefits from the use of continuous and pulsed corticosteroids in terms of seizure control and behavioural functioning (Gillberg and Neville 2010).

Outcome of Epilepsy in ASD

In the general population, 70–80 % of adults with new onset epilepsy will become seizure-free with current AEDs, although around half will experience adverse side effects (Schmidt and Schachter 2014). Seventy percent of patients with newly treated childhood onset epilepsy enter periods of remission of at least 5 years (Silanpää et al. 2010). A number of studies have suggested that remission rates of epilepsy in ASD are lower than in the epilepsy population without ASD. Danielsson et al. (2005) reported that the remission rate of epilepsy in individuals with ASD was only 16% in their community-based study of individuals with ASD followed up after 13–22 years. It was concluded that individuals with the combination of epilepsy, autism and IDD constitute a very severely disabled group usually with major brain dysfunction. Hara (2007) reported that only four of the 33 (12%) individuals with ASD and epilepsy met the International League against Epilepsy's (ILAE) definition of remission of epilepsy. Lower IQ and higher use of psychotropic drugs were noted in the epilepsy group and the authors conclude that epilepsy is not easy to control in ASD (Hara 2007). Sansa et al. (2011) reported that treatment-resistant epilepsy is common in ASD, particularly in those with early seizure onset. Furthermore, Sansa et al. (2011) reported on a small number of patients with ASD and epilepsy who had VNS and epilepsy surgery with relatively poor outcomes and suggested that surgical and VNS outcomes are less favourable than in those with treatment-resistant epilepsy without ASD.

Conclusion

Epilepsy is a common occurrence in ASD, particularly in individuals who are functioning in the IDD range. Studies that have included adults suggest a lifetime prevalence of epilepsy in individuals with ASD of 25–40%. Studies have not always employed criteria used for the diagnosis of epilepsy as described by ILAE or used terms to describe seizures accepted by the ILAE. With regard to diagnosis of ASD, studies have not always employed gold standard ASD diagnostic methods and it would appear that most studies have been biased towards those with ASD and IDD. As well as increased rates of seizures in children with ASD, there also appear to be elevated rates of EEG/epileptiform abnormalities without seizures, although prevalence rates have varied significantly, and there are no population-based studies to draw upon. There continues to be a need for population-based data using agreed-upon definitions of EEG/epileptiform abnormalities. The diagnosis of epilepsy in ASD should follow the same approach as diagnosis of epilepsy in those without ASD, although an awareness of the common manifestations of non-epileptic paroxysmal events in ASD will be helpful. Epilepsy may be a consideration in cases of children with ASD who regress, but in most cases ASD does not play a causative role.

Studies of seizure type in ASD have yielded mixed results and all seizure types can occur in ASD. While future studies will benefit from the use of internationally agreed seizure classification systems, it may be more useful to focus on particular epilepsy syndromes associated with ASD with respect to understanding potential relationships between epilepsy and ASD. A number of reviews have concluded that those with ASD and IDD are at higher risk for developing epilepsy than those with

ASD without IDD. Females with ASD appear more likely to have epilepsy than males although this relationship is moderated by the fact that females with ASD are also likely to have lower levels of cognitive functioning.

In ASD and epilepsy, there may be a different pattern of peak seizure onset compared with the non-ASD epilepsy population, but there is a need for more evidence particularly regarding peaks in adolescence and adult life. This potential difference between epilepsy in ASD and epilepsy in the non-ASD population needs further study as it might have implications regarding treatment of epilepsy in ASD and contribute to an understanding of pathophysiology of both disorders. There is limited research on outcomes in ASD post-childhood (Magiata et al. 2014), particularly in late adulthood. Future studies on the prevalence and manifestation of epilepsy in ASD in older adults may be helpful with regard to understanding the needs of those with ASD who have epilepsy. Epilepsy and ASD are both associated with significant behavioural, psychiatric and motor problems, and the limited research that has been carried out suggests that having ASD and epilepsy may be associated with a higher level of psychopathology and motor problems than ASD alone. Future studies of cognitive, behavioural and psychiatric difficulties in those with ASD and epilepsy may benefit from an early symptomatic syndromes eliciting neurodevelopmental clinical examinations (ESSENCE) approach which alerts clinicians to the likelihood of a child having difficulties in more than one domain of functioning (Gillberg 2010).

In terms of pathophysiology of epilepsy in ASD, there is likely to be an increased understanding of the neurobiology of the disorders arising from genetic studies. In both conditions, there is a need for an increased emphasis on translational research so that innovative findings in animal models can be translated into human trials. Environmental enrichment strategies, genetic and cellular therapeutic strategies and pharmacological therapeutic strategies need to be tested in humans with ASD, epilepsy and both conditions. The outcome of epilepsy in ASD would appear less favourable than in those with epilepsy without ASD. These may be due to the increased likelihood of the presence of cognitive impairment in ASD, but may also be due to other factors related to the development of ASD. Treatment of epilepsy in ASD is similar to treatment in those with ASD without epilepsy. There have been studies suggesting that the treatment of EEG/epileptiform abnormalities in the absence of epilepsy in those with ASD is warranted. However, such treatment remains controversial.

There is much that is still unknown regarding the relationship between epilepsy and ASD. Both disorders are heterogeneous in terms of aetiology and phenotype; this heterogeneity is increasingly being recognised by the use of the terms 'autisms' (Gillberg and Coleman 2012) and 'epilepsies' (Cross et al. 2013). This heterogeneity will increasingly be the basis for studies in both conditions with respect to understanding pathophysiological mechanisms and developing efficacious treatments. Individuals with the combination of ASD and epilepsy will continue to need individual diagnosis and treatment from collaborating professionals to ensure optimal outcome of both conditions.

References

Akshomoff, N., Farid, N., Courchesne, E., & Haas, R. (2007). Abnormalities on the neurological examination and EEG in young children with pervasive developmental disorders. *Journal of Autism and Developmental Disorders, 37,* 887–893.

Aman, M. G., Lam, K. S., & Collier-Crespin, A. (2003). Prevalence and patterns of use of psychoactive medicines among individuals with autism in the Autism Society of Ohio. *Journal of Autism and Developmental Disorders, 33,* 527–534.

American Psychiatric Association. (2000). *Diagnostic and statistical manual of mental disorders* (4th ed., text rev.). Washington, DC: Author.

American Psychiatric Association (APA). (2013). *Diagnostic and statistical manual of mental disorders* (5th ed.). Arlington: American Psychiatric Publishing.

Amiet, C., Gourfinkel-An, I., Bouzamondo, A., Tordjman, S., Baulac, M., Lechat, P., Mottron, L., & Cohen, D. (2008). Epilepsy in autism is associated with intellectual disability and gender: Evidence from a meta-analysis. *Biological Psychiatry, 64,* 577–582.

Arshad, S., Winterhalder, R., Underwood, L., Kelesidi, K., Chaplin, E., Kravariti, E., Anagnostopoulos, D., Bouras, N., McCarthy, J., & Tsakanikos, E. (2011). Epilepsy and intellectual disability: Does epilepsy increase the likelihood of co-morbid psychopathology? *Research in Developmental Disabilities, 32,* 353–357.

Baca, C. B., Vickrey, B. G., Caplan, R., Vassar, S. D., & Berg, A. T. (2011). Psychiatric and medical comorbidity and quality of life outcomes in childhood-onset epilepsy. *Pediatrics, 128,* e1532–e1543.

Baird, G., Simonoff, E., Pickles, A., Chandler, S., Loucas, T., Meldrum, D., & Charman, T. (2006a). Prevalence of disorders of the autism spectrum in a population cohort of children in South Thames: The special needs and autism project (SNAP). *Lancet, 368,* 210–215.

Baird, G., Robinson, R. O., Boyd, S., & Charman, T. (2006b). Sleep electroencephalograms in young children with autism with and without regression. *Developmental Medicine and Child Neurology, 48,* 604–648.

Ballaban-Gil, K., & Tuchman, R. (2000). Epilepsy and epileptiform EEG: Association with autism and language disorders. *Mental Retardation Developmental Disabilities Research Reviews, 6,* 300–308.

Belsito, K. M., Law, P. A., Kirk, K. S., Landa, R. J., & Zimmerman, A. W. (2001). Lamotrigine therapy for autistic disorder: A randomized, double-blind, placebo-controlled trial. *Journal of Autism and Developmental Disorders, 31,* 175–181.

Ben-Menachem, E. (2002) Vagus-nerve stimulation for the treatment of epilepsy, *Lancet Neurology, 1,* 477–482.

Berg, A., Berkovic, S. F., Brodie, M. J., Buchhalter, J., Cross, J. H., van Emde Boas, M., Engel, J., French, J., Glauer, T. A., Mathern, G. W., Moshé, S. L., Nordli, D., Plouin, P., & Schrffer, I. E. (2010). Revised terminology and concepts for organization of seizures and epilepsies: Report of the ILAE Commission on Classification and Terminology, 2005–2009. *Epilepsia, 51,* 676–685.

Besag, F. (2009). The relationship between epilepsy and autism: A continuing debate. *Acta Paediatrica, 98,* 618–620.

Bolton, P. F., Carcania-Rathwell, I., Hutton, J., Goode, S., Howlin, P., & Rutter, M. (2011). Epilepsy in autism: Features and correlates. *British Journal of Psychiatry, 198,* 289–294.

Brooks-Kayal, A. (2010). Epilepsy and autism spectrum disorders: Are there common developmental mechanisms. *Brain & Development, 32,* 731–738.

Camfield, C. S., Camfield, P. R., Gordon, K., Wirrell, E., & Dooley, J. M. (1996). Incidence of epilepsy in childhood and adolescence: A population based study in Nova-Scotia from 1987 to 1985. *Epilepsia, 37,* 19–23.

Canitano, R. (2007). Epilepsy in Autism Spectrum Disorders. *European Child & Adolescent Psychiatry, 16,* 61–66.

Canitano, R., Luchetti, A., & Zappella, M. (2005). Epilepsy, electroencephalographic abnormalities, and regression in children with autism. *Journal of Child Neurology, 20,* 27–31.

Cedurland, M., & Gillberg, C. (2004). One hundred males with Asperger syndrome: A clinical study of background and associated factors. *Developmental Medicine and Child Neurology, 46,* 652–660.

Chez, M. G., Chang, M., Krasne, V., Coughlan, C., Kominsky, M., & Schwartz. A. (2006). Frequency of epileptiform EEG abnormalities in a sequential screening of autistic patients with no known clinical epilepsy from 1996 to 2005. *Epilepsy & Behavior, 8,* 267–271.

Childs, J. A., & Blair, J. L. (1997). Valproic acid treatment of epilepsy in autistic twins. *Journal of Neuroscience Nursing, 29,* 244–248.

Commission on Classification & Terminology of the International League against Epilepsy. (1981). Proposal for revised clinical and electroencephalographic classification of epileptic seizures. From the Commission on Classification and Terminology of the International League Against Epilepsy. *Epilepsia, 22,* 489–501.

Cross, J. H., Kluger, G., & Lagae, L. (2013). Advancing the management of childhood epilepsies. *European Journal of Paediatric Neurology, 17,* 2334–2347.

Danielsson, S., Gillberg, I. C., Billstedt, E., Gillberg, C., & Olsson, I. (2005). Epilepsy in young adults with autism: A prospective population-based follow-up study of 120 individuals diagnosed in childhood. *Epilepsia, 46,* 918–923.

Danielsson, S., Gillberg, C., & Olsson, I. (2008). Lack of effects of vagus nerve stimulation on drug-resistant epilepsy in eight paediatric patients with autism spectrum disorders: A prospective 2-year follow-up study. *Epilepsy & Behavior, 12,* 298–304.

Danielsson, S., Viggedal, G., Steffenburg, S., Rydenhag, B., Gillberg, C., & Olsson, I. (2009). Psychopathology, psychosocial functioning, and IQ before and after epilepsy surgery in children with drug-resistant epilepsy. *Epilepsy & Behavior, 14,* 330–337.

Delorme, R., Ey, E., Toro, R., Leboyer, M., Gillberg, C., & Bourgeron, T. (2013). Progress toward treatments for synaptic defects in autism. *Nature Medicine, 19,* 685–694.

Deonna, T., & Roulet, E. (2006). Autistic spectrum disorder: Evaluating a possible contributing or causal role of epilepsy. *Epilepsia, 47*(Suppl 2), 79–82.

Deonna, T., & Roulet-Perez, E. (2005). *Cognitive and behavioral disorders of epileptic origin in children.* London: MacKeith Press.

Engel, J. (2001). Intractable epilepsy: Definition and neurobiology. *Epilepsia, 42*(Suppl 6), 3.

Evaneliou, A., Vlachonikolis, I., Mihailidou, H., Spiloti, M., Skarpalezou, A., Makaronas, N., Prokopiou, A., Christodoulou, P., Liapi-Adamidou, G., Helidonis, E., Sbyrakis, S., & Smeitink, J. (2003). Application of a ketogenic diet in children with autistic behavior: Pilot study. *Journal of Child Neurology, 18,* 113–118.

Fernell, E., Hedvall, A., Norrelgen, F., Eriksson, M., Höglund-Carlsson, L., Barnevik-Olsson, M., Svensson, L., Holm, A., Westerlund, J., & Gillberg. C. (2010). Developmental profiles in preschool children with autism spectrum disorders referred for intervention. *Research in Developmental Disabilities, 31,* 790–799.

Fernell, E., Hedvall, A., Westerlund, J., Höglund Carlsson, L., Eriksson, M., Barnevik Olsson, M., Holm, A., Norrelgen, F., Kjellmer, L., & Gillberg, C. (2011). Early intervention in 208 Swedish preschoolers with autism spectrum disorder. A prospective naturalistic study. *Research in Developmental Disabilities, 32,* 2092–2101.

Fong, C. Y., Baird, G., & Wraige, E. (2008). Do children with autism and developmental regression need EEG investigation in the absence of clinical seizures? *Archives of Disease in Childhood, 93,* 998–999.

Gabis, L., Pomeroy, J., & Andriola, M. R. (2005). Autism and epilepsy: Cause, consequence, comorbidity, or coincidence? *Epilepsy & Behavior, 7,* 652–656.

Gillberg, C. (1991). The treatment of epilepsy in autism. *Journal of Autism and Developmental Disorders, 21,* 61–77.

Gillberg, C. (2010). The ESSENCE in child psychiatry: Early Symptomatic Syndromes Eliciting Neurodevelopmental Clinical Examinations. *Research in Developmental Disabilities, 31,* 1543–1551.

Gillberg, C., & Coleman, M. (2012). *The autisms* (4th edn.). Oxford: Oxford University Press.
Gillberg, I. C., & Gillberg, C. (1989). Asperger syndrome-some epidemiological considerations: A research note. *Journal of Child Psychology and Psychiatry, 30,* 631–638.
Gillberg, C., & Neville, B. G. R. (2010). Autism and epilepsy: Comorbidity, coexistence or coincidence. In M. Bax & C. Gillberg (Eds.), *Comorbidities in developmental disorders. Clinics in developmental medicine no. 187* (pp. 89–100). London: Wiley.
Gillberg, C., & Schaumann, H. (1983). Epilepsy presenting as infantile autism? Two case studies. *Neuropediatrics, 14,* 206–212.
Green, D., Charman, T., Pickles, A., Chandler, S., Loucas, T., Simonoff, E., & Baird, G. (2009). Impairment in movement skills of children with autistic spectrum disorders. *Developmental Medicine and Child Neurology, 51,* 311–316.
Guerrini, R. (2006). Epilepsy in children. *Lancet, 367,* 499–524.
Hara, H. (2007). Autism and epilepsy: A retrospective follow-up study. *Brain & Development, 29,* 486–490.
Hemb, M., Velasco, T. R., Parnes, M. S., Wu, J. Y., Lerner, J. T., Matsumoto, J. H., Yudovin, S., Shields, W. D., Sankar, R., Salamon, N., Vinters, H. V., & Mathern, G. W. (2010). Improved outcomes in pediatric epilepsy surgery: The UCLA experience, 1986–2008. *Neurology, 74,* 1768–1775.
Hesdorffer, D. C., Logrosino, G., Benn, E. K., Katri, N., Cascino, G., & Hauser, W. A. (2011). Estimating risk for developing epilepsy: A population-based study in Rochester, Minnesota. *Neurology, 76,* 23–27.
Hindley, D., Ali, A., & Robson, C. (2006). Diagnoses made in a secondary care "fits, faints, and funny turns" clinic. *Archives of Disease in Childhood, 91,* 214–218.
Hirsch, E., Marescaux, C., Maquet, P., Metz-Lutz, M. N., Salmon, E., Franck, G., & Kurtz, D. (1990). Landau-Kleffner syndrome: A clinical and EEG study of five cases. *Epilepsia, 31,* 756–767.
Hrdlicka, M., Komarek, V., Propper, L., Kulisek, R., Zumrova, A., Faladova, L., Havovicova, M., Sedalacek, Z., Blatny, M., & Urbanek, T. (2004). Not EEG abnormalities but epilepsy is associated with autistic regression and mental functioning in childhood autism. *European Child and Adolescent Psychiatry, 13,* 209–213.
Humphrey, A., Neville, B. G. R., Clarke, A., & Bolton, P. (2006). Autistic regression associated with seizure onset in an infant with tuberous sclerosis. *Developmental Medicine and Child Neurology, 48,* 609–611.
Jensen, F. E. (2011). Epilepsy as a spectrum disorder: Implications from novel clinical and basic neuroscience. *Epilepsia, 52*(Suppl 1), 1–6.
Kanner, L. (1943). Autistic disturbances of affective contact. *Nervous Child, 2,* 217–250.
Kanner, L. (1971). Follow-up study of eleven autistic children originally reported in 1943. *Journal of Autism and Childhood Schizophrenia, 1–2,* 119–145.
Kim, S. H., Kim, H., Lim, B. C., Chae, J. H., Kim, K. J., Hwang, Y. S., & Hwang, H. (2012) Paroxysmal nonepileptic events in pediatric patients confirmed by long-term video-EEG monitoring-single tertiary centre review of 143 patients, *Epilepsy & Behavior, 24,* 336–360.
Kopp, S., & Gillberg, C. (2011). The autism spectrum screening questionnaire (ASSQ)-revised extended version (ASSQ-REV): An instrument for better capturing the autism phenotype in girls? A preliminary study involving 191 clinical cases and community controls. *Research in Developmetal Disabilities, 32,* 2875–2888.
Kopp, S., Beckung, E., & Gillberg, C. (2010). Developmental coordination disorder and other motor control problems in girls with autism spectrum disorder and/or attention-deficit/hyperactivity disorder. *Research in Developmental Disabilities, 31,* 350–361.
Kotagal, P., Costa, M., Wyllie, E., & Wolgamuth, B. (2002) Paroxysmal nonepileptic events in children and adolescents, *Pediatrics, 110,* e46.
Lesca, G., Rudolf, G., Labalme, A., Hirsch, E., Arzimanoglou, A., Genton, P., Motte, J., de Saint Martin, A., Valenti, M. P., Boulay, C., De Bellescize, J., Kéo-Kosal, P., Boutry-Kryza, N., Edery, P., Sanlaville, D., & Szepetowski, P. (2012). Epileptic encephalopathies of the Landau-

Kleffner and continuous spike and waves during slow-wave sleep types: Genomic dissection makes the link with autism. *Epilepsia, 53,* 1526–1538.

Levisohn, P. M. (2007). The autism-epilepsy connection. *Epilepsia, 48*(Suppl 9), 33–35.

Lotter, V. (1966). Epidemiology of autistic conditions in young children: I. Prevalence. *Social Psychiatry, 1,* 124–137.

Magiata, I., Tay, X. W., & Howlin, P. (2014). Cognitive, language, social and behavioural outcomes in adults with autism spectrum disorders: A systematic review of longitudinal follow-up studies in adulthood. *Clinical Psychology Review, 34,* 73–86.

Malow, B. A. (2006). Searching for autism symptomatology in children with epilepsy-a new approach to an established comorbidity. *Epilepsy Currents, 6,* 150–152.

Matson, J., & Neal, D. (2009). Seizures and epilepsy and their relationship to autism spectrum disorders. *Reseach in Autism Spectrum Disorders, 3,* 999–1005.

McLellan, A., Davies, S., Heyman, I., Harding, B., Harkness, W., Taylor, D., Neville, B. G., & Cross, J. H. (2005). Psychopathology in children with epilepsy before and after temporal lobe resection. *Developmental Medicine and Child Neurology, 47,* 666–672.

Millichap, J. G. (1997). *Progress in pediatric neurology III.* Chicago: PNB Publishers.

Mouridsen, S. E., Rich, B., & Isager, T. (2011). A longitudinal study of epilepsy and other central nervous system diseases in individuals with and without a history of infantile autism. *Brain & Development, 33,* 361–366.

Nabbout, R., & Dulac, O. (2003). Epileptic encephalopathies: A brief overview. *Journal of Clinical Neurophysiology, 20,* 393–397.

Neal, E. G., Chaffe, H., Schwartz, R. H., Lawson, M. S., Edwards, N., Fiztsimmons, G., Whitney, A., & Cross, J. H. (2008). The ketogenic diet for the treatment of childhood epilepsy: A randomised controlled trial. *Lancet Neurology, 7,* 500–506.

Neville, B. G. R., Harkness, W., Cross, J. H., Cass, H. C., Burch, V. C., Lees, J. A., & Taylor, D. C. (1997). Surgical treatment of severe autistic regression in childhood epilepsy. *Pediatric Neurology, 16,* 137–140.

Newschaffer, C. J., Croen, L. A., Daniels, J., Giarelli, E., Grether, J. K., Levy, S. E., Mandell, D. S., Miller, L. A., Pinto-Martin, J., Reaven, J., Reynolds, A. M., Rice, C. E., Schendel, D., & Windham, G. C. (2007). The epidemiology of autism spectrum disorders. *Annual Review of Public Health, 28,* 235–238.

Nomura, Y., Nagao, Y., Kimura, K., Hachimori, K., & Segawa, M. (2010). Epilepsy in autism: A pathophysiological consideration. *Brain & Development, 32,* 799–804.

O'Donoghue, M. F., Goodridge, D. M., Redhead, K., Sander, J. W., & Duncan, J. S. (1999). Assessing the psychosocial consequences of epilepsy: A community-based study. *The British Journal of General Practice, 49,* 211–214.

Olsson, I., Steffenburg, S., & Gillberg, C. (1988). Epilepsy in autism and autisticlike conditions. A population-based study. *Archives in Neurology, 45,* 666–668.

Park, Y. D. (2003). The effects of vagus nerve stimulation therapy on patients with intractable seizures and either Landau-Kleffner syndrome or autism. *Epilepsy & Behavior, 4,* 286–290.

Parmeggianai, A., Barcia, G., Posar, A., Raimondi, E., Santucci, M., & Scaduto, M. C. (2010). Epilepsy and EEG paroxysmal abnormalities in autism spectrum disorders. *Brain & Development, 32,* 783–789.

Payne, N. E., Cross, J. H., Sander, J. W., & Sisodiya, S. M. (2011). The ketogenic and related diets in adolescents and adults-a review. *Epilepsia, 52,* 1941–1948.

Plioplys, S. (1994). Autism: EEG abnormalities and clinical improvement with valproic acid. *Archives of Pediatrics and Adolescent Medicine, 148,* 220–222.

Posserud, M., Lundervold, A. J., Lie, S. A., & Gillberg, C. (2010). The prevalence of autism spectrum disorders: Impact of diagnostic instrument and non-response bias. *Social Psychiatry and Epidemiology, 45,* 319–327.

Rapin, I. (1995). Autistic regression and disintegrative disorder: How important the role of epilepsy? *Seminars in Pediatric Neurology, 2,* 278–285.

Reilly, C., Menlove, L., Fenton, V., & Das, K. B. (2013a). Psychogenic nonepileptic seizures in children: A review. *Epilepsia, 54,* 1715–1724.

Reilly, C., Neville, B. G. R., & Kent, E. (2013b). Psychopathology in childhood epilepsy. *Child and Adolescent Mental Health, 18,* 65–75.

Reilly, C., Atkinson, P., Das, K. B., Chin, R. M. F., Aylett, S. E., Gillberg, C., Burch, V., Scott, R. C., & Neville, B. G. R. (2014). A population-based study of neurobehavioral comorbidities in children with active epilepsy, *Pediatrics,* 133, e1586-93.

Riikonen, R., & Amnell, G. (1981). Psychiatric disorders in children with earlier infantile spasms. *Developmental Medicine and Child Neurology, 23,* 747–760.

Russ, S. A., Larson, K., & Halfon, N. (2012). A national profile of childhood epilepsy and seizure disorder. *Pediatrics, 129,* 256–264.

Saemundsen, E., Ludvigsson, P., & Rafnsson, V. (2007a). Autism spectrum disorders in children with a history of infantile spasms: A population-based study. *Journal of Child Neurology, 22,* 1102–1107.

Saemundsen, E., Ludvigsson, P., Hilmarsdottir, I., & Rafnsson, V. (2007b). Autism spectrum disorders in children with seizures in the first year of life— a population-based study. *Epilepsia, 48,* 1724–1730.

Sansa, G., Carlson, C., Doyle, W., Weiner, H. L., Bluvstein, J., Barr, W., & Devinsky, O. (2011). Medically refractory epilepsy in autism. *Epilepsia, 52,* 1071–1075.

Schmidt, D., & Schachter, S. C. (2014). Drug treatment of epilepsy in adults. *BMJ, 348,* g254.

Silanpää, M., Saarinen, M., & Schmidt, D. (2010). Long-term risks following first remission in childhood-onset epilepsy. A population-based study. *Epilepsy & Behavior, 25,* 145–149.

Smith, K. R., & Matson, J. L. (2010a). Behavior problems: Differences among intellectually disabled adults with co-morbid autism spectrum disorders and epilepsy. *Research in Developmental Disabilities, 31,* 1062–1069.

Smith, K. R., & Matson, J. L. (2010b). Social skills: Differences among adults with intellectual disabilities, co-morbid autism spectrum disorders and epilepsy. *Research in Developmental Disabilities, 31,* 1366–1372.

Speechio, N., Trivsano, M., Scott, R. C., & Ferrie, C. (2012). Epileptic encephalopathy. *Epilepsy Research and Treatment.* doi:10.1155/2012/460256.

Spence, S. J., & Schneider, M. T. (2009). The role of epilepsy and epileptiform EEGs in autism spectrum disorders. *Pediatric Research, 65,* 599–606.

Steffenburg, S., Gillberg, C., & Steffenburg, U. (1996). Psychiatric disorders in children and adolescents with mental retardation and active epilepsy. *Archives of Neurology, 53,* 904–912.

Surén, P., Bakken, I. J., Aase, H., Chin, R., Gunnes, N., Lie, K. K., Magnus, P., Reichborn-Kjennerud, T., Schjølberg, S., Øyen, A. S., & Stoltenberg, C. (2012). Autism spectrum disorder, ADHD, epilepsy, and cerebral palsy in Norwegian children. *Pediatrics, 130,* e152–e158.

Szabó, C. A., Wyllie, E., Dolske, M., Stanford, L. D., Kotagal, P., & Comair, Y. G. (1999). Epilepsy surgery in children with pervasive developmental disorder. *Pediatric Neurology, 20,* 349–353.

Talos, D. M., Sun, H., Zhou, X., Fitzgerald, E. C., Jackson, M. C., Klein, P. M., Lan, V. J., Joseph, A., & Jensen, F. E. (2012). The interaction between early life epilepsy and autistic-like behavioral consequences: A role for the mammalian target of rapamycin (mTOR) pathway. *PLoS One, 7,* e35995.

Taylor, D. C., Neville, B. G., & Cross, J. H. (1999). Autistic spectrum disorders in childhood epilepsy surgery candidates. *European Child and Adolescent Psychiatry, 8,* 189–192.

Tuchman, R. (2006). Autism and epilepsy: What has regression got to do with it? *Epilepsy Currents, 6,* 107–111.

Tuchman, R. F., & Rapin, I. (1997). Regression in pervasive developmental disorders: Seizures and epileptiform electroencephalogram correlates. *Pediatrics, 99,* 560–566.

Tuchman, R., & Rapin, I. (2002). Epilepsy in autism. *Lancet Neurology, 1,* 352–358.

Tuchman, R. F., Rapin, I., & Shinnar, S. (1991). Autistic and dysphasic children. II: Epilepsy. *Pediatrics, 88,* 1219–1225.

Tuchman, R., Alessandri, M., & Cuccaro, M. (2010). Autism spectrum disorders and epilepsy: Moving towards a comprehensive approach to treatment. *Brain & Development, 32,* 719–730.

Turk, J., Bax, M., Williams, C., Amin, P., Eriksson, M., & Gillberg, C. (2009). Autism spectrum disorder in children with and without epilepsy: impact on social functioning and communication, *Acta Paediatricia, 98,* 675–681.

Udall, P., Alving, J., Hansen, L. K., Kibaek, M., & Buchholt, J. (2006). The misdiagnosis of epilepsy in children admitted to a tertiary epilepsy centre with paroxysmal events, *Archives of Disease in Childhood, 91,* 219–221.

Uvebrant, P., & Bauzienė, R. (1994). Intractable epilepsy in children. The efficacy of lamotrigine treatment, including non-seizure-related benefits. *Neuropediatrics, 25,* 284–289.

Van Eeghen, A. M., Pulsifer, M. B., Merker, V. L., Neumeyer, A. M., Van Eeghen, E. E., Thibert, R. L., Cole, A. J., Leigh, F. A., Plotkin, S. R., & Thiele, E. A. (2012). Understanding relationships between autism, intelligence, and epilepsy: A cross-disorder approach. *Developmental Medicine and Child Neurology, 55,* 146–153.

Viscidi, E. W., Triche, E. W., Pescocolido, M. F., McLean, R. L., Joseph, R. M., Spence, S. J., & Morrow, E. M. (2013a). Clinical characteristics of children with autism spectrum disorder and co-occurring epilepsy. *PLoS ONE, 8,* e67797.

Viscidi, E. W., Johnson, A. L., Spence, S. J., Buka, S. L., Morrow, E. M., & Triche, E. W. (2013b). The association between epilepsy and autism symptoms and maladaptive behaviors in children with autism spectrum disorder. *Autism,* 2013 Oct 28. [Epub ahead of print].

Warwick, T. C., Griffith, J., Reyes, B., Legasse, B., & Evans, M. (2007). Effects of vagus nerve stimulation in a patient with temporal lobe epilepsy and Asperger syndrome: Case report and review of the literature. *Epilepsy & Behavior, 10,* 344–347.

Woolfenden, S., Sarkozy, V., Ridley, G., Coory, M., & Williams, K. (2012). A systematic review of two outcomes in autism spectrum disorder - epilepsy and mortality. *Developmental Medicine and Child Neurology, 54,* 306–312.

Chapter 11
Gastrointestinal Disorders

Geraldine Leader and Arlene Mannion

Research into gastrointestinal (GI) symptoms and disorders in autism spectrum disorder (ASD) is a relatively new area of study. This may be because GI symptoms can be very difficult to diagnose in individuals with ASD. Diagnosis can be especially difficult for individuals who are nonverbal or who have severe deficits in communicating their needs and wants. If an individual is in pain and cannot communicate this to caregivers, it makes it very difficult to recognize potential GI symptoms. GI symptoms in individuals with ASD may present themselves differently than in typically developing individuals. A person with ASD may not reach for their abdomen if in pain. Instead, they may display this pain through challenging behavior.

All too often, comorbid conditions such as GI symptoms are seen as being part of ASD, instead of being recognized as a separate comorbid condition. It is very important that we study and understand GI symptoms in ASD, as they may be potentially exacerbating symptoms of ASD such as repetitive behavior. GI symptoms have the potential to jeopardize interventions designed to reduce challenging behavior in children and adults with ASD, and interventions designed to teach new skills such as communication skills, academic skills, and self-help skills. An individual with ASD who has what appears to be difficulties with toileting or feeding may also have comorbid GI symptoms. If intervention just focuses on the presenting an issue such as challenging behavior or toilet training, practitioners may find that there are difficulties with teaching certain skills. These difficulties may be due to an individual with ASD experiencing pain and discomfort. It is imperative that we look at the environment for the individual with ASD, but that we also examine the whole body, including GI symptoms and disorders.

G. Leader (✉)
Irish Centre for Autism and Neurodevelopmental Research, School of Psychology, National University of Ireland, Galway, University Road, Galway, Ireland
e-mail: Geraldine.leader@nuigalway.ie

A. Mannion
Irish Centre for Autism and Neurodevelopmental Research, National University of Ireland, Galway, Galway, Ireland

Johnny L. Matson (ed.), *Comorbid Conditions Among Children with Autism Spectrum Disorders,* Autism and Child Psychopathology Series,
DOI 10.1007/978-3-319-19183-6_11

Definition

The most common GI symptoms reported in individuals with ASD are chronic constipation, abdominal pain with or without diarrhea, and encopresis as a consequence of constipation (Buie et al. 2010a). Buie et al. (2010a) also commented that other GI abnormalities include gastroesophageal reflux disease (GERD), abdominal bloating, disaccharidase deficiencies, inflammation of the GI tract and abnormalities of the enteric nervous system. Wang et al. (2011) noted that GI symptoms can include "constipation, diarrhea, abdominal pain, frequent vomiting, gaseousness, abnormal stool pattern, bloody stools, foul-smelling stools, abdominal bloating, feeding issues, food regurgitation, food selectivity, food intolerance, gastroesophageal reflux, encopresis and so on" (p. 351).

Gastrointestinal Symptoms and ASD Comorbidity

Prevalence

The reported prevalence of GI problems in children with ASD has ranged from 9 to 91 % (Coury et al. 2012; Ming et al. 2008; Black et al. 2002; Fombonne and Chakrabarti 2001; Ibrahim et al. 2009; Mannion and Leader 2014c; Molloy and Manning-Courtney 2003; Mouridsen et al. 2010; Nikolov et al. 2009; Taylor et al. 2002; Valicenti-McDermott et al. 2008; Horvath and Perman 2002; Wang et al. 2011; Parracho et al. 2005; Smith et al. 2009). Wang et al. (2011) commented on the factors that lead to differing rates of GI symptoms across studies. First, there are differences in the target population being studied. Some participants may have different diagnoses on the autism spectrum. Some studies use control groups, while others do not. Second, there are differences in how data are gathered, whether it is by medical records, physicians, or questionnaire-based research. Finally, there are different definitions used for what are considered GI symptoms (Wang et al. 2011). Wang et al. (2011) commented that these definitions can vary in frequency, duration, severity, and type of GI symptoms.

Importance of Studying Gastrointestinal Symptoms

There are many reasons GI symptoms in ASD need to be researched. First, given that a high prevalence of GI symptoms have been found in the literature, it is possible that GI symptoms affect a large proportion of those with ASD. Often these symptoms are just seen as part of ASD, rather than being a comorbid condition. Yet, GI symptoms are not core symptoms of ASD and should not been dismissed as such. Second, these symptoms may cause pain and discomfort. Individuals that are nonverbal or have little communication skills may not be able to tell parents or caregivers that they are in pain. The communication deficits of ASD can make GI symptoms very difficult for the individual who is in pain and unable to communicate this, as well as to the caregivers who are unsure of what the person is trying to communicate and how best to help this person. Third, it is important to recognize that abdominal pain or discomfort may act as a setting event for challenging behavior (Buie et al. 2010a). This discomfort and in turn, challenging behavior can get in the way of the individual acquiring new academic or self-help skills. Mulloy et al. (2010) commented on these biological motivating operations, whereby an upset stomach may act as a motivating operation affecting social consequences. Mulloy et al. (2010) gave the example that a child with an upset stomach may find academic work more demanding than if they did not have an illness. Therefore, they may engage in increasing levels of challenging behavior to escape the demand. It is essential that practitioners are aware of the co-occurrence of GI symptom in some individuals with ASD. By determining that a cause of challenging behavior may be biological rather than environmental, this may mean that appropriate treatment options can be considered. A practitioner could also then change the learning environment to best support the individual. This may include teaching an individual to identify and communicate the instance of pain. Furthermore, additional environmental supports could be put in place such as having a toilet nearby, decreasing demands or allowing frequent breaks to an individual who may be in pain. Finally, an individual's quality of life can be affected if they present with GI symptoms. Williams et al. (2010) found that children with ASD with GI symptoms had lower quality of life compared to children without GI symptoms. GI complaints are therefore associated with overall decreased health-related quality of life. If interventions seek to improve quality of life in individuals with ASD, it is important that GI symptoms are considered. The effect of treatment of GI symptoms needs to be considered. By treating GI symptoms, an individual's quality of life may be improved.

Difficulty of Diagnosis

GI symptoms are difficult to diagnose in individuals with ASD for several reasons. First, clinical practice guidelines in place for the diagnosis of ASD do not include routine consideration of potential GI or other medical conditions (Buie et al. 2010a). GI symptoms need to be routinely screened for. They need to not just be seen as part of ASD or affecting only a limited number of individuals as we know that this is not true. Second, many individuals with ASD are nonverbal or have communication difficulties. Because of this, they may not be able to express pain or discomfort in a typical manner. They may not be able to communicate their symptoms as clearly as those who are typically developing. Those who can verbally communicate may have difficulty describing subjective experiences or symptoms (Buie et al. 2010a). Third, those with ASD may present with GI symptoms in atypical ways. One may assume that if an individual has abdominal or other discomfort that they would touch their abdomen. However, this is not necessarily the case for those with ASD. GI disorders can present as non-GI problems (Buie et al. 2010a). For example, individuals may present with sleep problems or challenging behavior. When they present with vocal stereotypy or repetitive behavior, it could be incorrectly attributed to being symptoms of ASD. It is important to be aware of atypical presentations of GI symptoms. Fourth, diet may play a role in GI symptoms. Kuddo and Nelson (2003) commented that the insistence on sameness in ASD may lead children to demand stereotyped diets which are lacking in fibres, fluids, or other constitutes. Many children with ASD have difficulties with food selectivity and may be rigid in their routines about eating particular types of food. These feeding problems may lead to children exhibiting GI symptoms. Finally, if children are on medication, this can have side effects. Kuddo and Nelson (2003) comment that most medication administered to children with ASD can influence gut function. Children with ASD may be on medication for comorbid conditions such as attention deficit hyperactivity disorder (ADHD), epilepsy, or challenging behavior. Comorbid conditions do not just occur as one additional disorder with ASD. Some individuals may present with a multitude of comorbid symptoms and disorders.

Measures Used to Assess Gastrointestinal Symptoms

While some studies used medical history to assess GI symptoms (Molloy and Manning-Courtney 2003; Nikolov et al. 2009; Maenner et al. 2012), a variety of questionnaires have also been used. In addition to past medical history, Nikolov et al. (2009) used the Side Effects Review Form (Research Units on Pediatric Psychopharmacology). The form was designed to establish whether certain problems are present prior to drug exposure and to track changes. Side effects were rated as mild, moderate, or severe. A rating of mild was given when the problem was present, but not the source of impairment and there was no need for intervention; a rating of moderate was used if the problem caused some impairment or required intervention to prevent impairment, and a rating of severe was used when the problem caused impairment and required intervention (Nikolov et al. 2009). In the study by Nikolov et al. (2009), a pretreatment rating of moderate or severe on the Side Effects Review Form in response to one or more GI questions was classified as the presence of a GI symptom. Hansen et al. (2008) used the childhood autism risks from genetics and the environment (CHARGE) GI history form, which includes 10 items describing current GI symptoms as well as questions relating to food allergies and diet restrictions.

Valicenti-McDermott et al. (2008) developed The Gastrointestinal Questionnaire, derived from the Clinical Diagnostic Questionnaire for Pediatric Functional Gastrointestinal Disorders, as developed by the Committee on Childhood Functional Gastrointestinal Disorders Multinational Working Teams to Develop Criteria for Functional Disorders (Rome II). The GI Questionnaire includes questions on current GI symptoms, as well as lifetime GI or feeding problems. Gorrindo et al. (2012) used the Questionnaire on Pediatric Gastrointestinal Symptoms-Rome III Version (QPGS) which is a 71-item parent report instrument that assesses GI symptoms and classifies functional GI disorders (FGID) according to Rome III criteria. It is available online at http://romecriteria.org/. Gorrindo et al. (2012) also included clinical evaluation in their study. The authors found that parent report of any GI dysfunction in those with ASD was highly concurrent (92.1 %) with a clinical diagnosis of any GI dysfunction.

Chandler et al. (2013) constructed a 20-item GI symptom questionnaire. Questions were asked by current (past 3 months) and past (prior to the past 3 months' symptoms). The GI symptoms included persistent vomiting; stool consistency; abdominal pain; abdominal pain associated with food, bowel movement, or sleep; constipation; subjective difficulties with bowl movements, stool withholding, and soiling; diarrhea, weight loss, mouth ulcers, and presence of mucus or blood in the stools.

The Gastrointestinal Symptom Inventory (Autism Treatment Network 2005) is a 35-item questionnaire that was developed by the Autism Treatment Network (ATN). The ATN is the first network of hospitals and physicians dedicated to developing a model of comprehensive medical care for children and adolescents with autism through seventeen participating institutions in the USA and Canada. In the inventory, there are additional items should a participant exhibit certain symptomatology, and therefore includes 77 items in total. This tool has not been validated. It was based on previous questionnaires and on clinical symptom assessment for children with autism and identified GI disorders. It measures questions about the presence and duration of GI symptoms. The inventory is scored initially dichotomously, i.e., whether or not the child has any of the GI symptoms. The GI symptoms it measures are abdominal pain, nausea, bloating, diarrhea, or other GI symptom. The inventory also allows branching into specific areas of symptomatology: abdominal pain, abnormal bowel movements, reflux, and food insensitivity. These branches will allow determination of rates of these categories as well.

Mazurek et al. (2013b) used the GI Symptom Inventory in their research. It was also used in Williams et al. (2010); Williams et al. (2012a); Williams et al. (2012b), Mannion et al. (2013), and Mazefsky et al. (2014). The GI Symptom Inventory is no longer used by the ATN as part of its registry battery. Instead, questions are included about GI symptoms in the ATN Parent Baseline Assessment. The following symptoms are assessed: nausea/vomiting, reflux, diarrhea, constipation, and stomach/abdominal pain. Mazurek et al. (2013a) used the Parent Baseline Assessment in their research.

Relationships Between Gastrointestinal Symptoms in ASD and Other Variables

Regression

Valicenti-McDermott et al. (2008) investigated the relationship between GI symptoms and regression. Valicenti-McDermott et al. (2008) found that children with ASD who presented with language regression had more GI problems (84 %) than those without language regression (61 %). The authors also found that abnormal stool patterns were reported more frequently in the group with language regression

(42 vs. 12%). Niehus and Lord (2006) found that the medical records of children with ASD and regression indicated significantly more parental reports of bloody stools than those with ASD and no regression. Though nonsignificant, those with ASD and regression had more chronic diarrhea and stool complaints than those with ASD and no regression or those that were typically developing.

Baird et al. (2008) investigated factors associated with regression in children with ASD. Current GI symptoms varied across the three groups in the study; those with no regression, lower level regression, and definite language regression. Current GI symptoms varied across regression groups, but the rate was higher in the no regression group than the lower or definite regression groups. In terms of past GI symptoms, there was no group difference found between those with no regression, lower, or definite regression. This is supported by Chandler et al. (2013) who found that there were no differences between ASD children with and without a history of regression for current and past GI symptoms. Molloy and Manning-Courtney (2003) found that 24% of children with ASD had a history of at least one chronic GI symptom. It was found that 23.4% of the entire sample had a history of regression. However, in support of previous research, Molloy and Manning-Courtney (2003) found that developmental regression was not significantly associated with GI symptoms. Hansen et al. (2008) found no significant differences between the children with ASD with or without regression in terms of GI symptoms. More research is needed on regression, in general, and on the relationship, if any, between GI symptoms and regression. Previous research has indicated that up to one third of children with ASD regress; yet, little is known about why some children regress and why some do not. More research is needed to better understand regression and the long-term effect of regression on those with ASD.

Language and Communication

Gorrindo et al. (2012) examined expressive language and social responsiveness as communication variables in their study. They found that children with ASD and GI symptoms showed higher levels of social impairment than those with ASD only. However, social impairment was not associated with impaired language. In the ASD and GI symptoms group, there was no difference in social impairment in those that were verbal and non-verbal. Gorrindo et al. (2012) also investigated the risk factors for constipation as it was found to be the most common GI symptom in their study. The authors found that younger, more socially impaired, and nonverbal children had increased odds for constipation. Chandler et al. (2013) investigated parental reported GI symptoms in children with ASD, children with special educational needs but no ASD, and typically developing controls. It was found that 46.5% of the ASD group had at least one lifetime GI symptom compared to 29.2% of those with special educational needs, and 21.8% of the typically developing group. The ASD group had significantly increased past vomiting and diarrhea compared to those who were typically developing. They also had more abdominal pain that those with special educational needs. The ASD group had more current constipation and soiling than either the special educational needs group or the typically developing group. In contrast to Gorrindo et al. (2012), Chandler et al. (2013) did not find a difference between verbal ability in children with and without reported pain abdominal pain or constipation. This is supported by Williams et al. (2012b) who found that rates of GI complaints did not differ between four verbal ability groups: nonverbal, some words, phrase speech, and verbal.

Autism Severity

Wang et al. (2011) explored the relationship between GI symptoms and autism severity in children with ASD. They also compared children with ASD to their unaffected siblings. Wang et al. (2011) classified autism severity into three groups; full autism, almost autism, and not quite autism. Increased autism symptom severity was associated with increased odds of having significantly more GI problems being reported. Specifically, having full autism or almost autism was most highly associated with experiencing GI problems (Wang et al. 2011). However, Molloy and Manning-Courtney (2003) found that frequency of GI symptoms did not vary by age, gender, race, or severity of autism. In support of this finding, Nikolov et al. (2009) also found that those with GI problems were no different from those without GI problems in autism symptom severity, demographic characteristics, or measures of adaptive functioning. Mazefsky et al. (2014) found that children with high-functioning ASD who presented with and without GI problems did not differ in autism symptom severity. Chandler et al. (2013) found that there was no significant association between autism severity and current and past GI symptoms in the ASD group. Williams et al. (2010) found that presence of GI problems did not differ by gender, ASD subtype, race, or IQ. However, Williams et al. (2012b) found that chronic GI symptoms were more likely in children with Asperger's than autism. Future research needs to be conducted to understand if there is a relationship between autism severity and GI symptoms.

Challenging Behavior

Horvath et al. (1999) commented that unrecognized GI symptoms and disorders may contribute to the behavioral problems of nonverbal children with ASD, such as sudden irritability and aggressive behavior. Mazurek et al. (2013a) investigated the relationship between aggression and other variables, including GI symptoms in children with ASD. Children with aggression had significantly greater difficulties with GI problems than those without aggression. However, GI problems did not emerge as significant predictors of aggression. Mazefsky et al. (2014) found that children with high-functioning ASD, with and without GI symptoms did not differ in internalizing or externalizing problem behaviors.

Children with GI problems were more likely to present with argumentative, oppositional, or destructive behaviors than those without GI problems (Maenner et al. 2012). Tantrum behaviors were more common in those with GI problems than those without, but the association did not reach statistical significance. No association was found between presence of GI problems and stereotypic/repetitive behaviors or self-injurious behaviors (Maenner et al. 2012).

In contrast, Peters et al. (2014) found a relationship between GI symptoms and rigid-compulsive behavior. The authors found that rigid-compulsive behavior was significantly associated with constipation and diarrhea or soiling. Children with constipation and diarrhea or soiling were more likely to have a parental report of repetitive behavior and compulsive behavior and a parental report of an obsessive compulsive disorder (OCD) diagnosis. Children with constipation and diarrhea or soiling were also more likely to have a clinician report of rituals based on direct observation during the Autism Diagnostic and Observational Schedule (ADOS). Children with constipation only, who did not have diarrhea or soiling were more likely to have a parental report of an OCD diagnosis. Family history of OCD or anxiety or treatment with atypical antipsychotic medication was associated with constipation and diarrhea or underwear staining.

Chaidez et al. (2014) compared GI Symptoms in children with ASD, those with developmental delay, and typically developing children. Children with ASD were more likely to have at least one frequent GI symptom compared to children who are typically developing. The authors also investigated the relationship between GI symptoms and behavior problems. Children with ASD and frequent occurrences of constipation, diarrhea, abdominal pain, and gaseousness scored significantly higher on levels of irritability, social withdrawal, stereotypy, and hyperactivity than children with ASD and no frequent GI symptoms. Children with pain on passing stool, sensitivity to food, and difficulty swallowing scored higher on irritability, social withdrawal, and stereotypy.

Comorbid Psychopathology

In their review of comorbid psychopathology in ASD, Mannion et al. (2014) discussed the relationship between comorbid psychopathology and GI symptoms. Williams et al. (2010) found that children aged 1–5 years with GI symptoms had higher total scores on the Child Behavior Checklist (CBCL) (Achenbach and Roscorla 2000) and for the emotionally reactive, anxious/depressed, somatic complaints, internalizing problems, affective problems, anxiety problems subscales. The authors also found that children aged 6 to 18 years had higher total scores on the Child Behavior Checklist (CBCL) (Achenbach and Roscorla 2001) and on all subscales. Maenner et al. (2012) found that mood disturbances were more common in children with GI problems than those without but this association did not reach statistical significance. In terms of other comorbid disorders, children with ASD and GI problems were significantly more likely than those without GI problems to have co-occurring cerebral palsy and seizure-like activity (Maenner et al. 2012). Mazefsky et al. (2014) found that children with high-functioning ASD with GI problems had significantly higher levels of affective problems than those without GI problems. Future research needs to be conducted on the relationship between GI symptoms and depression in individuals with ASD.

Mannion and Leader (2013a) investigated predictors of GI symptoms in children with ASD. In the study, total number of GI symptoms predicted total scores on the autism spectrum disorder-comorbid for children (ASD-CC) (Matson and González 2007). The ASD-CC is a questionnaire used to assess comorbid psychopathology in those with ASD. Specifically, abdominal pain and constipation also predicted conduct behavior. Diarrhea predicted tantrum behavior. Nausea predicted worry/depressed behavior, avoidant behavior, and conduct behavior. The worry/depressed subscale and the avoidant behavior subscale of the ASD-CC form a measure of anxiety (Davis et al. 2011).

Other authors have also investigated the relationship between GI problems and anxiety. Nikolov et al. (2009) found that when compared to children without GI problems, those with GI problems showed greater symptom severity on measures of irritability, anxiety, and social withdrawal. Williams et al. (2012b) found that clinical anxiety is associated with chronic GI symptoms in children with ASD. Chronic GI complaints were greater in children with clinical anxiety compared to those with no anxiety.

Mazurek et al. (2013b) found that children with ASD who presented with each type of GI symptom had significantly higher rates of anxiety. The following GI symptoms were included: chronic constipation, chronic diarrhea, chronic abdominal pain, chronic bloating, and chronic nausea. A relationship was found between the number of GI symptoms and anxiety. Those with more chronic GI problems had higher anxiety scores than those with no chronic GI problems. Those with no chronic GI problems had significantly lower anxiety scores than those with only one GI problem, those with two problems or those with three or more problems. Anxiety contributed to the prediction of chronic constipation, chronic bloating, chronic nausea, and chronic abdominal pain, but not to the prediction of chronic diarrhea.

In typically developing children, Shelby et al. (2013) found that functional abdominal pain (FAP) in childhood was associated with high risk of anxiety disorders in adolescence and young adulthood. During follow-up in adolescence and young adulthood, 51 % of those with a childhood history of FAP met criteria for an anxiety disorder during their lifetime and 30 % currently met criteria for an anxiety disorder. Lifetime risk of depressive disorder was significantly higher in those with FAP than control participants.

Sleep Problems

Mannion and Leader (2014d) discussed the relationship between GI symptoms and sleep problems in their literature review on sleep problems in ASD. Horvath et al. (1999) commented that unrecognized GI symptoms may lead to nighttime awakenings in nonverbal children with ASD. Maenner et al. (2012) found that children with sleep abnormalities were more likely to have a medically documented history of GI problems, than those without. Williams et al. (2010) found that sleep problems occurred most frequently in those with GI problems (50 %) than those without (37 %). Williams et al. (2012a) found that 24.5 % of children with ASD had sleep problems and chronic GI symptoms, while 25.2 % had neither sleep nor GI problems. It was found that 42.5 % had sleep problems only, while 7.8 % had a chronic GI complaint only. Sleep problems occurred in 84 % of children with chronic nausea, 82 % of children with chronic diarrhea, 81 % of children with chronic bloating, 79 % of children with chronic constipation, and 78 % of children with chronic abdominal pain.

Mannion et al. (2013) investigated predictors of sleep problems in children with ASD. The total number of GI symptoms predicted higher rates of sleep problems. Under-eating, avoidant behavior, and GI symptoms predicted sleep problems. Specifically, abdominal pain predicted sleep anxiety. Under-eating, avoidant behavior, and the five GI symptoms (constipation, diarrhea, nausea, abdominal pain and bloating) predicted parasomnias and daytime sleepiness.

This finding of GI symptoms predicting sleep problems is supported by Hollway et al. (2013). Hollway et al. (2013) found that GI problems including constipation and diarrhea predicted total scores on the Children's Sleep Habits Questionnaire (CSHQ), which was the same measure used by Mannion et al. (2013). GI symptoms predicted sleep anxiety in Hollway et al.'s (2013) research. This is supported by Mannion et al.'s (2013) finding of the relationship between GI symptoms and sleep anxiety. The relationship between sleep problems and GI symptoms is supported by Williams et al. (2012a). The authors reported that abdominal pain predicted sleep anxiety.

Mannion and Leader (2013a) found that sleep problems predicted GI symptoms. Specifically, sleep-disordered breathing and daytime sleepiness predicted both abdominal pain and bloating. Sleep anxiety predicted abdominal pain. It was found that 67.8 % of individuals had both sleep problems and GI symptoms, while only 8 % had neither sleep problems nor GI symptoms. Sleep problems occurred in 92.3 % of those with nausea and in 91.1 % of those with abdominal pain. Sleep problems occurred in 90.9 % of those with bloating. Sleep problems occurred in 90 % of those with diarrhea and in 83.7 % of those with constipation. It was found that 11.5 % had GI symptoms only, while 12.6 % had sleep problems only.

Kang et al. (2014) investigated the association between GI dysfunction and other comorbidity. They found that children with ASD with any symptoms of GI disorder exhibited significantly higher rates of sleep disorders. The authors commented that "Sleep could be disrupted by any of the GI symptoms and, therefore, it is not surprising to observe the association between the two" (p. 5). The relationship between sleep problems and GI symptoms is one that needs to be further explored in future research.

Sensory Issues

Mazurek et al. (2013b) investigated the relationship between sensory over-responsivity and GI problems. They found that those with chronic GI problems had higher levels of sensory over-responsivity. Increasing numbers of GI problems were associated with higher levels of sensory over-responsivity. Sensory over-responsivity also predicted chronic GI problems. The relationship between sensory problems and GI symptoms needs to be further examined in future research.

Parental Stress and Psychological Distress

Silva and Schalock (2012) investigated parenting stress and focused on comorbid behavioral and physical symptoms as well as the core symptoms of ASD. The researchers investigated bowel problems, including constipation and diarrhea as a comorbid physical condition. Bowel problems were found to be stressful for 31.8 % of parents of children with ASD, compared to 5 % of parents of typically developing children and 17.9 % of parents of children with other developmental disabilities. Parents of children with ASD who exhibited bowel problems differed significantly from parents of typically developing children in parenting stress levels. However, no significant differences were found between parents of children with ASD and parents of children with other developmental disabilities for bowel problems. Future research needs to examine the relationship between GI symptoms in ASD and parental stress.

Adaptive Behavior

Little research has focused on the relationship between GI symptoms and adaptive behavior in individuals with ASD. Nikolov et al. (2009) found that there was no difference between children with ASD with and without GI symptoms on measures of adaptive functioning. Mazefsky et al. (2014) investigated the association between emotional and behavioral problems and GI symptoms among children with high-functioning autism. The authors hypothesized that children with GI symptoms would have lower mean adaptive behavior than children without any GI symptoms. However, the study found that participants with and without GI symptoms did not differ in overall adaptive behavior. Future research should further investigate the relationship between GI symptoms and adaptive behavior in individuals with low-functioning ASD as well as in individuals with high-functioning ASD and Asperger's syndrome.

Social Responsiveness and Social Problems

Mazefsky et al. (2014) included social responsiveness as a variable in their study with children with high-functioning ASD. They found that there was no difference between those with and without GI symptoms in terms of social responsiveness. However, the authors found that social problems were significantly associated with the number of GI symptoms. In analyzing this relationship, the authors commented that those with and without GI problems did not differ in their mean social problems scores, and that a similar number of participants in the GI and non-GI groups exceeded the borderline clinical level of social problems.

Gorrindo et al. (2012) used the Social Responsiveness Scale (SRS; Constantino and Gruber 2005) to measure social responsiveness. Gorrindo et al. (2012) found that children with both ASD and GI dysfunction showed more severe social impairment compared to children with ASD alone or children with GI dysfunction alone. The researchers also found that more socially impaired children with ASD had increased odds of functional constipation. It was found that there was a 5 % increase in odds of constipation for each point increase in the SRS T-score.

Quality of Life

The relationship between GI symptoms in individuals with ASD and quality of life is one in which very little research has been conducted in the past. Williams et al. (2010) investigated the relationship between GI symptoms and quality of life in children with ASD. The authors found that children with ASD with GI symptoms had lower quality of life compared to children without GI symptoms. The authors commented on the need for future research to clarify this association.

Physical functioning is often studied as an aspect of quality of life. Previous research has examined the relationship between physical functioning in individuals with ASD. Kuhlthau et al. (2010) compared children with ASD to children with chronic conditions. The authors found that children with ASD did not differ from children with chronic conditions in their physical health. Williams et al. (2010) commented on the need for further investigation on whether treatment of GI disorders improves quality of life in children with ASD. Similarly, Chaidez et al. (2014) commented that "Appropriate treatment of GI symptoms may help alleviate at least some problematic behaviors and improve the quality of life in children with ASD along with their families" (p. 1125). Future research needs to further investigate the relationship between GI symptoms and quality of life in individuals with ASD.

Attention Deficit Hyperactivity Disorder (ADHD)

Mannion and Leader (2014a) discussed the relationship between GI symptoms and comorbid attention deficit hyperactivity Disorder (ADHD). McKeown et al. (2013) investigated the association of constipation and fecal incontinence with ADHD. Children with ADHD had an increased prevalence of constipation (4.1 % of children with ADHD versus 1.5 % of children without ADHD) and fecal incontinence (0.9 % of children with ADHD versus 0.15 % of children without ADHD). The rate of constipation and fecal incontinence was the same for children with ADHD who were prescribed medication, as those not prescribed medication. We know GI symptoms are common in children with ASD. We also know that ADHD and ASD are comorbid conditions. However, we do not yet know about the relationship between ADHD and GI symptoms in individuals with ASD.

Epilepsy

Mannion and Leader (2014b) discussed GI symptoms in their literature review on epilepsy in ASD. Turk et al. (2009) found that those with ASD and epilepsy showed greater incontinence, such as not being clean and dry in day and at night, than those with ASD alone. Gobbi (2005) conducted a review on coeliac disease, epilepsy, and cerebral calcifications. It is unknown if this association is a coincidence or a genetic condition. Research is needed to determine if there is a relationship between GI symptoms and epilepsy, both in typically developing populations and in individuals with ASD.

Feeding Problems

Feeding problems have been identified as a common comorbid condition in individuals with ASD (Mannion and Leader 2013b). Parmeggiani (2014) discussed the relationship between feeding and GI disorders in ASDs. The author commented on how GI disorders can be causes of feeding problems. These GI disorders include gastroesophageal reflux, food allergies, gastritis, colitis, and celiac disease. Parmeggiani (2014) also commented that "Feeding problems may cause GI disorders, which, in turn, can be responsible for other clinical problems, such as sleep disorders and impaired behavior in ASDs" (p. 2041).

Sharp et al. (2013) conducted a literature review and meta-analysis on feeding problems and nutrient intake in children with ASD. The authors commented that future research should determine the long-term health burden associated with atypical patterns of intake on a population level as well as the relationship with other areas of functioning, such as GI issues and quality of life. Kral et al. (2013) conducted a review for nurses on eating behaviors, diet quality, and GI symptoms in children with ASD. The authors concluded that "an assessment of co-occurring medical conditions is a necessary first step in a comprehensive medical evaluation to address concerns about eating behaviors, diet, and limited food variety" (p. 555).

Levy et al. (2007) investigated the relationship between dietary intake and GI symptoms in children with ASD. The researchers found that GI symptoms are not significantly related to abnormal patterns of dietary intake of carbohydrates, proteins, or fats. The researchers also examined stool consistency. No relationship was observed between stool consistency and dietary intake. The authors concluded that future research needs to "describe the relationship between nutritional intake and GI symptoms, determine nutritional risk factors for children with ASD and selective diets, and determine the etiology of GI dysfunction in children with ASD" (p. 495).

Ming et al. (2008) found that food intolerance was associated with GI dysfunction in children with ASD. Kang et al. (2014) found that children with ASD who presented with any symptoms of GI disorder exhibited significantly higher rates of food intolerance than children without GI symptoms. The relationship between GI symptoms and feeding problems needs to be further explored in future research.

Family Medical History and Autoimmune Diseases

Stigler et al. (2009) conducted a review of autism and immune factors. The review discussed GI factors as a possible immune factor. Similarly, Brown and Mehl-Madrona (2011) conducted a review on the possible links between autism, immune system dysfunctions, and GI symptoms in a subgroup of children with ASD. Brown and Mehl-Madrona (2011) concluded that "sufficient evidence exists to support the hypothesis that at least a subgroup of children diagnosed with ASD suffers from altered immune function and GI disturbance" (p. 472). The authors suggested a number of areas in which research could be conducted within the next 5 years with children with ASD and GI symptoms. First, they recommended identifying autism subgroups so that the diagnosis could eventually have pathophysiological differentiation with specific subdiagnosis criteria. Second, GI symptom criteria to screen for food sensitivities could be created. Third, GI symptom criteria could be used to screen for specific subjects rather than indiscriminately selecting subjects from the greater pool of children with ASD. Fourth, it should be determined if this GI symptom-prone group has higher rates of food sensitivities, food allergies, lactose intolerance, celiac disease, and/or other GI enzyme deficiencies or autoimmunities. Fifth, the effectiveness of dietary therapy, including an elimination diet, should be determined in alleviating GI and/or behavioral symptoms. Sixth, the prevalence of GI symptoms in all autoimmune conditions should be determined and not just autism. Finally, the effectiveness of a dietary therapy in reducing GI symptoms should be determined in all autoimmune conditions.

Mouridsen et al. (2007) examined autoimmune disease in the parents of children diagnosed with infantile autism and a matched control group of parents during an observation period of 27 years. It was found that 10.8% of mothers of children diagnosed with infantile autism had an autoimmune disease compared to 9.1% of mothers in the control group. The researchers found that 8.6% of fathers of children diagnosed with infantile autism had an autoimmune disease compared to 4.6%. Type 1 diabetes was found in significantly more fathers of children with infantile autism compared to controls. Ulcerative colitis was found in significantly more mothers of children with infantile autism. It was found that 2.7% of mothers of children with infantile autism had a diagnosis of ulcerative colitis, compared to 0.3% of controls.

Valicenti-McDermott et al. (2006) examined the association of GI symptoms with a family history of autoimmune disease. Family history of autoimmune disease was reported in 38% of the ASD group and in 34% of control participants.

The researchers found that there was no association between family history of autoimmune disease and GI symptoms in children with ASD. A family history of cognitive or psychiatric problems was not associated with an increased risk of GI symptoms.

Valicenti-McDermott et al. (2008) found an association between language regression, a family history of autoimmune disease, and GI symptoms. Children with language regression were more likely to exhibit an abnormal stool pattern, had an increased family family history of celiac disease or inflammatory bowel disease, and of rheumatoid arthritis. Of all of the children with a family history of autoimmune disease, an abnormal stool pattern was reported more frequently in those with language regression than those without language regression. An abnormal stool pattern was found in 78 % of those with a family history of autoimmune disease and language regression and, compared to 15 % of those with a family history of autoimmune disease, but without language regression. Peters et al. (2014) commented that obtaining a family history of GI symptoms "could be useful in establishing a genetic or familial component to bowel symptoms" (p. 1431).

Gastrointestinal Symptoms Throughout the Lifespan

Ibrahim et al. (2009) conducted a long-term population-based retrospective study of the incidence of GI symptoms in children with ASD, compared to matched controls. The participants were followed from their date of birth to their last follow-up before the age of 21 years. Significant differences were found for the incidence of constipation before the age of 20 years, in those with ASD (33.9 %) compared to 17.6 % of controls. There was a significant difference between feeding issues in those with and without ASD, with there being a higher incidence of feeding problems in those with ASD. No significant association was found for those with ASD and overall incidence of GI symptoms, diarrhea, gastroesophageal reflux/vomiting, or abdominal bloating/discomfort/irritability.

Mouridsen et al. (2010) conducted a longitudinal study of GI diseases in individuals diagnosed with autism as children. The research was conducted using medical records. The participants were observed over an average of a 30-year time period. The mean age at the end of the observation period was 42.7 years, with participants ranging from 27 to 57 years of age. It was found that 30.5 % of those with infantile autism had received a diagnosis of a disease of the digestive tract, while 30.7 % of those in the control group received a diagnosis of a disease of the digestive tract. Therefore, individuals with infantile autism were found to be no more likely to be diagnosed with a GI disease.

Kral et al. (2013) commented on the need for longitudinal studies conducted over an extended period of time to assess children's dietary intake and GI and bone health. Future longitudinal studies are needed to examine if GI symptoms change over time. If so, do they improve or do they get worse as children and adolescents with ASD grow into adulthood?

Mouse Model Studies

Hsiao et al. (2013) conducted research using the maternal immune activation (MIA) mouse model. The offspring of these mice display autism-like symptoms including communicative, social, and stereotyped impairments. The offsprings of immune-activated mothers were found to exhibit GI symptoms of human ASD. The researchers found that adult offsprings of immune-activated mothers exhibited increased gut permeability and abnormal intestinal cytokine profiles. The researchers targeted the gut microbiota by administering *Bacteroides fragilis* to the mice. *Bacteroides Fragilis* was found to relate to specific microbiota changes in the MIA offspring. The *Bacteroides Fragilis*-treated offspring exbited improved communicative, repetitive, anxiety-like, and sensori-motor behavior. However, deficits in sociability and social preference remained. The authors concluded that microbiome-mediated therapies may be an effective treatment for neurodevelopmental disorders.

Desbonnet et al. (2014) studied the contributions of microbiota to social behavior in mice. They examined the effects of germ-free (GF) rearing conditions through early life and adolescence on social behavior in adulthood. They found that GF mice spent a decreased proportion of time engaging in social investigation, and spent a greater proportion of time engaged in repetitive self-grooming behavior during social interaction. The behaviors were normalized following GF bacterial colonization. This demonstrated the role of microbiota in social behaviors. The authors concluded that microbiota are important for normal social behaviors, including social motivation and preference for social novelty.

Mouse model studies are an effective way of better understanding the biological mechanisms of GI symptoms. In addition to examining the autism-like symptoms in mice, researchers can examine how these symptoms affect the entire body, including the gut. Levels of bacteria can be researched in the gut. If treating the gut with certain types of bacteria proves effective in animal models, this gives hope of probiotic treatment for GI symptoms in ASD. Some mouse model studies look at treating ASD and treating the behavioral manifestations of ASD in mice. However, research also needs to focus on how the GI symptoms can be treated in the first place. Furthermore, the effect treating GI symptoms has on behavioral symptoms then needs to be understood. We need to first understand the basic animal models of research before focusing on how the basic research can be applied to individuals with ASD.

Genetic and Environmental Risk Factors

Campbell et al. (2009) found that there was a genetic risk based on the association of *MET* in families with co-occurring ASD and GI conditions. MET is a pleiotropic receptor that functions in both brain development and GI repair. A *MET* gene variant was associated with both ASD and GI conditions. The authors suggested that disrupted *MET* signalling may contribute to increased risk for ASD that includes familial GI dysfunction. The researchers also suggested that future research could focus on families with co-occurring ASD and GI symptoms versus ASD alone.

Hsiao (2014) conducted a review of GI issues in ASD, and discussed the potential GI manifestations of genetic and environmental risk factors for ASD. The author discussed *MET* and also discussed that *SLC6A4* is another susceptibility gene that may be linked to GI dysfunction. SLCA4 encodes the integral membrane transporter for the neurotransmitter, serotonin (SERT). The author noted that the endocrine cells of the GI tract are known to produce over 90 % of the body's SERT. Hsiao (2014) discussed how maternal autoreactive antibody production may be a risk factor for ASD with GI abnormalities. Hsiao (2014) discussed possible environmental risk factors for comorbid ASD and GI abnormalities. MIA is one possible risk factor. The author discussed how research has been conducted on mice, but research on humans with ASD is still needed.

We need to better understand the genetics of ASD as well as the genetic risk factors of comorbid conditions such as GI symptoms. It is promising that research is being conducted into the genetics of GI symptoms. We can therefore better understand why some individuals present with GI symptoms and others do not. We need to learn more about familial risk factors, including family medical history as well as genetic risk factors of GI symptoms in families of individuals with ASD. More research is needed to better understand how environmental risk factors play a role in ASD and how they interact with GI symptoms. Mouse model studies are useful for understanding possible environmental risk factors such as the MIA. However, this basic research needs to be expanded and transferred to humans for applied research in the future.

Neuroimaging Research

Breece et al. (2013) compared the frequencies of dendritic cells in children with ASD and typically developing controls. The authors commented on the role of dendritic cells in innate immunity. It was found that myeloid dendritic cell frequencies increase in children with ASD. The researchers collected information on parental report of the GI symptoms of constipation and diarrhea to determine if there were associations with dendritic cell frequencies. Myeloid dendritic cells were associated with the severity of GI symptoms. Increased frequency of mDC2 was positively associated with increased frequency of symptoms of constipation.

Neuroimaging technologies are a state-of-the-art way of better understanding the brain. Neuroimaging studies structural differences in the brain. More research is needed on how the brain structure and anatomy is different in individuals with ASD. By understanding structural neurological research, we can understand the effect that differences in the brain have on the entire human body including the GI tract. We need to better understand the gut-brain connection in ASD in order to conduct important research. By understanding this connection, we can also understand how treatment will be most effective.

Celiac Disease

Buie (2013) conducted a review of the relationship of autism and gluten. Buie (2013) commented that most people who have GI symptoms do not have celiac disease but have a different reaction to gluten. The author also commented that there are several non-GI manifestations of celiac disease including cerebellar ataxia, peripheral neuropathy, epilepsy, dementia, and depression. Lau et al. (2013) assessed immune reactivity to gluten in children with ASD to evaluate the potential link between autism and celiac disease. The researchers found that a subset of children displayed increased immune reactivity to gluten in a manner unrelated to that of celiac disease. Children with GI symptoms were found to have significantly higher levels of IgG antibody to gliadin when compared to those without GI symptoms. However, no association was observed between the elevated anti-gliadin antibody level and the presence of markers of celiac disease. The authors concluded that the majority of individuals with ASD with elevated antibody to gliadin do not have celiac disease but this subset of individuals may have "non-celiac gluten sensitivity" (p. 66155). The authors also commented that the increased anti-gliadin antibody response may involve immunological and/or intestinal permeability abnormalities in children with ASD.

Special Diets

Perrin et al. (2012) investigated complementary and alternative medicine (CAM) use in children with ASD. Parents of children with ASD were asked if their children use any of the following treatments: acupuncture, chelation, chiropractic, or hyperbaric oxygen therapy; dietary supplements (vitamin supplements, probiotics, antifungal agents, digestive enzymes, glutathione, sulfation, amino acids, or essential fatty acids); and special diets(classified as gluten free, casein free, Feingold, no processed sugars, no salicylates, or other). Special diet usage versus no CAM usage was investigated in the study too. Parents reported higher rates of CAM usage in general and for special diets when they also reported GI problems. The authors commented that families seek to address problematic behaviors or symptoms using CAM and that parents whose children have GI symptoms may try both dietary changes and other CAM treatments to improve their child's nutrition and symptoms.

Whitehouse (2013) reviewed CAM for ASDs and included a discussion of the gluten-free, casein-free (GFCF) diet. Whitehouse (2013) concluded that "Currently, there is a lack of evidence to support the use of GFCF diets as an effective intervention for children with ASD" (p. 439). Pennesi and Klein (2012) investigated the effectiveness of the GFCF diet in children with ASD. The authors found the diet to be effective in improving ASD behaviors, physiological behaviors, and social behaviors for children with GI symptoms (specifically, constipation and diarrhea) compared to children with no GI symptoms. The authors suggested that children predisposed to GI abnormalities might particularly benefit more from a GFCF dietary intervention. However, the authors also commented that the findings reported may be highly sensitive to parental perceptions and that the high effectiveness ratings may be explained by a placebo effect. In terms of future research, the authors stated that the priority of future research should be to define the immunological and GI diagnoses and symptoms that best predict those individuals who will be most responsive to the GFCF diet.

Mulloy et al. (2010) conducted a systematic review on GFCFdiets in the treatment of ASD. The authors concluded that the published studies they located do not support the use of GFCF diets in the treatment of ASD. The authors commented on negative consequences of the use of the GFCF diet, such as the use of treatment resources, stigmatization, and reduced cortical bone thickness. The authors recommended that should a child with ASD experience behavioral changes seemingly associated with change in diet, practitioners should consider testing the child for allergies and food intolerances and eliminate identified allergens or irritants from their environment.

Cognitive Behavior Therapy

van der Veek et al. (2013) conducted a randomized controlled trial of cognitive behavior therapy (CBT) for pediatric FAP in typically developing children. Six sessions of CBT were compared to six visits to a pediatrician for the intensive medical care (IMC). Abdominal pain measured was reported on questionnaires and diaries. Other outcomes were measured including GI complaints, functional disability, other somatic complaints, anxiety, depression, and quality of life. It was found that both CBT and IMC resulted in a significant decrease in abdominal pain. CBT was found to be as effective as IMC. Both treatments were also equally effective at reducing GI complaints, functional disability and other somatic complaints, and increasing quality of life. CBT was found to be more effective than IMC for decreasing anxiety and depression symptoms at a 6-month follow-up, but there was no difference between CBT and IMC at a 12-month follow-up. The researchers commented that future research should focus on determining the working mechanisms of CBT. As this research was conducted with typically developing children, it may be a fruitful line of research to determine if the effectiveness of CBT for abdominal pain can be transferred to children with high-functioning ASD who present with GI pain and symptoms. Future research should also examine the use of CBT for abdominal pain in high-functioning adolescents and adults with ASD.

Meta-analysis of Gastrointestinal Symptoms in Autism Spectrum Disorder

McElhanon et al. (2014) conducted a meta-analysis of GI symptoms in ASD. The authors analyzed all studies with a non-ASD comparison group. It was found that GI status was assessed by a caregiver report in 73 % of the studies, while medical chart review was used in 27% of the studies. It was found that the odds of GI symptoms in children with ASD were four times more prevalent than in children without ASD. There was an increase of three times more diarrhea and constipation in children with ASD. There was a two-fold increase of abdominal pain in children with ASD. The authors commented on the need for future research to examine "factors such as immune abnormalities, mucosal barrier dysfunction, GI mobility, feeding and toileting concerns, and the gut microbiome" (p. 881).

Recommendations for Treatment

Buie et al. (2010b) commented that children with ASD can benefit from the adaptation of general pediatric guidelines for diagnosing GI symptoms. The authors provided a review of guidelines to diagnose and treat GI symptoms using current general pediatric guidelines, until specific guidelines are designed for those with ASD. Information on differential diagnosis, evaluation, and treatment considerations are provided for chronic abdominal pain, constipation, chronic diarrhea and, GERD, in children with ASD.

Furuta et al. (2012) developed an algorithm to help health-care providers identify, evaluate, and manage constipation in children with ASD. The consensus among the authors is that (1) subtle or atypical symptoms might indicate the presence of constipation; (2) screening, identification, and treatment through a deliberate approach to identify underlying causes of constipation is appropriate; (3) diagnostic–therapeutic intervention can be provided when constipation is documented; and (4) careful follow-up after any intervention be performed to evaluate effectiveness and tolerance of the therapy (Furuta et al. 2012). According to the algorithm, any child with atypical behaviors should be evaluated for constipation. Examples of these behaviors include self-injurious behavior, posturing, grimacing, holding the abdomen, squeezing the legs together, or walking around with a narrow gait to hold the stool in (Furuta et al. 2012).

Buie et al. (2010a) commented that integrating behavioral and biomedical roles can be advantageous. First, functional behavioral assessments can be used in order to interpret the function of challenging behavior. Second, it is important to be aware that pain and discomfort can function as a setting event for challenging behavior. Third, functional communication skills may be taught. Buie et al. (2010a) commented that it would be useful for diagnosis to teach a child to identify the location and type of pain they are experiencing. Finally, the individual could be taught skills for coping with a task demand appropriately during moments of pain or discomfort (Buie et al. 2010a).

Future Research

Coury et al. (2012) developed a research agenda for GI conditions. They defined four priority areas for research: epidemiology of GI conditions in ASD; underlying pathology; treatment and outcome; and nutrition. There is a need for rigorously designed prevalence studies to identify risk factors including clinical and behavioral indicators of GI problems, atypical presentations of GI disorders in ASD, and subpopulations within ASD that have GI symptoms (Coury et al. 2012).

As evidenced by the lack of papers on adults with ASD discussed in this chapter, there is a real need for more research to be conducted on adults with ASD to investigate the relationship between GI problems and ASD in adults. Edwards et al. (2012) found that in the intervention research on ASD, only 1.7% of participants were 20 years or more. In ASD research, in general, there is a need for adult research and this is especially so in relation to GI symptoms.

Longitudinal studies are needed to determine if GI symptoms change over time. We need to understand if GI symptoms continue on to adolescence, adulthood, and older adulthood. Do these symptoms get better? Do they get worse? Do symptoms remain constant over time? These are questions that we not know the answer to, as of now. Future research needs to investigate these questions.

Research is needed on the relationship between GI symptoms and other comorbid conditions in ASD, such as sleep problems, anxiety, and depression. The relationship between GI symptoms and outcome variables such as quality of life, behavior problems, social functioning, and adaptive behavior needs to be better understood. We need to understand what effect GI symptoms have on an individual's level of functioning. We need to better understand treatment options for these GI symptoms in animal models as well as in humans with ASD. Furthermore, the effects that treating these GI symptoms have on an individual's quality of life, behavior problems, social functioning, and adaptive behavior need to be determined.

The animal model research gives us an underlying understanding of the biological mechanisms that interact with the GI symptoms. This research is in the early stages but a greater understanding of the biological mechanisms will allow us to investigate and design effective treatment models in the future. Future treatment may include the use of dietary interventions such as probiotics. While special diets or nutritional therapy may be found to be a possible treatment option in the future, it is important that dietary intervention is not just seen as a treatment for all individuals with ASD. Instead, we need to better understand what symptoms can best predict the individuals who will be most responsive to special diets such as the GFCF diet.

We now know that GI symptoms and disorders are a prevalent comorbid condition in ASD. However, they are difficult to diagnose due to the communication deficits in ASD. It may be difficult to determine if individuals are in pain if they cannot communicate this verbally, or instead communicate it through challenging behavior. We know that GI symptoms may present in atypical ways, such as through aggression, repetitive behavior, or sleep disturbances. We need to better understand how to diagnose these GI symptoms that present atypically. GI symptoms can exacerbate the core symptoms of ASD and can cause a variety of other behaviors that are not the core symptoms of ASD. GI symptoms need to be screened by medical practitioners, so that treatment can be provided.

Researchers need to understand that GI symptoms may be an exacerbating variable in ASD research, whereby GI symptoms affect an individual with ASD and their behavior. Often GI symptoms are not considered or controlled for in ASD research. Practitioners need to be aware of how GI symptoms may interfere with an individual's learning environment. A key skill that practitioners need to focus on in teaching is to identify and communicate pain to parents, caregivers, or teachers. In conclusion, an awareness and understanding of GI symptoms is essential for practitioners and researchers alike.

References

Achenbach, T. M., & Rescorla, L. A. (2000). *Manual for the ASEBA preschool forms and profiles.* Burlington: University of Vermont Department of Psychiatry.

Achenbach, T. M., & Rescorla, L. A. (2001). *Manual for the ASEBA school-age forms and profiles.* Burlington: University of Vermont, Research Center for Children, Youth, and Families.

Autism Treatment Network. (2005). *GI symptom inventory questionnaire, vers. 3.0.* New York: Autism Speaks.

Baird, G., Charman, T., Pickles, A., Chandler, S., Loucas, T., Meldrum, D., et al. (2008). Regression, developmental trajectory and associated problems in disorders in the autism spectrum: The SNAP study. *Journal of Autism and Developmental Disorders, 38,* 1827–1836.

Black, C., Kaye, J. A., & Jick, H. (2002). Relation of childhood gastrointestinal disorders to autism: Nested case-control study using data from the UK general practice database. *British Medical Journal, 325,* 419–421.

Breece, E., Paciotti, B., Nordahl, C. W., Ozonoff, S., Van de Water, J. A., Rogers, S. J., et al. (2013). Myeloid dendritic cells frequencies are increased in children with autism spectrum disorder and associated with amygdala volume and repetitive behaviors. *Brain, Behavior, and Immunity, 31,* 69–75.

Brown, A. C., & Mehl-Madrona, L. (2011). Autoimmune and gastrointestinal dysfunctions: Does a subset of children with autism reveal a broader connection? *Expert Review of Gastroenterology & Hepatology, 5*(4), 465–477.

Buie, T. (2013). The relationship of autism and gluten. *Clinical Therapeutics, 35*(5), 578–583.

Buie, T., Campbell, D. B., Fuchs, G. J. III, Furuta, G. T., Levy, J., VandeWater, J., et al. (2010a). Evaluation, diagnosis, and treatment of gastrointestinal disorders in individuals with ASDs: A consensus report. *Pediatrics, 125,* S1–S18.

Buie, T., Fuchs, G. J. III, Furuta, G. T., Kooros, K., Levy, J., Lewis, J. D., et al. (2010b). Recommendations for evaluation and treatment of common gastrointestinal problems in children with ASDs. *Pediatrics, 124,* S19–S29.

Campbell, D. B., Buie, T. M., Winter, H., Bauman, M., Sutcliffe, J. S., Perrin, J. M., et al. (2009). Distinct genetic risk based on association of *MET* in families with co-occurring autism and gastrointestinal conditions. *Pediatrics, 123,* 1018–1025.

Chaidez, V., Hansen, R. L., & Hertz-Picciotto, I. (2014). Gastrointestinal problems in children with autism, developmental delays or typical development. *Journal of Autism and Developmental Disorders, 44,* 1117–1127.

Chandler, S., Carcani-Rathwell, I., Charman, T., Pickles, A., Loucas, T., Meldrum, D., et al. (2013). Parent-Reported gastro-intestinal symptoms in children with autism spectrum disorders. *Journal of Autism and Developmental Disorders, 43,* 2737–2747.

Constantino, J. N., & Gruber, C. P. (2005). *Social responsiveness scale: Manual.* Torrance: Western Psychological Services.

Coury, D. L., Ashwood, P., Fasano, A., Fuchs, G., Geraghty, M., Kaul, A., et al. (2012). Gastrointestinal conditions in children with autism spectrum disorder: developing a research agenda. *Pediatrics, 130*(Suppl. 2.), 160–168.

Davis, T. E., Moree, B. N., Dempsey, T., Reuther, E. T., Fodstad, J. C., Hess, J. A., et al. (2011). The relationship between autism spectrum disorders and anxiety: The moderating effect of communication. *Research in Autism Spectrum Disorders, 5,* 324–329.

Desbonnet, L., Clarke, G., Shanahan, F., Dinan, T. G., & Cryan, J. F. (2014). Microbiota is essential for social development in the mouse. *Molecular Psychiatry, 19,* 146–148.

Edwards, T. L., Watkins, E. E., Lotfizadeh, A. D., & Poling, A. (2012). Intervention research to benefit people with autism: How old are the participants? *Research in Autism Spectrum Disorders, 6,* 996–999.

Fombonne, E., & Chakrabarti, S. (2001). No evidence for a new variant of measles-mumps-rubella-induced autism. *Pediatrics, 108*(4), e58.

Furuta, G. T., Williams, K., Kooros, K., Kaul, A., Panzer, R., Coury, D. L., et al. (2012). Management of constipation in children and adolescents with autism spectrum disorders. *Pediatrics, 130*(Suppl. 2), S98–S105.

Gobbi, G. (2005). Coeliac disease, epilepsy and cerebral calcifications. *Brain & Development, 27,* 189–200.

Gorrindo, P., Williams, K. C., Lee, E. B., Walker, L. S., McGrew, S. G., & Levitt, P. (2012). Gastrointestinal dysfunction in autism: Parental report, clinical evaluation, and associated factors. *Autism Research, 5*(2), 101–108.

Hansen, R. L., Ozonoff, S., Krakowiak, P., Angkustsiri, K., Jones, C., Deprey, L. J., et al. (2008). Regression in Autism: Prevalence and associated factors in the CHARGE study. *Ambulatory Pediatrics, 8*(1), 25–31.

Hollway, J. A., Aman, M. G., & Butter, E. (2013). Correlates and risk markers for sleep disturbance in participants of the autism treatment network. *Journal of Autism and Developmental Disorders, 43,* 2830–2843.

Horvath, K., & Perman, J. A. (2002). Autistic disorder and gastrointestinal disease. *Current Opinion in Pediatrics, 14,* 583–587.

Horvath, K., Papadimitriou, J. C., Rabsztyn, A., Drachenberg, C., & Tyson Tildon, J. (1999). Gastrointestinal abnormalities in children with autistic disorder. *The Journal of Pediatrics, 135*(5), 559–563.

Hsiao, E. Y. (2014). Gastrointestinal issues in Autism Spectrum Disorder. *Harvard Review of Psychiatry, 22*(2), 104–111.

Hsiao, E. Y., McBride, S. W., Hsien, S., Sharon, G., Hyde, E. R., McCue, T., et al. (2013). Microbiota modulate behavioral and physiological abnormalities associated with neurodevelopmental disorders. *Cell, 155*(7), 1451–1463.

Ibrahim, S. H., Voigt, R. G., Katusic, S. K., Weaver, A. L., & Barbaresi, J. (2009). Incidence of gastrointestinal symptoms in children with autism: A population based study. *Pediatrics, 124,* 680–686.

Kang, V., Wagner, G. C., & Ming, X. (2014). Gastrointestinal dysfunction in children with autism spectrum disorders. *Autism Research.* In Press. doi:10.1002/aur.1386.

Kral, T. V. E., Eriksen, W. T., Souders, M. C., & Pinto-Martin, J. A. (2013). Eating behaviors, diet quality, and gastrointestinal symptoms in children with autism spectrum disorders: A brief review. *Journal of Pediatric Nursing, 28,* 548–556.

Kuddo, T., & Nelson, K. B. (2003). How common are gastrointestinal disorders in children with autism? *Current Opinion in Pediatrics, 15,* 339–343.

Kuhlthau, K., Orlich, F., Hall, T. A., Sikora, D., Kovacs, E. A., Delahaye, J., et al. (2010). Health-related quality of life in children with autism spectrum disorders: Results from the Autism Treatment Network. *Journal of Autism and Developmental Disorders, 40,* 721–729.

Lau, N. M., Green, P. H. R., Taylor, A. K., Hellberg, D., Ajamian, M., Tan, C. Z., et al. (2013). Markers of celiac disease and gluten sensitivity in children with autism. *PLoS ONE, 8*(6), e66155–e66155.

Levy, S. E., Souders, M. C., Ittenbach, R. F., Giarelli, E., Mulberg, A. E., & Pinto-Martin, J. A. (2007). Relationship of dietary intake to gastrointestinal symptoms in children with autistic spectrum disorders. *Biological Psychiatry, 61,* 492–497.

Maenner, M. J., Arneson, C. L., Levy, S. E., Kirby, R. S., Nicholas, J. S., & Durkin, M. S. (2012). Brief report: Association between behavioral features and gastrointestinal problems among children with autism spectrum disorder. *Journal of Autism and Developmental Disorders, 42,* 1520–1525.

Mannion, A., & Leader, G. (2013a). An analysis of the predictors of comorbid psychopathology, gastrointestinal symptoms and epilepsy in children and adolescents with autism spectrum disorder. *Research in Autism Spectrum Disorders, 7*(12), 1663–1671.

Mannion, A., & Leader, G. (2013b). Comorbidity in autism spectrum disorder: A literature review. *Research in Autism Spectrum Disorders, 7*(12), 1595–1616.

Mannion, A., & Leader, G. (2014a). Attention-deficit/hyperactivity disorder in autism spectrum disorder. *Research in Autism Spectrum Disorders, 8*(4), 432–439.

Mannion, A., & Leader, G. (2014b). Epilepsy in autism spectrum disorder. *Research in Autism Spectrum Disorders, 8*(4), 354–361.

Mannion, A., & Leader, G. (2014c). Gastrointestinal symptoms in autism spectrum disorder: A literature review. *Review Journal of Autism and Developmental Disorders, 1*(1), 11–17.

Mannion, A., & Leader, G. (2014d). Sleep problems in autism spectrum disorder: A literature review. *Review Journal of Autism and Developmental Disorders, 1*(2), 101–109.

Mannion, A., Leader, G., & Healy, O. (2013). An investigation of comorbid psychological disorders, sleep problems, gastrointestinal symptoms and epilepsy in children and adolescents with autism spectrum disorder. *Research in Autism Spectrum Disorders, 7*, 35–42.

Mannion, A., Brahm, M., & Leader, G. (2014). Comorbid psychopathology in autism spectrum disorder. *Review Journal of Autism and Developmental Disorders, 1*(2), 124–134.

Matson, J. L., & González, M. L. (2007). *Autism Spectrum Disorders—Comorbidity—Child Version*. Baton Rouge: Disability Consultants, LLC.

Mazefsky, C. A., Schreiber, D. R., Olino, T. M., & Minshew, N. J. (2014). The association between emotional and behavioral problems and gastrointestinal symptoms among children with high-functioning autism. *Autism: the international journal of research and practice, 18*(5), 493–501.

Mazurek, M. O., Kanne, S. M., & Wodka, E. L. (2013a). Physical aggression in children and adolescents with autism spectrum disorders. *Research in Autism Spectrum Disorders, 7*, 455–465.

Mazurek, M. O., Vasa, R. A., Kalb, L. G., Kanne, S. M., Rosenberg, D., Keefer, A., et al. (2013b). Anxiety, sensory over-responsivity, and gastrointestinal problems in children with autism spectrum disorders. *Journal of Abnormal Child Psychology, 41*, 165–176.

McElhanon, B. O., McCracken, C., Karpen, S., & Sharp, W. G. (2014). Gastrointestinal symptoms in autism spectrum disorder: A meta-analysis. *Pediatrics, 133*(5), 872–883.

McKeown, C., Hisle-Gorman, E., Eide, M., Gorman, G. H., & Nylund, C. M. (2013). Association of constipation and fecal incontinence with attention-deficit/hyperactivity disorder. *Pediatrics, 132*, e1210–e1215.

Ming, X., Brimacombe, M., Chaaban, J., Zimmerman-Bier, B., & Wagner, G. C. (2008). Autism spectrum disorders: Concurrent clinical disorders. *Journal of Child Neurology, 23*, 6–13.

Molloy, C. A., & Manning-Courtney (2003). Prevalence of chronic gastrointestinal symptoms in children with autism and autistic spectrum disorders. *Autism: The International Journal of Research and Practice, 7*, 165–171.

Mouridsen, S. E., Rich, B., Isager, T., & Nedergaard, N. J. (2007). Autoimmune diseases in parents of children with infantile autism: A case control study. *Developmental Medicine & Child Neurology, 49*, 429–432.

Mouridsen, S. E., Rich, B., & Isager, T. (2010). A longitudinal study of gastrointestinal diseases in individuals diagnosed with infantile autism as children. *Child: Care, Health and Development, 36*(3), 437–443.

Mulloy, A., Lang, R., O' Reilly, M., Sigafoos, J., Lancioni, G., & Rispoli, M. (2010). Gluten-free and casein-free diets in the treatment of autism spectrum disorders: A systematic review. *Research in Autism Spectrum Disorders, 4*, 328–339.

Niehus, R., & Lord, C. (2006). Early medical history of children with autism spectrum disorders. *Developmental and Behavioral Pediatrics, 27*(2), S120–S127.

Nikolov, R. N., Bearss, K. E., Lettinga, J., Erickson, C., Rodowski, M., Aman, M. G., et al. (2009). Gastrointestinal symptoms in a sample of children with pervasive developmental disorders. *Journal of Autism and Developmental Disorders, 30*, 405–413.

Parmeggiani, A. (2014). Gastrointestinal disorders and autism. In V. B. Patel, V. R. Preedy, & C. R. Martin (Eds.), *Comprehensive guide to autism*. New York: Springer.

Parracho, H. M. R. T., Bingham, M. O., Gibson, G. R., & McCartney, A. L. (2005). Differences between the gut microflora of children with autistic spectrum disorders and that of healthy children. *Journal of Medical Microbiology, 54*(10), 987–991.

Pennesi, C. M., & Klein, L. C. (2012). Effectiveness of the gluten-free, casein-free diet for children diagnosed with autism spectrum disorder: Based on parental report. *Nutritional Neuroscience, 15*(2), 85–91.

Perrin, J. M., Coury, D. L., Hyman, S. L., Cole, L., Reynolds, A. M., & Clemons, T. (2012). Complementary and alternative medicine use in a large pediatric autism sample. *Pediatrics, 130*(Suppl. 2), S77–S82.

Peters, B., Williams, K. C., Gorrindo, P., Rosenberg, D., Lee, E. B., Levitt, P., et al. (2014). Rigid-compulsive behaviors are associated with mixed bowel symptoms in autism spectrum disorder. *Journal of Autism and Developmental Disorders, 44,* 1425–1432.

Sharp, W. G., Berry, R. C., McCracken, C., Nuhu, N. N., Marvel, E., Saulnier, C. A., et al. (2013). Feeding problems and nutrient intake in children with autism spectrum disorders: A meta-analysis and comprehensive review of the literature. *Journal of Autism and Developmental Disorders, 43,* 2159–2173.

Shelby, J. D., Shirkey, K. C., Sherman, A. L., Beck, J. E., Haman, K., Shears, A. R., et al. (2013). Functional abdominal pain in childhood and long-term vulnerability to anxiety disorders. *Pediatrics, 132,* 475–482.

Silva, L. M. T., & Schalock, M. (2012). Autism Parenting Stress Index: Initial Psychometric Evidence. *Journal of Autism and Developmental Disorders, 42,* 566–574.

Smith, R. A., Farnworth, H., Wright, B., & Allgar, V. (2009). Are there more bowel symptoms in children with autism compared to normal children and children with other developmental and neurological disorders? A case control study. *Autism, 13*(4), 343–355.

Stigler, K. A., Sweeten, T. L., Posey, D. J., & McDougle, C. J. (2009). Autism and immune factors: A comprehensive review. *Research in Autism Spectrum Disorders, 3,* 840–860.

Taylor, B., Miller, E., Lingam, R., Andrews, N., Simmons, A., & Stowe, J. (2002). Measles, mumps, and rubella vaccination and bowel problems or developmental regression in children with autism: Population study. *British Medical Journal, 324,* 393–396.

Turk, J., Bax, M., Williams, C., Amin, P., Eriksson, M., & Gillberg, C. (2009). Autism spectrum disorder in children with and without epilepsy: Impact on social functioning and communication. *Acta Pœdiatrica, 98,* 675–681.

Valicenti-McDermott, M. D., McVicar, K., Rapin, I., Wershil, B. K., Cohen, H., & Shinnar, S. (2006). Frequency of gastrointestinal symptoms in children with autistic spectrum disorders and association with family history of autoimmune disease. *Developmental and Behavioral Pediatrics, 27*(2), s128–s136.

Valicenti-McDermott, M. D., McVicar, K., Cohen, H. J., Wershil, B. K., & Shinnar, S. (2008). Gastrointestinal symptoms in children with an autism spectrum disorder and language regression. *Pediatric Neurology, 39*(6), 392–398.

van der Veek, S. M. C., Derkx, B. H. F., Benninga, M. A., Boer, F., & de Hann, E. (2013). Cognitive Behavior Therapy for Pediatric Functional Abdominal Pain: A randomised controlled trial. *Pediatrics, 132*(5), e1163–e1172.

Wang, L. W., Tancredi, D. J., & Thomas, D. W. (2011). The prevalence of gastrointestinal problems in children across the United States with Autism Spectrum Disorders from families with multiple affected members. *Journal of Developmental and Behavioral Pediatrics, 32,* 351–360.

Whitehouse, A. J. O. (2013). Complementary and alternative medicine for autism spectrum disorders: Rationale, safety and efficiency. *Journal of Paediatics and Child Health, 49,* E438–E442.

Williams, K. C., Fuchs, G. J., Furuta, G. T., Marcon, M. A., & Coury, D. L. (2010). Clinical features associated with GI symptoms in Autism Spectrum Disorders (ASD). *Gastroenterology, 138*(5), (Suppl. 1), S–74.

Williams, K. C., Christofi, F. L., Clemmons, T., Rosenberg, D., & Fuchs, G. J. (2012a). Association of chronic gastrointestinal symptoms with sleep problems may help identify distinct subgroups of autism spectrum disorders. *Gastroenterology, 142*(5), (Suppl. 1), S–714.

Williams, K. C., Christofi, F. L., Clemmons, T., Rosenberg, D., & Fuchs, G. J. (2012b). Chronic GI symptoms in children with autism spectrum disorders are associated with clinical anxiety. *Gastroenterology, 142*(5), (Suppl. 1), S-79–S-80.

Chapter 12
Intellectual Disability

Nienke Peters-Scheffer, Robert Didden and Russell Lang

Introduction

Autism spectrum disorder (ASD) and intellectual disability (ID) often co-occur and severity of symptom presentation in ASD seems to strongly correlate with the degree of ID. Specifically, the lower a child's intelligence quotient (IQ), the more severe the ASD symptoms. For example, the severity of diagnostic characteristics (i.e., communication impairment, social interaction deficits, and excessive stereotypic behavior) and associated features such as challenging behavior and medical conditions are often more severe in children with profound ID and ASD than in children with ASD and mild ID throughout the individual's lifespan (Matson and Shoemaker 2009; O'Brien and Pearson 2004). In addition, these co-occurring disorders have a negative impact on treatment efficacy and overall development (Ben-Itzchak et al. 2008; Eikeseth 2009). Although ID is characterized as a global delay, ASD is characterized by both delay and deviance. Therefore, diagnosing ASD in children with ID may be challenging as symptoms of both disorders overlap because children with ID often display autistic behaviors such as absent or delayed speech, stereotyped movements, and poor social connectedness (Hartley and Sikora 2010).

N. Peters-Scheffer (✉) · R. Didden
Behavioural Science Institute, Radboud University,
P.O. Box 9104, Nijmegen, 6500 HE, The Netherlands
e-mail: n.peters@pwo.ru.nl

N. Peters-Scheffer
Driestroom Elst, Nijmegen, The Netherlands

R. Lang
College of Education, Texas State University, San Marcos, TX, USA

Johnny L. Matson (ed.), *Comorbid Conditions Among Children with Autism Spectrum Disorders,* Autism and Child Psychopathology Series,
DOI 10.1007/978-3-319-19183-6_12

In this chapter, we discuss the prevalence, core symptoms, and prognosis of children with comorbid ASD and ID. Furthermore, we describe challenging behavior, and psychiatric and comorbid conditions in children with ASD and ID. Finally, we discuss the treatment, the diagnosis, and the parenting of individuals with comorbid ASD and ID.

Prevalence

Reported prevalence rates of ASD vary, but are estimated at 62 per 10,000 (Elsabbagh et al. 2012). Prevalence studies defining the size of the population of individuals with comorbid ASD and ID are limited and their results are even more variable across reports. Results of several studies suggest that a substantial number of individuals with ASD evince ID. In approximately 50–70 % of the individuals with ASD, an ID is present (Matson and Shoemaker 2009). Between 28 and 40 % of the individuals with ID have an ASD (Bryson et al. 2008; LaMalfa et al. 2004; Morgan et al. 2002). The severity of ID is correlated with the rate of ASD (LaMalfa et al. 2004; Morgan et al. 2002). Prevalence of ASD among individuals with severe or profound ID has been found to be higher than the prevalence reported in individuals with mild and moderate ID. For example, LaMalfa et al. (2004) report that the prevalence of ASD in individuals with mild, moderate, severe, and profound ID is 8.3, 24.1, 37.1, and 59.6 %, respectively. This relationship seems to indicate the more severe the ID, the higher the prevalence of ASD.

Associated medical conditions, particularly neurological or chromosomal disorders, are estimated to be present in approximately 10–25 % of all individuals with ASD and this estimated percentage may be even higher in individuals with ASD and ID (Gillberg and Billdstedt 2000; O'Brien and Pearson 2004). Tuberous sclerosis, Cornelia de Lange syndrome, and Fragile X syndrome are some of the examples of genetic syndromes that are high-risk factors for ASD (e.g., Bailey et al. 2000; Moss et al. 2008; Smalley 1998).

Core Symptoms of Comorbid ASD and ID

ASD is characterized by impairments in the domains of communication, social interaction, and repetitive and stereotyped behaviors, while ID is characterized by a significant impairment in cognitive (i.e., an IQ below 70) and adaptive functioning. These impairments emerge early and persist in development even though their precise manifestation varies across individuals and changes over the course of development (American Psychiatric Association 2013). Matson et al. (2008) investigated whether the level of IQ had an effect on the expression of ASD symptoms (i.e., communication, social interaction, and stereotypic behavior) in individuals with ID by comparing a group with comorbid ID and ASD to group with ID only. As expected, individuals with autism and ID displayed a higher number of symptoms than those with pervasive developmental disorder-not otherwise specified (PDD-NOS) and ID on all three domains, while individuals with ID only evinced far fewer symptoms than both groups. They found that a lower IQ was related to larger deficits in communication and social interaction and a greater presentation of stereotypic behavior and further noticed that symptom severity was affected very little by IQ in individuals with autistic disorder, moderately influenced ASD symptom severity in individuals with PDD-NOS, and that ASD symptom severity was affected most severe by IQ in individuals with ID only.

Communication and Social Skills

In both children with ASD and children with ID, verbal and nonverbal communications are impaired to some degree, and development of speech and language is highly correlated with IQ. Some children never acquire functional speech (Lord and Paul 1997). Given the strong correlation between IQ and verbal ability, most nonverbal children with ASD are also diagnosed with ID. Comorbidity of ASD and ID further increases the complexity and severity of communication deficits because communication development is not only delayed due to the ID but may also be atypical as a result of ASD (Noens and Van Berckelaer-Onnes 2004).

In addition, children with ID, as well as those with ASD, have significant deficits in social skills, (i.e., skills used to facilitate interaction with others; Smith and Matson 2010; Matson et al. 2009). Children with comorbid ASD and ID present with greater impairments in social skills than those with ASD or ID only (Matson et al. 2003; Wilkins and Matson 2009). Severity of ID is associated with degree of social impairment, with children with severe and profound ID displaying the greatest level of social impairment (Sevin et al. 1995).

Repetitive and Stereotypic Behavior

Children with ASD also have a restricted repertoire of activities and interests and may evince stereotypic behaviors (American Psychiatric Association 2013). Stereotypic behaviors are repetitive actions or movements with the whole body, parts of the body or objects that the individual engages in repeatedly over short periods of time. Stereotypic behaviors are associated with ASD as well as ID and research suggests distinct symptom profiles based on IQ. Children with an IQ below 70 display more stereotyped motor behavior (e.g., hand flapping) while children with an IQ above 70 may display more complex repetitive behaviors such as circumscribed interests or rituals (O'Brien and Pearson 2004).

Adaptive Behavior

Adaptive behaviors include the skills required to support personal and social self-sufficiency that range from basic self-help skills (e.g., dressing and preparing meals) to competitive employment and self-advocacy (Palmen et al. 2012). Adaptive behaviors are a key determinant of overall functioning and adjustment (Matson et al. 2009a) and may serve as an important indicator for the level of education that can be attained in normal development and ID (De Bildt et al. 2005).

A delay in adaptive functioning is a defining aspect of ID and known to be related to IQ in individuals with ID, especially in the lower ranges of ID. Children with ASD also have an overall lower level of adaptive functioning with the social aspect of adaptive behavior being most affected (e.g., De Bildt et al. 2005). As ASD symptoms increase, the level of adaptive behavior decreases with adaptive skills related to social interaction being most impaired (Carpentieri and Morgan 1996; Matson et al. 2009a, b; Smith and Matson 2010). In general, children with comorbid ASD and ID display less adaptive behavior across all domains (i.e., communication, daily living skills, and socialization) than children with only ID or only ASD.

Deficits in adaptive behavior are a major barrier to independent living (Soenen et al. 2009) and without intervention, these difficulties tend to persist throughout the individual's life (Chadwick et al. 2005; De Bildt et al. 2005). Given the lower levels of adaptive behavior seen in children with ASD and ID treatment needs to focus on improving the adaptive skills using evidence-based methods appropriate for children with comorbid ASD and ID. Reviews by Matson et al. (2012) and Palmen et al. (2012) conclude that applied behavior analysis-based (ABA) interventions have the strongest supporting evidence base supporting for teaching adaptive living skills in individuals with ASD and ID.

Challenging Behavior and Behavioral Problems

Challenging behaviors are defined by Emerson (1995) as behaviors that are culturally abnormal and of such intensity, frequency, or duration that the physical safety of the individual or others is at risk, or behaviors which are likely to limit or block an individual's access to normal community environments.

Challenging behaviors, such as aggression, property destruction, tantrums, and self-injurious behaviors are frequently observed in children with ID. In addition, the presence of ASD is associated with an increased risk of developing challenging behavior and children with comorbid ASD and ID display significantly more challenging behaviors than children with ID alone (Horowitz et al. 2013; Lang et al. 2013; Matson and Rivet 2008). For example, McCarthy and colleagues (2010) found that challenging behavior is four times more likely in individuals with comorbid ASD and ID as compared to individuals with ID only in a study involving a total of 686 adults.

Although results across studies are inconsistent, a growing corpus of studies suggest that—next to cognitive functioning and autism severity—adaptive functioning, age (more challenging behavior is seen among adolescents and young adults as compared with older adults), and male gender are the biggest risk factors for the presence of challenging behavior in individuals with ID and/or ASD (e.g., Holden and Gitlesen 2006; Lang et al. 2013; Matson and Nebel-Schwalm 2007; Matson and Rivet 2008).

Challenging behavior often persists over time. In a 12-year follow-up study, Murphy and colleagues (2005) found that persons with the highest ratings of challenging behavior still had the highest ratings later in life. This is worrisome as challenging behavior puts the individual at risk for abuse, poor social adjustment, exclusion from social situations, inappropriate treatment (e.g., overuse off label medication, restraint, seclusion, and aversive positive punishment), referral to facilities, and results in more caregiver stress than the core symptoms of ASD and ID (Emerson et al. 2001; Matson and Horovitz 2010; Murphy et al. 2005).

Psychiatric and Comorbid Conditions

The presence and severity of ASD and ID are associated with an increased risk of psychiatric conditions in children and adolescents (Lovullo and Matson 2009). For instance, Totsika et al. (2011) found that the related behavioral and emotional problems were more frequent among children with comorbid ASD and ID, followed by children with ASD and children with ID only as compared with their typically developing peers.

Adults with comorbid ASD and ID display fewer psychiatric symptoms than children with comorbid ASD and ID (Bhaumik et al. 2008; Holden and Gitlesen 2006; Totsika et al. 2010). Studies investigating adults with comorbid ASD and ID suggest that the presence of ASD is not a risk factor for psychiatric disorders. For example, Tsakanikos et al. (2006) compared psychiatric comorbidity in 147 adults with comorbid ASD and ID to 605 adults with ID but without ASD and found no differences in psychopathology as measured by psychiatric diagnosis and by the Psychiatric Assessment Schedules for Adults with Developmental Disabilities (PAS-ADD) checklist (Moss et al. 1996). However, they found that nearly 70 % of the individuals with comorbid ASD and ID were taking psychotropic medication and it might be that any psychopathology was well-controlled. Results of Tsakanikos et al. (2006) are in line with those of Totsika et al. (2010) who found no differences between adults of 50 years and older with comorbid ASD and ID and a group of adults with ID only in behavior problems, psychiatric disorder, and quality of life.

Conclusions on the relationship between psychiatric comorbidity in individuals with comorbid ASD and ID cannot yet be drawn in the light of diagnostic difficulties, methodological limitations of relevant studies, and possible overlap between autistic behaviors and those relating to other disorders.

Prognosis

The presence and severity of both ASD and ID negatively affect learning and development (O'Brien and Pearson 2004). However, outcomes do vary and, with appropriate intervention and educational services, some individuals demonstrate substantial improvement. Unfortunately, in the absence of research-based treatment, others experience deterioration in functioning. For most adults with ASD, IQ remains relatively stable and the three core autism symptoms tend to persist into adulthood (Seltzer et al. 2003; Shattuck et al. 2007).

Individuals with comorbid ASD and ID show greater impairments in communication, social skills, stereotyped behavior, and adaptive behavior as compared to individuals with ASD only or ID only. Consequently, the presence of comorbid ID is associated with poorer outcomes and chronicity of core ASD symptoms and challenging behaviors. For example, Eaves and Ho (2008) found that worse outcomes related to work, friendships, and independence were correlated with lower IQ and more severe autism while better outcomes were correlated with higher IQ. Furthermore, behavioral problems are related to poorer outcome and may diminish the likelihood of being placed in least restrictive environments. Next to factors such as autism severity and cognitive functioning, the prognosis is further influenced by physical disability, self-perception, absence or presence of communicative speech before the age of 6 and environmental factors such as parental and family coping, service engagement, and societal acceptances (see for a review O'Brien 2001).

Diagnosis in Individuals with Comorbid ASD en ID

Diagnosis of ASD and ID within the same individual is complicated by a number of factors. First, the range and variety of behavioral and cognitive characteristics associated with ASD and ID make diagnostic assessments difficult to create and, after being created, difficult to implement. In addition, behaviors used to distinguish between these two diagnoses vary in terms of frequency, intensity, and topography both between individuals and within the same individual over time (Howlin 2000; Lang et al. 2013). Second, a biological marker for ASD has not been identified and may not exist and, therefore, diagnosis is based on the behavioral phenotype (American Psychiatric Association 2013; Fombonne 2009). As many of the behaviors that typify ASD overlap with behaviors common in ID, diagnosing ASD in individuals with ID is difficult, especially when the level of ID is in the severe to profound range (Siklos and Kerns 2007). Finally, traditional instruments and methods for assessing psychiatric disorders often rely on self-report and interviews, and due to delays in expressive and comprehensive language levels it is difficult to use such measures in individuals with ID and, even higher functioning individuals with

ASD, may struggle to engage in the introspection required to accurately participate in such procedures (Lang et al. 2010)

Because many children with an ID will show the typical triad of autistic impairments, distinguishing between ASD-specific symptoms and ID is challenging. The absence of social and communication skills and stereotyped and repetitive behavior may be attributed to the overall cognitive impairment or to the ASD. As stated by Howlin (2000), the care and outcome of children with ID is dominated by the severity of ID, making the diagnosis of ASD to some extent a theoretical matter. Therefore, differential diagnosis is more important for children with severe to mild ID since ASD intervention should be even more individualized, specialized, and structured than the intervention in children with the same severity of ID but without ASD.

Given the general level of development, absence of skills in the areas of communication and social interaction are more indicative of ASD in children with ID than deviance in these skills. However, other factors, such as aversion to some common forms of sensory stimuli (e.g., specific textures and noises) or abuse may also contribute to explanations as to why children with ID show delays or absences communication and social interaction. In addition, the presence of behavioral problems (e.g., self-injurious behaviors and aggression), epilepsy, psychiatric disorders, and environmental factors may further complicate the diagnostic process. Furthermore, children with ID might not have yet reached the developmental level required to achieve a particular skill and the repetitive behaviors frequently seen in children with ID may function to preclude opportunities for skill development in certain areas. For example, a child who engages in stereotypy might not learn to play in a way that is recognizable to other children and play opportunities with other children may be limited as a result; ultimately, this lack of opportunity for social interaction during play may further exacerbate the social deficits inherent to both ID and ASD (e.g., Lang et al. 2014).

Hence, assessing children with comorbid ASD and ID is multifactorial and complex because of the overlap in symptoms. However, several (screening) instruments have been developed for assessing ASD in individuals with ID. Examples of screening instruments are the *Scale of Pervasive Developmental Disorder in Mentally Retarded Persons* (PDD-MRS; Kraijer and de Bildt 2005), the *Autism Behaviour Checklist* (Krug et al. 1980), the *Social Communication Questionnaire* (SCQ; Rutter et al. 2003), and the *Diagnostic Assessment for the Severely Handicapped* (DASH; Matson et al. 1996). Interview formats such as the *Autism Diagnostic Interview Revised* (ADI-R; Le Couteur et al. 2003) and the *Diagnostic Interview for Social and Communication Disorders* (DISCO; Wing et al. 2002) are recommended to gather information from parents, teachers, and/or caregivers in a standardized way. In addition, the *Childhood Autism Rating Scale* (Schopler et al. 2007) and the *Autism Diagnostic Observation Schedule* (Lord et al. 1999) are commonly used to assist professionals in reaching a diagnosis of ASD in individuals with ID.

In individuals with ASD, the level of ID can be assessed with careful selection of measures. For children, the Mullen Scale of Early Learning (Mullen 1995) can be used to asses early cognitive and motor development, and IQ may be measured with the Merrill-Palmer (Roid and Sampers 2004), the Kaufman Assessment Battery for Children (Kaufman and Kaufman 1983), the Griffiths Scales (Griffiths 1984), the Differential Ability Scales (Elliot 1990), and various versions of the Wechsler Scales, including the Wechsler Preschool and Primary Scale of Intelligence (WPPSI) Testing for preschool children (Wechsler 2002), and the Wechsler Intelligence Scale for Children (WISC-III; Wechsler 1991). The latter is used for children 6 years of age and older and is intended primarily for children with an IQ above 70. For older individuals with ASD, the Wide Range Achievement Test-Revised (WRAT-R; Jastak and Wilkinson 1984) and the Wechsler Adult Intelligence Scale (Wechsler 1997) have been frequently used (O'Brien and Pearson 2004).

Although indirect and standardized measures can yield valuable information about individuals with comorbid ASD and ID, definitive diagnosis should not be made based on these instruments alone. Assessing individuals with ASD and ID should include direct observation and caregiver report. For differential diagnosis, the diagnostic team needs to have knowledge of both atypical and normal developmental patterns to consider whether the observed behaviors are appropriated for the individual's chronological age, developmental age, and language age (Howlin 2000). Given the complex interaction between individual characteristics and symptoms inherent to both diagnoses, delays in diagnosing and consequently treatment of individuals with comorbid ASD plus ID are still common.

Treatment

Because of the often idiosyncratic profiles of children with comorbid ASD and ID, treatment is also often complex and specialized. Overall, the more severe the ID, the more resistant the child is to treatment (Ben-Itzchak and Zachor 2007; Wolery and Garfinkle 2002). Treating children with comorbid ASD and ID is further complicated by comorbid psychopathology, challenging behaviors, and social deficits.

Based on the deficits often seen in ASD and ID and based on the child's pattern of skills and difficulties treatment programs need to be individualized. However, according to Howlin (2000), successful comprehensive treatments involve: (1) a combination of behavioral, developmental, and educational approaches adapted to the individual's skills and deficits; (2) a focus on the development of social communication and play activities; (3) recognize the need for structured teaching programs and provide the individuals with a predictable and understandable environment; (4) acknowledge that obsessions and rituals are an underlying cause of many behavior problems, help the individual to reduce anxiety and might be used to motivate and reinforce desired behavior; (5) focus on skill enhancement as an effective way to reduce difficult or disruptive behavior; (6) use a family-centered rather than an exclusively client-centered approach; and (7) use procedures that can be implemented consistently without excessive sacrifice of resources related to family life (e.g., money and time). Nevertheless, meaningful clinically significant change can be achieved in many cases without all of these components present.

A large number of interventions have been developed for children with ASD and/or ID including: (a) biomedical (e.g., medication, supplements, and diets), (b) physiological (e.g., sensory integration therapy and auditory integration therapy), (c) relationship-based interventions, (d) skill-based interventions such as applied behavior analysis (ABA), and (e) combined programs incorporating a range of procedures such as Treatment and Education of Autistic and related Communication handicapped Children (TEACCH; Heflin and Simpson 1998; Odom et al. 2010). Although some treatments initially appeared promising, only a few have been subjected to outcome research and are empirically supported (Foxx 2008; Schechtman 2007). Interventions based on the principles and procedures of ABA, however, gathered substantial scientific support (e.g., Matson et al. 1996; Peters-Scheffer et al. 2011).

A basic assumption of ABA is that everything that people do can be considered behavior (including verbal and nonverbal communication) and that the consequences of behavior can either strengthen or weaken it (i.e., make specific behaviors more or less likely to occur again in the future when circumstances are similar). By systematically arranging the environment and programming reinforcing or non-reinforcing contingencies (e.g., extinction or punishment procedures) for specific behaviors, the probability of future behavior increases or decreases (Granpeesheh et al. 2009).

Several early intervention programs based on ABA have appeared and although slight differences between programs exist, all programs involve operant teaching procedures including error-correction, prompt fading, functional analysis, incidental teaching, modeling, prompting, reinforcement, shaping, stimulus and response generalization, and task analysis (see e.g., Duker et al. 2004). To address preacademic skills (e.g., attending, imitation, and matching), daily living skills, language, social skills, and behavioral problems (e.g., stereotypy and self-injury) in these programs, comprehensive curricula are used which are individualized to each child's strengths and deficits. Although great variability in children's gains within and between studies has been reported, early intervention programs based on ABA result in significant improvement in cognitive, adaptive, social and communication skills, and in reductions in challenging behavior (Eldevik et al. 2009; Makrygianni and Reed 2010; Reichow and Wolery 2009; Spreckley and Boyd 2009; Peters-Scheffer et al. 2011). Two examples of early intervention programs based on ABA are discrete trial teaching (DTT) and pivotal response treatment (PRT).

Most early intervention programs were initially primarily comprised of DTT. DTT is a structured teaching format for individualizing and simplifying instruction to enhance children's learning. Multiple discrete trials (i.e., small units of instruction) are presented across the session. A discrete trial consists of five components; (1) the discriminative stimulus (i.e., a brief, clear instruction or question), (2) a prompt (i.e., assistance to help the child in responding correctly to the cue), (3) a response of the child (i.e., the child gives a correct or incorrect answer to the cue), (4) a consequence (i.e., reinforcement after a correct response and a correction after an incorrect response), and (5) the intertrial interval (i.e., a brief pause before presenting the cue for the next trial). DTT is first implemented in a distraction free environment. In many programs, DTT is supplemented with less structured teaching formats in which skills are taught in the natural environment of the child using formats that more closely resemble the typical daily activities that a young child may encounter (Smith 2001). Usually, DTT is implemented intensively (20–40 h per week during 1–3 years), although less intensive DTT (5–10 h per week during 1–3 years) also has been proven to be effective (e.g., Peters-Scheffer et al. 2013).

PRT is a naturalistic behavioral approach originally based upon DTT. In contrast to DTT, PRT focuses on the pivotal areas motivation, social initiations, responding to multiple cues, and self-management. Pivotal areas are targeted behaviors that result in collateral improvements in a variety of symptoms of the disability and result in improvements in the overall quality of social–communicative interactions (Koegel and Koegel 2006; Koegel et al. 2001). PRT is implemented in the natural environment (e.g., home, school, and community) by the parents and teachers of the child (e.g., school and home) to foster generalization and maintenance of skills over situations, persons, and time. Therefore, specific PRT procedures such as embedded interests and shared control (i.e., child choice), clear opportunities for the child to respond by displaying the target behavior and contingent and natural reinforcement are taught to the parents and teachers using instruction, (video)modelling, role-play, and (video)feedback (Koegel and Koegel 2006).

A substantial amount of research has also been conducted on ABA treatment for older children, adolescents, and adults with ASD and/or ID. In general, the scope and the duration of these treatment programs are narrower and these programs often emphasize high-priority short-term goals which are addressed in a relative short period of time (i.e., 1 or 2 months). A wide variety of skills have been targeted during interventions based on ABA, including aggression, adaptive skills, self-stimulatory behavior, play, communication, and academics (see for reviews Granpeesheh et al. 2009; Matson et al. 2012). Programs are often implemented using a consultative model and used to solve behavioral problems or help the individual to acquire a particular and pivotal skill (e.g., communication and toilet training). A large and growing body of peer-reviewed research has demonstrated that ABA can achieve treatment goals related to these areas for individuals with ASD and/or ID (Matson et al. 1996).

Although many treatments lack scientific support or even have been proven to be ineffective, surprisingly many of them continue to be used by clinicians and parents. Green et al. (2006) found that parents use on an average of seven treatments and have used eight different treatments in the past. More treatments were used when the child had severe ASD, while fewer treatments were used when the child was described as having a less severe ASD (Asperger syndrome). Green and colleagues concluded that the type or severity of the child's disability appeared to influence the number and categories of treatments used.

Parenting

Parenting a child with comorbid ASD and ID is associated with more parental stress than parenting typically developing children or children with other development disabilities (Griffith et al. 2010; Osborne et al. 2008). As many children with comorbid ASD and ID require intensive care and treatment, parents often must contribute substantially to their children's treatment and are frequently and actively involved in their child's therapy. Also selecting, coordinating, and advocating treatment can be cumbersome (Johnson and Hastings 2002; Peters-Scheffer et al. 2011). Finally, families are often faced with financial hardships associated with having a child with comorbid ASD and ID due to therapy costs and lifestyle changes that may cause heightened stress levels (Sharpe and Baker 2007).

Because of the nature of ASD and ID, parenting a child with comorbid ASD and ID may present parents with unique challenges. Anxiety, sleeping and eating disturbances, temper tantrums, self-injury and aggressive behavior, social isolation, and difficulties in self-care are frequently seen in ASD and ID, causing considerable challenges to parents on a daily basis (e.g., Cotton and Richdale 2010; Matson and Shoemaker 2009; Rodrigue et al. 1991; Schreck et al. 2004; White et al. 2009). Many parents experience the period in which their child obtains the diagnosis as particularly stressful, especially when there is a lack of clarity about the diagnosis, the diagnosis is set comparatively late, and when there is a delay between the first concerns and the final diagnosis (Brogan and Knussen 2003; Howlin and Moore 1997; Moh and Magiati 2012). Concerns about the future of their child, his or her level of cognitive and communicative impairment, physical health and needs and abilities to get accepted in the community, to function independently, and to obtain help may even further elevate stress (Koegel et al. 1992; Konstantareas and Homatidis 1989; Ogston et al. 2011).

Several studies have linked specific variables to increased levels of parental stress (Ornstein Davis and Carter 2008). Most studies found that challenging behavior is a more reliable predictor of increased parental stress than the severity of the disability itself (e.g., Peters-Scheffer et al. 2012). However, results of studies on the relationship between maternal stress and other variables related to diagnosis are inconclusive. For example, Mori et al. (2009) found no relationship between parental stress and IQ, and results about the relationship between maternal stress and impaired adaptive behavior are mixed (Beck et al. 2004; Lecavalier et al. 2006). On the other hand, several studies report that higher parental stress is associated with more severe autism symptom scores (Hastings and Johnson 2001; Konstantareas and Homatidis 1989; Konstantareas and Papageorgiou 2006). Other child factors associated with increased parental stress include: (1) the severity of social deficits, such as a lack of social skills (Baker-Ericzen et al. 2005), limited responsiveness to social initiations, and poor social relatedness (Ornstein Davis and Carter 2008; Kasari and Sigman 1997), (2) temperament (i.e., high activity level, low flexibility, and low mood scores; Konstantareas and Papageorgiou 2006), and (3) repetitive and self-injurious behavior (Konstantareas and Homatidis 1989).

Parental stress also appears to be related to parent characteristics. Specifically, the parents age and coping styles (e.g., an emotional-oriented coping style is associated with higher parental stress; Dabrowska and Pisula 2010). Higher reported levels of social and professional support result in lower reported levels of parental stress (Bromley et al. 2004; Dabrowska and Pisula 2010; Hastings and Johnson 2001). In addition, the interrelationships between mothers, fathers, and other family members influence parental stress. For example, child behavioral problems and father's mental health (i.e., anxiety and depression) were associated with mother's stress (Hastings 2003).

Multiple studies show that parental stress and treatment outcome are interrelated (Birnbauer and Leach 1993; Eisenhower et al. 2005; Griffith et al. 2010; Osborne et al. 2008). Although treatments, such as early intensive behavioral treatment programs, may decrease parental stress in the long term (e.g., Birnbrauer and Leach 1993), higher parental stress is also associated with lower treatment outcome (Osborne et al. 2008). Because parental stress associated with caring for a child with ASD seems receptive to treatment (Bristol et al. 1993), it is important that parents reduce their stress levels before commencing treatment or at the beginning of the treatment because parents with high stress levels are less able to contribute to their child's treatment. As indicated by several studies, emotional and behavioral problems contribute significantly more to parental stress than ID or (severity of) ASD, and therefore need to be identified and addressed with priority in the treatment with ASD and ID.

Conclusion

ASD and ID often co-occur at high rates and the relationship between the two conditions is complex. Children with comorbid ASD and ID differ distinctly from children with only ASD or only ID and may have other needs. The study of ASD in children with ID is a relatively new phenomenon and much of the recent advances in ASD research have been with children without ID limiting the ability to generalize study findings to children with comorbid ASD and ID (Matson and Shoemaker 2009). Further research regarding intervention for this population, as well as research aiming to understand these co-occurring disorders is warranted to improve assessment, diagnosis, and treatment of children with comorbid ASD and ID.

References

American Psychiatric Association. (2013). *Diagnostic and statistical manual of mental disorders: Fifth edition*. Arlington: American Psychiatric Publishing.

Bailey, D., Hatton, D., Mesibov, G., Ament, N., & Skinner, M. (2000). Early development, temperament, and functional impairment in autism and fragile X syndrome. *Journal of Autism and Developmental Disorders, 30,* 49–59.

Baker-Ericzen, M. J., Brookman-Frazee, L., & Stahmer, A. (2005). Stress levels and adaptability in parents of toddlers with and without autism spectrum disorders. *Research and Practice for Persons with Severe Disabilities, 30,* 194–204.

Beck, A., Hastings, R. P., Daley, D., & Stevenson, J. (2004). Pro-social behavior and behavior problems independently predict maternal stress. *Journal of Intellectual and Developmental Disability, 29,* 339–349.

Ben-Itzchak, E., & Zachor, D. A. (2007). The effects of intellectual functioning and autism severity on outcome of early behavioral intervention for children with autism. *Research in Developmental Disabilities, 28,* 287–303.

Ben-Itzchak, E., Lahat, E., Burgin, R., & Zachor, D. A. (2008). Cognitive, behavior and intervention outcome in young children with autism. *Research in Developmental Disabilities, 29,* 447–458.

Bhaumik, S., Tyrer, F. C., McGrother, C., & Ganghadaran, K. (2008). Psychiatric service use and psychiatric disorders in adults with intellectual disability. *Journal of Intellectual Disability Research, 52,* 986–995.

Birnbauer, J. S., & Leach D. J. (1993). The murdoch early intervention program after 2 years. *Behaviour Change,* 10, 63–74.

Bristol, M. M., Gallagher, J. J., & Holt, K. D. (1993). Maternal depressive symptoms in autism: Response to psycho educational intervention. *Rehabilitation Psychology, 38,* 3–10.

Brogan, C. A., & Knussen, C. (2003). The disclosure of a diagnosis of an autistic spectrum disorder: Determinants of satisfaction in a sample of Scottish parents. *Autism, 7,* 31–46.

Bromley, J., Hare, D. J., Davison, K., & Emerson, E. (2004). Mothers supporting children with autistic spectrum disorders: Social support, mental health status and satisfaction with services. *Autism, 8,* 409–423.

Bryson, S. E., Bradley, E. A., Thompson, A., & Wainwright, A. (2008). Prevalence of autism among adolescents with intellectual disabilities. *Canadian Journal of Psychiatry, 53,* 449–459.

Carpentieri, S., & Morgan, S. B. (1996). Adaptive and intellectual functioning in autistic and non-autistic retarded children. *Journal of Autism and Developmental Disorders, 26,* 611–620.

Chadwick, O., Cuddy, M., Kusel, Y., & Taylor, E. (2005). Handicaps and the development of skills between childhood and early adolescence in young people with severe intellectual disabilities. *Journal of Intellectual Disability Research, 49,* 877–888.

Cotton, S. M., & Richdale, A. L. (2010). Sleep patterns and behaviour in typically developing children and children with autism, Down syndrome, Prader-Willi syndrome and intellectual disability. *Research in Autism Spectrum Disorders, 4,* 490–500.

Dabrowska, A., & Pisula, E. (2010). Parenting stress and coping styles in mother and fathers of pre-school children with autism and Down syndrome. *Journal of Intellectual Disability Research, 54,* 266–280.

De Bildt, A., Sytema, S., Kraijer, D., Sparrow, S., & Minderaa, R. (2005). Adaptive functioning and behaviour problems in relation to level of education in children and adolescents with intellectual disability. *Journal of Intellectual Disability Research, 49,* 672–681.

Duker, P., Didden, R., & Sigafoos, J. (2004). *One-to-one training: Instructional procedures for learners with developmental disabilities*. Austin: Pro-Ed.

Eaves, L. C., & Ho, H. H. (2008). Young adult outcome of autism spectrum disorders. *Journal of Autism and Developmental Disorders, 38,* 739–747.

Eikeseth, S. (2009). Outcome of comprehensive psycho-educational interventions for young children with autism. *Research in Developmental Disabilities, 30,* 158–178.

Eisenhower, A. S., Baker, B. L., & Blacher, J. (2005). Pre school children with intellectual disability: Syndrome specificity, behaviour problems, and maternal well-being. *Journal of Intellectual Disability Research, 9,* 657–671.

Eldevik, S., Hastings, R. P., Hughes, J. C., Jahr, E., Eikeseth, S., & Cross, S. (2009). Meta-analysis of early intensive behavioral intervention for children with autism. *Journal of Clinical Child and Adolescent Psychology, 38,* 439–450.

Elliott, C. D. (1990). *Differential abilities scales*. San Antonio: The Psychological Corporation.

Elsabbagh, M., Divan, G., Koh, Y., Kim, Y. S., Kauchali, S., Marcín, C., et al. (2012). Global prevalence of autism and other pervasive developmental disorders. *Autism Research, 5, 160–179.*

Emerson, E. (1995). *Challenging behaviour: Analysis and intervention in people with learning disabilities*. Cambridge: Cambridge University Press.

Emerson, E., Kiernan, C., Alborz, A., Reeves, D., Mason, H., Swarbrick, R., et al. (2001). The prevalence of challenging behaviors: A total population study. *Research in Developmental Disabilities, 22,* 77–93.

Fombonne, E. (2009). Epidemiology of pervasive developmental disorders. *Pediatric Research, 65,* 591–598.

Foxx, R. M. (2008). Applied behavior analysis treatment of autism: The state of art. *Child and Adolescent Psychiatric Clinics of North America, 17,* 821–834.

Gillberg, C., & Billstedt, E. (2000). Autism and Asperger syndrome: Coexistence with other clinical disorders. *Acta Psychiatrica Scandinavica, 102,* 321–330.

Granpeesheh, D., Tarbox, J., & Dixon, D. R. (2009). Applied behavior analytic interventions for children with autism: A description and review of treatment research. *Annals of Clinical Psychiatry, 21,* 162–173.

Green, V. A., Pituch, K. A., Itchon, J., Choi, A., O'Reilly, M., & Sigafoos, J. (2006). Internet survey of treatments used by parents of children with autism. *Research in Developmental Disabilities, 27,* 70–84.

Griffith, G. M., Hasting, R. P., Nash, S., & Hill, C. (2010). Using matched groups to explore child behavior problems and maternal well-being in children with Down syndrome and autism. *Journal of Autism and Developmental Disorders, 40,* 610–619.

Griffiths, R. (1984). *The abilities of young children: A comprehensive system of mental measurement for the first eight years of life*. Bucks: The Test Agency.

Hartley, S. L., & Sikora, D. M. (2010). Detecting autism spectrum disorder in children with intellectual disability: Which DSM-IV-TR criteria are most useful? *Focus on Autism and Other Developmental Disabilities, 25,* 85–97.

Hastings, R. P. (2003). Child behaviour problems and partner mental health as correlates of stress in mothers and fathers of children with autism. *Journal of Intellectual Disability Research, 47,* 231–237.

Hastings, R. P., & Johnson, E. (2001). Stress in UK families conducting intensive home-based behavioral interventions for their young child with autism. *Journal of Autism and Developmental Disabilities, 31,* 327–336.

Heflin, L. J., & Simpson, R. L. (1998). Interventions for children and youth with autism. *Focus on Autism and Other Developmental Disabilities, 13,* 194–211.

Holden, B., & Gitlesen, J. P. (2006). A total population study of challenging behaviour in the county of Hedmark, Norway: Prevalence, and risk markers. *Research in Developmental Disabilities, 27,* 456–465.

Horowitz, M., Matson, J. L., Hattier, M. A., Tureck, K., & Bamburg, J. W. (2013). Challenging behaviour in adults with intellectual disability: The effect of race of autism spectrum disorders. *Journal of Mental Health Research in Intellectual Disabilities, 6,* 1–13.

Howlin, P. (2000). Autism and intellectual disability: Diagnostic and treatment issues. *Journal of the Royal Society of Medicine, 93,* 351–355.

Howlin, P., & Moore, A. (1997). Diagnosis in autism: A survey of over 1200 patients in the UK. *Autism: The International Journal of Research and Practice, 1,* 135–162.

Jastak, S., & Wilkinson, G. (1984). *The wide range achievement test: Manual of instructions*. Wilmington: Jastak Associates.

Johnson, E., & Hastings, R. P. (2002). Facilitating factors and barriers to the implementation of intensive home-based behavioural intervention for young children with autism. *Child: Care, Health and Development, 28,* 123–129.

Kasari, C., & Sigman, M. (1997). Linking parental perceptions to interactions in young children with autism. *Journal of Autism and Developmental Disorders, 27,* 39–57.

Kaufman, A. S., & Kaufman, N. L. (1983). *Kaufman Assessment Battery for Children*. Circle Pines: American Guidance Service.

Koegel, R. L., & Koegel, L. K. (2006). *Pivotal response treatments for autism: Communication, social, & academic development*. Baltimore: Paul H. Brookes.

Koegel, R. L., Schreibman, L., Loos, L. M., Dirlich-Wilhelm, H., Dunlap, G., Robbins, F. R., et al. (1992). Consistent stress profiles in mothers of children with autism. *Journal of Autism and Developmental Disorders, 22,* 205–216.

Koegel, R. L., Koegel, L. K., & McNerney, E. K. (2001). Pivotal areas in intervention for autism. *Journal of Clinical Child & Adolescent Psychology, 30,* 19–32.

Konstantareas, M. M., & Homatidis, S. (1989). Assessing child symptom severity and stress in parents of autistic children. *Journal of Child Psychology and Psychiatry, 30,* 459–470.

Konstantareas, M. M., & Papageorgiou, V. (2006). Effects of temperament, symptom severity and level of functioning on maternal stress in Greek children and youth with ASD. *Autism, 10,* 593–607.

Kraijer, D., & de Bildt, A. (2005). The PDD-MRS: An instrument for identification of autism spectrum disorders in persons with mental retardation. *Journal of Autism and Developmental Disorders, 35,* 499–513.

Krug, D. A., Arick, J., & Almond, P. (1980). Behavior checklist for identifying severely handicapped individuals with high levels of autistic behavior. *Journal of Child Psychology and Psychiatry, 21,* 221–229.

LaMalfa, G., Lassi, S., Bertelli, M., Salvini, R., & Placidi, G. F. (2004). Autism and intellectual disability: A study of prevalence on a sample of the Italian population. *Journal of Intellectual Disability Research, 48,* 262–267.

Lang, R., Regester, A., Lauderdale, S., Ashbaugh, K., & Haring, A. (2010). Treatment of anxiety in autism spectrum disorders using cognitive behavior therapy: A systematic review. *Developmental Neurorehabilitation, 13,* 53–63.

Lang, R., Sigafoos, J., van der Meer, L., O'Reilly, M. F., Lancioni, G. E., & Didden, R. (2013). Early signs and early behavioral intervention of challenging behavior. In R. Hastings & J. Rojahn (Eds.), *Challenging behavior. International review of research in developmental disability, 44* (pp. 1–35). London: Elsevier (Academic Press).

Lang, R., Machalicek, W., Rispoli, M., O'Reilly, M., Sigafoos, J., Lancioni, G., et al. (2014). Play skills taught via behavioral intervention generalize, maintain, and persist in the absence of socially-mediated reinforcement in children with autism. *Research in Autism Spectrum Disorders, 8,* 860–872.

Le Couteur, A., Lord, C., & Rutter, M. (2003). *The autism diagnostic interview-revised (ADI-R)*. Los Angeles: Western Psychological Services.

Lecavalier, L., Leone, S., & Wiltz, J. (2006). The impact on behaviour problems on caregiver stress in young people with autism spectrum disorder. *Journal of Intellectual Disability Research, 50,* 172–183.

Lord, C., & Paul, R. (1997). Language and communication in autism. In D. J. Cohen & F. R. Volkmar (Eds.), *Handbook of autism and pervasive developmental disorders* (pp. 195–225). New York: Wiley.

Lord, C., Rutter, M., Dilavore, P. C., & Risi, S. (1999). *Autism Diagnostic Observation Schedule (ADOS): Manual*. Los Angeles: Western Psychological Services.

Lovullo, S. V., & Matson, J. L. (2009). Comorbid psychopathology in adults with autism spectrum disorders and intellectual disabilities. *Research in Developmental Disabilities, 30,* 1288–1296.

Makrygianni, M. K., & Reed, P. (2010). A meta-analytic review of the effectiveness of behavioural early intervention programs for children with autistic spectrum disorders. *Research in Autism Spectrum Disorders, 4,* 577–593.

Matson, J. L., & Horovitz, M. (2010). Stability of autism spectrum disorders symptoms over time. *Journal of Developmental and Physical Disabilities, 22,* 331–342.

Matson, J. L., & Nebel-Schwalm, M. S. (2007). Comorbid psychopathology with autism spectrum disorder in children: An overview. *Research in Developmental Disabilities, 28,* 341–353.

Matson, J. L., & Rivet, T. T. (2008). Characteristics of challenging behaviours in adults with autistic disorder, PDD-NOS, and intellectual disability. *Journal of Intellectual and Developmental Disability, 33,* 323–329.

Matson, J. L., & Shoemaker, M. (2009). Intellectual disability and its relationship to autism spectrum disorders. *Research in Developmental Disabilities, 30,* 1107–1114.

Matson, J. L., Benavidez, D. A., Compton, L. S., Paclawskyj, T., & Baglio, C. (1996). Behavioral treatment of autistic persons: A review of research from 1980 to the present. *Research in Developmental Disabilities, 17,* 433–465.

Matson, J. L., Baglio, C. S., Smirolodo, B. B., Hamilton, M., & Packlowskj, T. (1996). Characteristics of autism as assessed by the diagnostic assessment for the severely handicapped-II (DASH-II). *Research in Developmental Disabilities, 17,* 135–143.

Matson, J. L., Mayville, E. A., Lott, J. D., Bielecki, J., & Logan, R. (2003). A comparison of social and adaptive functioning in persons with psychosis, autism and severe or profound mental retardation. *Journal of Developmental and Psychical Disabilities, 15,* 57–65.

Matson, J. L., Demsey, T., LoVullo, S. V., & Wilkins, J. (2008). The effects of intellectual functioning on the range of core symptoms of autism spectrum disorders. *Research in Developmental Disabilities, 29,* 341–350.

Matson, J. L., Demsey, T., & LoVullo, S. V. (2009). Characteristics of social skills for adults with intellectual disability, autism, and PDD-NOS. *Research in Autism Spectrum Disorders, 3,* 207–213.

Matson, J. L., Rivet, T. T., Fodstad, J. C., Dempsey, T., & Boisjoli, J. A. (2009a). Examination of adaptive behavior differences in adults with autism spectrum disorders and intellectual disability. *Research in Developmental Disabilities, 30,* 1317–1325.

Matson, J. L., Dempsey, T., & Fodstad, J. C. (2009b). The effect of autism spectrum disorders on adaptive independent living skills in adults with severe intellectual disability. *Research in Developmental Disabilities, 30,* 1203–1211.

Matson, J. L., Hattier, M. A., & Belva, B. (2012). Treating adaptive living skills of persons with autism using applied behavior analysis: A review. *Research in Autism Spectrum Disorders, 6,* 271–276.

McCarthy, J., Hemmings, C., Kravariti, E., Dworzynski, K., Holt, G., Bouras, N., et al. (2010). Challenging behaviour and co-morbid psychopathology in adults with intellectual disability and autism spectrum disorders. *Research in Developmental Disabilities, 31,* 362–366.

Moh, T. A., & Magiati, I. (2012). Factors associated with parental stresss and satisfaction during the process of diagnosis of children with autism spectrum disorders. *Research in Autism Spectrum Disorders, 6,* 293–303.

Morgan, C. N., Roy, M., Nasr, A., Chance, P., Hand, M., Mlele, T., et al. (2002). A community survey establishing the prevalence rate of autistic disorder in adults with learning disability. *Psychiatric Bulletin, 26,* 127–130.

Mori, K., Ujiie, T., Smith, A., & Howlin, P. (2009). Parental stress associated with caring with Asperger's syndrome or autism. *Paediatrics International, 51,* 364–370.

Moss, S. C., Prosser, H., Costello, H., Simpson, N., & Patel, P. (1996) *PAS-ADD Checklist.* Manchester: Hester Adrian Research Centre, University of Manchester.

Moss, J., Oliver, C., Wilkie, L., Berg, K., Kaur, G., & Cornish, K. (2008). Prevalence of autism spectrum phenomenology in Cornelia de Lange and Cri du Chat syndromes. *American Journal of Mental Retardation, 113,* 278–291.

Mullen, E. M. (1995). *Mullen's scale of early learning.* Circle Pines: American Guidance Service.

Murphy, G. H., Beadle-Brown, J., Wing, L., Gould, J., Shah, A., & Holmes, N. (2005). Chronocity of challenging behaviours in people with severe intellectual disabilities and/or autism: A total population sample. *Journal of Autism and Developmental Disorders, 35,* 405–418.

Noens, I., & Van Berckelaer-Onnes, I. (2004). Making sense in a fragmentary wordl. *Autism: The International Journal of Research and Practice, 8,* 197–218.

O'Brien, G. (2001). Adult outcome of childhood disability. *Developmental Medicine and Child Neurology, 43,* 634–638.

O'Brien, G., & Pearson, J. (2004). Autism and learning disability. *Autism, 8,* 125–140.

Odom, S. L., Boyd, B. A., Hall, L. J., & Hume, K. (2010). Evaluation of comprehensive treatment models for individuals with autism spectrum disorders. *Journal of Autism and Developmental Disorders, 40,* 425–436.

Ogston, P. L., Mckintosh, V. H., & Myers, B. (2011). Hope and worry in mothers of children with an autism spectrum disorders or Down syndrome. *Research in Autism Spectrum Disorders, 5,* 1378–1384.

Ornstein Davis, N., & Carter, A. S. (2008). Parenting stress in mothers and fathers of toddlers with autism spectrum disorders: Associations with child characteristics. *Journal of Autism and Developmental Disorders, 38,* 1278–1291.

Osborne, L. A., McHugh, L., Saunders, J., & Reed, P. (2008). Parenting stress reduces the effectiveness of early teaching interventions for autistic spectrum disorders. *Journal of Autism and Developmental Disorders, 38,* 1092–1103.

Palmen, A., Didden, R., & Lang, R. (2012). A systematic review of behavioral intervention research on adaptive skill building in high-functioning young adults with autism spectrum disorder. *Research in Autism Spectrum Disorders, 6,* 602–617.

Peters-Scheffer, N., Didden, R., Korzilius, H., & Sturmey, P. (2011). A meta-analytic study on the effectiveness of comprehensive ABA-based early intervention programs for children with autism spectrum disorders. *Research in Autism Spectrum Disorders, 5,* 60–69.

Peters-Scheffer, N. C., Didden, R., & Korzilius, H. (2012). Characteristics of children with autism spectrum disorders and intellectual disability predicting maternal stress. *Research in Autism Spectrum Disorders, 6,* 696–706.

Peters-Scheffer, N. C., Didden, R., Mulders, M., & Korzilius, H. P. L. M. (2013). Effectiveness of low intensity behavioral treatment for children with autism spectrum disorder and intellectual disability. *Research in Autism Spectrum Disorders, 7,* 1012–1025.

Reichow, B., & Wolery, M. (2009). Comprehensive synthesis of early intensive behavioral interventions for young children with autism based on the UCLA Young Autism Project model. *Journal of Autism and Developmental Disorders, 39,* 23–41.

Rodrigue, J. R., Morgan, S. B., & Geffken, G. R. (1991). A comparative evaluation of adaptive behavior in children and adolescents with autism, Down syndrome and normal development. *Journal of Autism and Developmental Disorders, 21,* 187–196.

Roid, G. H., & Sampers, J. L. (2004). *Merrill-Palmer-revised scales of development.* Wood Dale: Stoelting Co.

Rutter, M., Bailey, A., & Lord, C. (2003). *Social communication questionnaire.* Los Angeles: Western Psychological Services.

Schechtman, M. A. (2007). Scientifically unsupported therapies in the treatment of young children with autism disorders. *Psychiatric Annals, 37,* 639–645.

Schopler, E., Reichler, R. J., & Rochen Renner, B. (2007). *The childhood autism rating scale.* Los Angeles: Western Psychology Services.

Schreck, K. A., Williams, K., & Smith, A. F. (2004). A comparison of eating behaviors between children with and without autism. *Journal of Autism and Developmental Disorders, 34,* 433–438.

Seltzer, M. M., Krauss, M. W., Shattuck, P. T., Orsmond, G., Swe, A., & Lord, C. (2003). The symptoms of autism spectrum disorders in adolescence and adulthood. *Journal of Autism and Developmental Disorders, 33,* 565–581.

Sevin, J. A., Matson, J. L., Coe, D., Love, S. R., Matese, M. J., & Benavidez, D. A. (1995). Empirically derived subtypes of pervasive developmental disorders: A cluster analytic study. *Journal of Autism and Developmental Disorders, 25,* 561–578.

Sharpe, D. L., & Baker, D. L. (2007). Financial issues associated with having a child with autism. *Journal of Family Economic Issues, 28,* 247–264.

Shattuck, P. T., Mailick Seltzer, M., Greenberg, J. S., Orsmond, G. I., Bolt, D., Kring, S., et al. (2007). Change in autism symptoms and maladaptive behaviors in adolescents and adults with an autism spectrum disorder. *Journal of Autism and Developmental Disorders, 37,* 1735–1747.

Siklos, S., & Kerns, K. A. (2007). Assessing the diagnostic experiences of a small sample of parents of children with autism spectrum disorders. *Research in Developmental Disabilities, 28,* 9–22.

Smalley, S. L. (1998). Autism and tuberous sclerosis. *Journal of Autism and Developmental Disorders, 28,* 407–414.

Smith, T. (2001). Discrete trial training in the treatment of autism. *Focus on Autism and Other Developmental Disabilities, 16,* 86–92.

Smith, K. R. M., & Matson, J. L. (2010). Social skills: Differences among adults with intellectual disabilities, co-morbid autism spectrum disorders and epilepsy. *Research in Developmental Disabilities, 31,* 1366–1372.

Soenen, S., Van Berckelaer-Onnes, I., & Scholte, E. (2009). Patterns of intellectual, adaptive and behavioral functioning in individuals with mild mental retardation. *Research in Development Disabilities, 30,* 433–444.

Spreckley, M., & Boyd, R. (2009). Efficacy of applied behavioral intervention in preschool children with autism for improving cognitive, language, and adaptive behavior: A systematic review and meta-analysis. *The Journal of Pediatrics, 154,* 338–344.

Totsika, V., Felce, D., Kerr, M., & Hastings, R. P. (2010). Behavior problems, psychiatric symptoms, and quality of life for older adults with intellectual disability with and without autism. *Journal of Autism Developmental Disorders, 40,* 1171–1178.

Totsika, V., Hastings, R. P., Emerson, E., Berridge, D. M., & Lancaster, G. A. (2011). Behavioural problems at 5 years of age and mental health in autism and intellectual disability. *Jouranal of abnormal child psychology 39,* 1137–1147.

Tsakanikos, E., Costello, H., Holt, G., Bouras, N., Sturmey, P., & Newton, T. (2006). Psychopathology in adults with autism and intellectual disability. *Journal of Autism and Developmental Disorders, 36,* 1123–1129.

Wechsler, D. (1991). *Wechsler Intelligence Scale for children (WISC-III).* San Antonio: Psychological Corp.

Wechsler, D. (1997). *Wechsler Adult Intelligence Scale-III (WAISIII).* San Antonio: Psychological Corp.

Wechsler, D. (2002). *WPPSI-III: Technical and Interpretive Manual.* San Antonio: The Psychological Corporation.

White, S. W., Oswald, D., Ollendick, T., & Scahill, L. (2009). Anxiety in children and adolescents with autism spectrum disorders. *Clinical Psychology Review, 29,* 216–229.

Wilkins, J., & Matson, J. L. (2009). A comparison of social skills profiles in intellectually disabled adults with and without ASD. *Behavior Modification, 33,* 143–155.

Wing, L., Leekam, S. R., Libby, S. J., Gould, J., & Larcombe, M. (2002). The diagnostic interview for social and communication disorders: Background, inter-rater reliability and clinical use. *Journal of Child Psychology and Psychiatry, 43,* 307–325.

Wolery, M., & Garfinkle, A. N. (2002). Measures in intervention research with young children who have autism. *Journal of Autism and Developmental Disorders, 32,* 463–478.

Part IV
Motor Movement and Activity

Chapter 13
Developmental Coordination Disorder

John Cairney and Sara King-Dowling

> (The)so-called clumsy child, the child who is awkward in his movements, poor at games, hopeless in dancing and gymnastics, a bad writer, and defective in concentration. He is inattentive, cannot sit still, leaves his shoelaces untied, does buttons wrongly, bumps into furniture, breaks glassware, slips off his chair, kicks his legs against the desk, and perhaps reads badly. Some, she says, tend to make large sweeping movements when writing, to write with the whole body, with the tongue protruding and travelling from one side of the mouth to the other. Some are worse when they are anxious and being watched. Reprimands merely make the child worse and lead to a variety of behaviour problems-truancy, insecurity, aggressiveness, bullying, encopresis, enuresis, and day-dreaming. He cannot help it.(British Medical Journal 1962, p. 1665).

The quote mentioned above comes from an editorial that appeared in the *British Medical Journal* in 1962. Earlier references to "clumsy" children can also be found in the published literature (Langford 1955; Orton 1937; Strauss and Lehtinen 1947). Collectively, these works reveal a long-standing interest in the field of developmental neurology and pediatrics regarding the so-called clumsy child—one who is motorically uncoordinated in the absence of known neurological or psycho-behavioral pathology.

Recognizing the frequent co-occurrence of other developmental problems in children with poor coordination, some approaches have considered motor coordination only as a domain within a broader developmental condition. Proposed diagnostic entities, such as "minimal brain dysfunction" and "deficits in attention, motor control and perception," for example, grouped motor functioning with cognitive, behavioral, or perceptual impairments. The current research and clinical consensus, while acknowledging the high levels of comorbidity with other disor-

J. Cairney (✉)
Department of Psychiatry and Behavioral Neuroscience Family Medicine, Kinesiology and CanChild, Center for Childhood Disability Research, McMaster University, Hamilton, ON, Canada
e-mail: cairnej@mcmaster.ca

S. King-Dowling
Department of Kinesiology, McMaster University, Hamilton, ON, Canada

Johnny L. Matson (ed.), *Comorbid Conditions Among Children with Autism Spectrum Disorders,* Autism and Child Psychopathology Series,
DOI 10.1007/978-3-319-19183-6_13

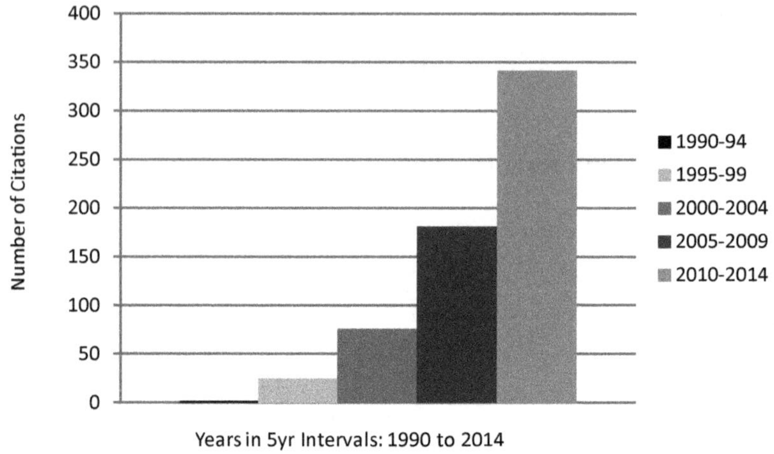

Fig. 13.1 Number of citations in PubMed using the search term "Developmental Coordination Disorder"

ders of childhood, views developmental coordination disorder (DCD) as a separate condition. Its essential feature is simply motor functioning that is poorer than expected. Other diagnostic criteria are concerned with the need to establish that the resulting impairment is significant, is developmental (rather than acquired, due to, for example, a traumatic brain injury), and is not the result of another condition.

Historically, many labels have been attached to this condition namely: clumsy child syndrome (Gubbay 1975), congenital maladroitness (Ford 1944), and developmental dyspraxia (Cermak 1985), to name only a few. However, "developmental coordination disorder" (DCD) has emerged as the preferred diagnostic label (Polatajko et al. 1995). Consensus guidelines on diagnosis and treatment use this name (Blank et al. 2012), as does the Diagnostic and Statistical Manual of Mental Disorders (American Psychiatric Association 2013), which lists the most widely-accepted set of diagnostic criteria. Over the past 20 years, there has been increasing attention to DCD in the published, scientific and medical literature. This is illustrated in Fig. 13.1, which shows the number of citation hits using the term "developmental coordination disorder" in PubMed has increased exponentially since the 1990s. DCD is fast becoming a neurodevelopmental disorder of interest in the field of developmental pediatrics, pediatric neurology and psychiatry, and rehabilitation.

DCD: Prevalence and Risk Factors

Although many sources, including the DSM-V, report a prevalence of 5 %, estimates in the scientific literature vary widely. Measurement of the prevalence of DCD is complicated by a number of factors. First, as noted above, the different labels and definitions used historically have hindered both the practice and synthesis of research. Second, even when studies agree on the definition of the condition, they often use different standardized tests, different thresholds, and different populations. Finally, studies have differed in their operationalization of diagnostic criteria. These factors have been the focus of several publications, two consensus statements (Polatajko et al. 1995; Sugden 2006) and, more recently, a set of clinical guidelines endorsed by the European Academy of Childhood Disability (Blank et al. 2012) that specifies clinical assessment tools and cut-points. In light of this, the best evidence we have on prevalence comes from the AVON longitudinal study of parents and children (Lingam et al. 2009). This study directly follows the criteria endorsed by these publications. Based on their work, it would appear that 4.7% of children have significantly impaired motor function, not attributable to existing neurological conditions (e.g., cerebral palsy and muscular dystrophy), but that only 1.7% of children meet criterion B, showing demonstrably problems in activities of daily living. However, it should be noted that these authors took a very conservative approach with regard to the estimation of ADLs. This highlights an on-going concern with diagnostic criteria, which require impairment in day-to-day life, but do not give a clear guidance on how this should be defined or measured. Although there is an agreement that practical impairment is important, there is far less consensus on how best to measure it in this context (Cairney 2010a).

As with other developmental disorders, the etiology of DCD is imperfectly understood. DCD is frequently associated with other developmental and behavioral conditions, including attention deficit hyperactivity disorder (ADHD) and learning difficulties, and it also shares risk factors with these and other developmental conditions. Research has consistently shown an increased risk among males, with boys outnumbering girls by a ratio of 2:1 or more in clinical settings (Zwicker et al. 2012). Low birth weight—which is itself etiologically complex—is also associated with greater risk (Holsti et al. 2002; Lingam et al. 2009). Recent work has also demonstrated that perinatal factors, including those related to oxygen perfusion at birth, are also relevant (Pearsall-Jones et al. 2009). Although the genetics and epigenetics of DCD have received less attention than those of other developmental conditions, recent work has demonstrated shared risk with both ADHD and autism spectrum disorder (ASD) (Lichtenstein et al. 2010).[1] Much more research is required to identify risk factors for this disorder.

Notwithstanding controversies in case definition and methodological challenges, even a conservative lower bound estimate of 1.7% suggests that DCD is a common disorder, affecting large number of children.

Objectives of this Chapter

In this chapter, our concern is less with prevalence and risk than with the clinical presentation of DCD and with its relation to other neurodevelopmental disorders of childhood. Specifically, our objectives are as follows: (1) to review recent

[1] There is a small but growing body of research in genetics, which supports the idea of shared or common pathways, particularly between DCD and ADHD (Martin et al. 2006) and DCD and ASD (Lichtenstein et al. 2010). Lichtenstein et al.'s twin study, for example, found a genetic correlation between ASD and DCD of 0.71.

diagnostic criteria for DCD found in the Diagnostic and Statistical Manual of the American Psychiatric Association (APA), 5th edition (American Psychiatric Association 2013); (2) to consider some of the challenges, in both research and clinical contexts, associated with assessing each criterion; (3) to review the associations between DCD and other developmental conditions, particularly ADHD; (4) to consider, in more detail, the association between DCD and ASD; (5) to review current treatment approaches to DCD and discuss some of the challenges in providing services to children with DCD and associated conditions.

Diagnostic Criteria for DCD

Although DCD first appeared in the DSM-IIIR back in late 1980s, as our understanding of DCD has evolved diagnostic criteria have changed commensurately. The most significant changes, however, are recent, reflected in the newest edition of the DSM (American Psychiatric Association 2013). These criteria are outlined in Table 13.1 below.

The column labeled "description" includes the exact text from the DSM-V (American Psychiatric Association 2013). The criterion column, however, includes labels we have created to describe each of the criterion based on general content. We will provide a detail review below.

Table 13.1 DSM-V diagnostic criteria for DCD

Criterion	Description
General features (Criterion A)	The acquisition and execution of coordinated motor skills is substantially below that expected given the individual's chronological age and opportunity for skill learning and use. Difficulties are manifested as clumsiness (e.g., dropping or bumping into objects) as well as slowness and inaccuracy of performance of motor skills (e.g., catching an object, using scissors or cutlery, handwriting, riding a bike, or participating in sports)
Impact of disorder (Criterion B)	The motor skills deficit in criterion A significantly and persistently interferes with activities of day-to-day living appropriate to chronological age (e.g., self-care and self-maintenance) and also impacts academic/school productivity, prevocational and vocational activities, leisure, and play
Developmental onset (Criterion C)	Onset of symptoms is in the early developmental period
Exclusion considerations (Criterion D)	The motor skills deficits are not better explained by intellectual disability (intellectual developmental disorder) or visual impairment and are not attributable to a neurological condition affecting movement (e.g., cerebral palsy, muscular dystrophy, degenerative disorder)

Criterion A: General Features

This criterion reflects some common, core features of the disorder at a clinical and functional level. Of principal import, the child's motor skill ability must be assessed to be substantially below that of his/her peers. Practically, this is accomplished using a standardized test of motor coordination, appropriate for a child's developmental age. At present, there is no single, universal, or gold standard measure for assessing motor coordination in children. The most commonly used instruments include the Movement Assessment Battery for Children (2nd Edition) or M-ABC-2 (Henderson et al. 2007); the Bruininks-Oseretsky Test of Motor Proficiency (2nd Edition) or BOT-2 (Bruininks and Bruininks 2005); and the McCarron Assessmentt of Neuromusculr Development or MAND (McCarron 1997). All of these tests are standardized, and age norms have been determined. Although there are significant differences in items across tests, they all include, broadly, tasks involving fine motor skills or manual dexterity, static and dynamic balance, and gross motor movement skills involving control, such as throwing and catching. The BOT-2 also includes items related to running speed and agility and strength (e.g., push-ups). Regardless of the test, scoring of individual items involves accuracy and/or timing, dependent upon the task and the age of the child. Notwithstanding similarities in domain content and administration, there are notable and significant differences between these measures. For example, the M-ABC-2 was developed specifically to identify children with motor coordination difficulties, indeed, the test developers are considered as leading experts in the field of DCD. As a result, the tasks included in this measure are generally more effective at discriminating between poor and normal motor ability children. The BOT-2 conversely, was designed to produce accurate assessments across the full range of motor proficiency. Perhaps in part for this reason, studies have reported moderate agreement between these measures (Crawford et al. 2001; Spironello et al. 2010; Tan et al. 2010).

The absence of a true gold standard and the modest agreement between instruments commonly used for assessment have led to considerable debate about how DCD should be diagnosed. Recent years have produced a general consensus, reflected in published guidelines. First, increasingly, the M-ABC-2 is the preferred criterion measure for assessing motor impairment in children where DCD is suspected as most experts agree there is reasonable evidence for the reliability and validity of this tool when used for this purpose (Blank et al. 2012). Second, administration of any test of motor ability should be accompanied by clinical evaluation to rule out other medical conditions; an assessment of impact on daily functioning and scholastic achievement; an assessment of cognitive function; and, when possible, administration of multiple or repeated tests of motor coordination to track change and reduce the possibility of false positives resulting from child behavorial issues or other concerns. In other words, wherever possible, additional data both on motor and on related criteria needs to be collected before diagnosis. This goes some way to overcoming inherent challenges in the absence of a gold standard. At the same time, however, the use of multiple tests, all with less than perfect accuracy, introduces other problems (Veldhuizen and Cairney 2015). In clinical settings, these can be overcome by sensible evaluation of the evidence by clinicians, but they remain a challenge in research, where a formal protocol must be followed.

It should be noted that the DSM is mute with regard to specific clinical cut-points on these tests to determine diagnosis. Adoption of the M-ABC-2 as the criterion standard brings with it the test's own criteria for case ascertainment as follows: children scoring below the 6th percentile are considered to have significant motor impairment; children scoring between the 6th and the 16th, are considered "borderline," and it is recommended that these children be monitored closely. These thresholds, however, are close to those recommended in published guidelines, which suggest that the bottom 5% of the population distribution should be considered to have poor motor functioning.

Finally, it should be noted that the presentation of motor coordination problems in children with DCD is heterogeneous. Attempts at motor skills classifications or subtyping have not as yet been successful (Visser 2003). Children with DCD present with a myriad of motoric challenges is related to performance of fine motor skills, gross motor skills, motor planning, and visual-spatial reasoning (Wilson et al. 2013). As with other developmental conditions, "DCD" is a useful label that subsumes a variety of motor impairments with numerous possible etiologies. Future work may come to consider motor functioning, like ASD, as a "spectrum" rather than a unitary disorder.

Impact of the Disorder

According to the DSM-V, the presence of poor motor coordination is necessary but insufficient for diagnosis. There must be evidence of impaired functioning. Children with poor motor coordination must experience "significant" and "persistent" difficulties in one or more of the following domains: age-appropriate day-to-day activities (e.g., tying shoelaces and buttoning shirts); school work and participation; work; and leisure and play (American Psychiatric Association 2013). As noted previously, however, the measurement of functioning presents a difficult problem, particularly in research contexts. In the research literature, studies have often elected to not measure functional impact, either explicitly or tacitly adopting a position that this particular criterion is of less import than motor skill ability itself. Others have, in the absence of explicit consensus criteria, defined their own. One example of this we have already mentioned (Lingam et al. 2009). In their study, they operationalized criterion B of the DSM-IV by using administrative school record data to identify children scoring below acceptable standards on standardized assessments of handwriting. Still other studies have used qualitative interviews, where any evidence of functional impact is accepted as sufficient for meeting this criterion (Missiuna et al. 2011).

Our own position on this has been described in previous publications (Veldhuizen and Cairney 2015). Briefly, we have argued that at least for research purposes, there is a compelling case to be made for not applying criterion B for case ascertainment.

First, in the absence of any agreed upon standard for assessment, any imposition of such criteria is arbitrary. Second, excluding "cases" by failing to find evidence of functional impact may homogenize the sample in a way that negatively impacts our ability to understand social, behavioral, or/and biological adaptations to the condition. For example, consider the frequently reported findings that, on average, children with poor or low-motor coordination are much less likely to participate in organized physical activities and sport, and also in open or free play activities relative to typically developing children (Rivilis et al. 2011). On the surface, this body of work supports criterion B, as poor motor coordination would seem to be negatively associated with leisure and play participation. However, not all children with DCD have been shown to withdraw or avoid physical activity altogether, including structured or organized participation in sports. An interesting question that flows from this observation is, why are some children participating and others are not? If we were to exclude children who were participating to fulfill the criteria, we run the risk of biasing the sample toward the extreme or more severe end of the functioning continuum. The consequence is that we may also miss the opportunity to understand differences in coping or resilience that may help to explain not only differential participation, but also provide important insight into behavioral and social strategies that could be employed to better manage the condition.

It is important to note that, although "impairment" in diagnostic criteria refers to immediate functional problems, DCD has much more far-reaching consequences. Balance or postural problems that do not produce obvious problems in day-to-day life, for example, may still negatively affect participation in active play, and this may contribute to poor cardiorespiratory fitness, obesity, and increased risk for heart disease in adulthood (Cairney et al. 2005; Cairney et al. 2007; Zhu et al. 2011). Children with DCD have also been shown to be at greater risk for social-emotional problems, such as depression and anxiety. This may represent shared risk due to, for example, genetic factors or developmental insults, but it has also been linked to greater exposure to negative interpersonal stressors and strains (Cairney et al. 2013; Cairney et al. 2010b). Once again, this highlights the somewhat thorny problem of including impact as part of the definition of the disorder. Although to incorporate these consequences into diagnostic criteria would perhaps be to conflate symptoms and outcomes, the absence of important, but more distal, consequences from the disorder definition should not lead to their neglect.

Developmental Onset

Another change from the DSM-IIIR and DSM-IV criteria is DCD is now required to emerge in early childhood. Although somewhat vague, this criterion underscores the fact that the disorder is developmental—that it is present early in life and is characterized by a trajectory of atypical motor development, such that the child will probably present significantly behind her motorically typically developing peers at all points in development from early childhood through adolescence into adulthood.

Two things flow from this: First, DCD is not "acquired" (Veldhuizen and Cairney 2015). Second, DCD is persistent. Although characterized this way frequently in the literature, there is evidence to show that some children who present with symptoms of DCD in early childhood, in fact show marked improvement in motor ability by mid-adolescence and early adulthood (Cantell et al. 2003). It is not yet clear that is this due to initial misclassification (i.e., these children never had DCD in the first place) or to problems related to measuring functioning at other time points, or whether it represents genuine improvement. At present, we lack measures capable of producing reliable and valid assessments of motor coordination in adults: Existing tools used in childhood have upper age bounds of 16 (M-ABC) and 21 BOT-2). This makes it extremely difficult to track motor coordination problems into later life. There is at least some qualitative data, however, which does suggests that symptoms of DCD persists well into adulthood (Missiuna et al. 2008).

Exclusion Considerations

Finally, DCD is a residual diagnosis, one that is made after alternate diagnoses have been ruled out. The most obvious ones are other neurological conditions which would impact gross and/or fine motor coordinations, such as cerebral palsy and muscular dystrophy. Clinically, however, one would have to also pay attention to the potential of neurological trauma (e.g., head injury) and other pathologies (e.g., tumor) that might be underlying causes. A full neurological examination is essential to clinical diagnosis of this condition. Another consideration is intellectual ability. If it is suspected that motor problems are due to the presence of intellectual disability, then a diagnosis of DCD should not be given. It has been recommended that a threshold IQ of 70 be used as a cut-off; children scoring below 70 would be excluded from the diagnosis (Blank et al. 2012; Smits-Engelsman and Hill 2012). This approach has often been followed in research studies.

Together, these four components define current diagnostic criteria for DCD. In the sections that follow, we consider DCD in relation to two other neurodevelopmental disorders namely: ADHD/ADD and ASD. It should also be noted that DCD has been found to be associated with specific learning disorders, to speech/language delay, and to social and emotional problems (Dewey et al. 2002; Visscher et al. 2007). We focus on these two particular disorders for three reasons. One, given that the current volume is concerned with ASD, and given that recent changes to the DSM-V allow for the first time children with ASD to be also diagnosed with DCD, it seems imperative that we consider this particular comorbidity. Second, ADHD/ADD is the most frequently co-occurring disorder with DCD; given the high prevalence of both conditions in the general population, it is difficult to describe one without reference to the other. Finally, a consideration of the overlap in symptoms among ASD, ADHD/ADD, and DCD also highlights a core problem: that of disentangling what we might call "pure" motor coordination problems, from, for example, problems of inattention that result in poor motor performance.

DCD and Attention Deficit Hyperactivity Disorder

ADHD is among the most prevalent psychiatric or developmental disorders of childhood. The disorder is characterized by inattention, impulsivity, and hyperactivity (Treuting and Hinshaw 2001). According to the DSM-V, these core symptoms must be persistent, developmentally inappropriate, and maladaptive (American Psychiatric Association 2013). Similar to DCD, the expression of ADHD is not uniform across cases. Unlike DCD, however, subtypes have been identified and accepted—either inattention or hyperactivity-impulsivity may predominate, and the DSM-IV lists three subtypes of the disorder namely: ADHD-Predominantly Inattentive type, ADHD-Predominantly Hyperactive-Impulsive type, and ADHD-Combined type, in which both symptoms are prominent (American Psychiatric Association 2000).

Rates of comorbidity between ADHD/ADD and DCD have been estimated to be as high as 50% (Kadesjo and Gillberg 1999). This figure, however, should be qualified, because estimates are significantly influenced by the method of clinical investigation. Simply put, studies reporting the highest rates of comorbidity tend to come from clinical samples of children already identified as having, or being at risk for, ADHD/ADD, who are subsequently tested for DCD (Piek et al. 1999; Pitcher et al. 2003). Studies that use a general population screening approach tend to show much lower levels of comorbidity (Missiuna et al. 2011). It is tempting therefore to conclude that clinical referral bias may be one reason why the rates of comorbidity are so high in some studies.

In addition to sampling, however, the challenges of disentangling these disorders arise from the nature of the symptoms present in both. A child who is impulsive will surely at times appear clumsy, especially while playing with other children. A child who has problems with inhibitory control will find it difficult to concentrate on a task like printing, especially when distractions are present. A child with DCD, conversely, may act out due to frustration at being unable to participate, or in an attempt to distract attention from problems doing motor-based activities, thereby appearing to be inattentive, disruptive, or hyperactive. It is only under carefully controlled conditions, and with experienced clinical (or highly-trained research) professionals, that one can start to disentangle problems of inattention or motivation from problems better characterized as motor coordination deficits. One wonders how much of the referral bias previously described is due to the fact that children with DCD may be more likely to be referred to clinics for what are perceived to be problems with inattention or impulsivity. Research on the miss-classification of ADHD/ADD in children with DCD, though certainly difficult to do, is required.

DCD and Autism Spectrum Disorders

In this section, we review clinical and research articles concerning the relationship between DCD and ASD. One of the most notable changes in diagnostic criteria from DSM-IV to DSM-V concern elimination of pervasive developmental delay

(PDD) as an exclusion criterion. In the DSM-IV, a child with PDD, which includes such disorders as autism disorder or Asperger's syndrome, would not have received a diagnosis of DCD. As we observed with ADHD/ADD, some level of motor dysfunction or atypical presentation of motor behavior is an inherent part of the diagnostic criteria for ASD. It stands to reason, therefore, given that atypical presentation of movement is bound up in the diagnostic criteria, one would expect a level of motoric dysfunction in this population that might render a separate diagnosis unnecessary. Yet, there is good reason for the removal of PDD as an exclusion for the diagnosis of DCD.

Diagnostic Criteria for ASD

ASD is characterized by impairments in social communication and interaction, as well as restricted, repetitive patters of behavior, interests or activities (American Psychiatric Association 2013). The motor components of the ASD diagnosis are focused on stereotypies, such as hand flapping or body rocking (Goldman et al. 2009). These repetitive motor movements are a criterion for ASD diagnosis. Gross and fine motor delays, as well as problems with the execution of motor skills and tasks—although recognized as a common feature—are not an essential or defining characteristic (Green et al. 2002). The removal of the PDD exclusion opens the door to more research into comorbidities and intervention strategies that target aspects of both disorders.

Motor Coordination Problems in ASD

Early research by Kanner (1943) and Asperger (1944) documented general sensory-motor deficits in children with what is now known as ASD. Since then, research has consistently found that the majority of children with ASD, present with fine motor and gross motor problems, irrespective of the motor assessment conducted (e.g., M-ABC-2, BOT-2, etc.) (Dewey et al. 2007; Ghaziuddin and Butler 1998; Green et al. 2002, 2009; Miyahara 1997). These findings tend to hold true across the entire autism spectrum and across a wide range of child ages, and are independent of gender (Berkeley and Zittel 2010; Fournier et al. 2010; Kopp et al. 2010; Lloyd et al. 2013; Miyahara 2013; Staples and Reid 2009; Whyatt and Craig 2011). In addition, evidence suggests that these deficits remain even when intellectual/cognitive development and receptive vocabulary are taken into account (Green et al. 2009; Staples and Reid 2009; Whyatt and Craig 2011). Further, longitudinal work indicates that these motor deficits widen over time in children with ASD (Landa and Garrett-Mayer 2006; Lloyd et al. 2013; Van Waelvelde et al. 2010), meaning that these children tend to fall further and further behind norms for their chronological age as they get older.

Much like DCD, our concern with motor development in children with ASD lies in the important role that fundamental motor skill plays in overall development. Fundamental motor skills, such as running, jumping, hopping, balance, ball skills and others, are the necessary building blocks for long-term engagement in physical active play, exercise, and participation in sport. Since most of childhood is spent in play that requires competencies in both fine and gross motor skills, our concern is that when such competencies are absent, the child's overall development, especially in relation to peer interactions and in the execution of motor tasks associated with formal learning (e.g., printing), is further impaired. This is especially the case for children at the less severe end of the ASD spectrum.

The development of fundamental motor skills is complex and involves a complex interaction between the task itself (e.g., walking), the inherent capabilities of the child with respect to characteristics, such as temperament and biological (genetic) endowment, and the environment (Chambers and Sugden 2006). With regard to the last component, in particular, it is commonly held that fundamental motor skills are generally learned as part of normal growth and development through interaction with others (e.g., imitation, exploration, direct instruction, unstructured play) (Clark 2005). As the play and social engagement necessary for building these movement patterns are constrained in children with ASD, it is plausible that the interaction between delayed motor skills and limited social interactions negatively impact each other and lead to greater and greater deficits over time (Bhat et al. 2011; Lloyd et al. 2013). Preliminary work has supported this hypothesis, finding that weaker motor skills are associated with greater social communicative deficits and poorer future outcomes (MacDonald et al. 2013, 2014; Piek and Dyck 2004; Sutera et al. 2007). In addition, when visual–spatial organization and motor coordination abilities are both impaired, ASD symptoms seem to be the most severe (Piek and Dyck 2004). Whether impairments in one area cause worsening of problems in another, however, has not been established. Longitudinal research would help to establish precedence, and may provide evidence on whether improvements in motor skills can positively impact social development and other ASD symptoms over time.

ASD and DCD: Comorbid or Separate Disorders

Not only does the existing ASD literature find consistent deficits in motor abilities but these are also severe enough that many of the children with ASD also meet the criteria for a diagnosis of motor impairment (Green et al. 2002). Such a diagnosis, it should be remembered, requires coordination deficits in excess of those to be expected given a child's cognitive functioning. In fact, when comparing children with ASD against children with DCD, the children with ASD tend to have the weakest motor skills and show the least improvements over time (Dewey et al. 2007; Green et al. 2002; Van Waelvelde et al. 2010; Wisdom et al. 2007). The pervasiveness of these motor coordination deficits in children with ASD has led to an argument that motor coordination problems be considered as a cardinal feature of the ASD diagnosis (Fournier et al. 2010). The nature of motor involvement in ASD, however, remains the subject of debate. This in fact is not limited to discussions of ASD and DCD, as we have seen. It stems from a long-standing debate about the nature of the associations among neurodevelopmental problems.

In the early 1980s the notion of generalized atypical brain development made a resurgence in the clinical neurological and psychiatric literatures, largely on the basis of research conducted in Northern Europe on the high rate of co-occurrence of problems related to sensory, motor, and behavioral problems in children. The concept of "DAMP" (deficits in attention, motor control, and perception), alluded to earlier, was introduced to describe the high rate of comorbidity between DCD, ADHD, and ASD symptoms (Gillberg and Kadesjo 2003). Bonnie Kaplan and her colleagues similarly used the concept of "atypical brain development" as an overarching explanation for the myriad of neurological deficits seen in children with ADHD and DCD (Kaplan et al. 1998). Arguments continue to be made along these lines, all hinging on overlapping symptoms (Wisdom et al. 2007).

A pervasive brain dysfunction hypothesis is most useful from a research perspective if it directs inquiry into specific mechanisms or interventions. It is unclear to us that a direct link between the concept of "atypical brain development" and more recent research in developmental neurosciences can be made. Nevertheless, it is true that convergent lines of research into the function of the cerebellum and its relationship to other areas of the brain associated with cognitive abilities (executive functioning) (Diamond 2000), as well as the growing body of research that links the cerebellum to a number of developmental disorders including autism (Mostofsky et al. 2009), learning disabilities, such as dyslexia (Nicolson et al. 2001), and ADHD/ADD (Visser 2003), suggests investigation of cerebellar dysfunction may aid our understanding of the etiology of these neurodevelopmental disorders—particularly in terms of elucidating common underlying pathways.

At a purely clinical or descriptive level, however, a compelling case can be made for rejecting this paradigm in favor of keeping distinct diagnostic categories, such as ASD and DCD, intact (Cairney et al. 2010a). Specifically, keeping existing clinical diagnoses, even if there is a common mechanism linking them together, is useful because, at least in theory, it facilities comprehensive evaluation of the child difficulties or challenges (and strengths), which in turn provides a roadmap for targeted interventions to address each cluster of symptoms. At the present time, it would seem prudent to maintain discrete diagnostic categories for both the purpose of classification and treatment, while continuing to search for common pathways that ultimately lead to more effective treatments and/or prevention strategies (Cairney et al. 2010a).

Regardless of etiology or clinical utility, what we do know is this—children with comorbid DCD, whether it is with ADHD/ADD or ASD, have worse outcomes than children who do not have comorbid motor coordination problems (Gillberg and Kadesjo 2003; Missiuna et al. 2014).

Implications for Intervention

Easily the single most important question for parents of children with DCD, and for clinicians involved in identification of the disorder, is what can be done for children with this condition? Historically, the literature has identified two sets of interventions, for which there is at least some empirical evidence regarding efficacy. The first are referred to as "bottom-up" approaches. These interventions are designed to target the fundamental abilities that govern motor control and movement skill. The theory being, if we can identify (and understand) the underlying mechanisms that produce motor coordination problems, we can intervene effectively. Examples in this area include the work of Ayres and her sensory-motor integration approach (Ayres 1972; Ayres et al. 1979), Laszlo's kinaesthetic training (Laszlo and Bairstow 1985; Laszlo et al. 1988), and Lord and Hulme's perceptual motor intervention (Lord and Hulme 1987a, b). Although theoretically appealing, evidence for efficacy is wanting: replication of the results of these studies has produced at best equivocal findings, and several meta-analyses and systematic reviews suggest that existing bottom-up approaches produce, at best, minimal improvement (Hillier 2007; Polatajko and Cantin 2005; Wilson and Lipsey 2007).

The other approach, so-called "top-down" interventions, are rooted in the principles of dynamics systems theory (Thelen 1995) and motor learning (Mandich et al. 2001). The emphasis is on the acquisition of particular motor skills, and the role of the therapist is to instruct, encourage, and model. Two approaches, Neuromotor Task Training (NTT) (Niemeijer, Smits-Engelsman and Schoemaker 2007) and Cognitive Orientation to daily Occupational Performance (CO-OP) (Levac et al. 2009), are among the preferred interventions for children with DCD. An important difference between the two concerns the level of participation of the child. In NTT, learning is more directed, whereas, in CO-OP, the child is more actively involved, both in selecting tasks and setting goals (Schoemaker and Smits-Engelsman 2005). CO-OP also uses a cognitive strategy approach, with focus and attention directed toward specific components of the target motor skill with which the child is having the most difficulty (Missiuna et al. 2015). Evidence for the efficacy and effectiveness of these interventions is considerably more compelling than that for "bottom-up" approaches (Sugden 2007).

Available evidence would suggest, then, that targeting function, rather than underlying deficits, is the better approach for intervention at the present time (Sugden 2007). However, there is no evidence from either approach that the core problems or symptoms of DCD can be completely corrected. Moreover, these interventions are typically provided one-on-one, and may continue for long periods of time. Therefore, it has been noted that, given the large number of children with DCD in the population, the demand for these interventions will far exceed the capacity of the health system to provide them (Deloitte 2010; Dunford et al. 2004; Missiuna et al. 2015). As a result, Missiuna and her colleagues have argued for a population health approach to problem of early identification and management of children with DCD. Termed Partnering for Change (P4C), the model incorporates occupational therapists directly into school support services to consult and advise teachers on management strategies, not to provide one-on-one therapy. Through a response-to-intervention approach (Shores and Bender 2007), teachers systematically try environmental and behavioral modifications to accommodate the motor challenges of the child. Only when successive attempts fail a child is referred to specialized services. The OT guides and consults continuously throughout the process. A somewhat radical proposition is embedded into this model—the focus is not on correction of motor problems at the child level, but in providing adequate environmental modifications to support the child's needs. In other words, the environment and the task (e.g., writing), as well as the child, are all the foci of the intervention. Evaluation of the approach is ongoing but initial results in terms of feasibility and acceptability of the program in schools are promising (Missiuna et al. 2015).

There is limited research on the efficacy of these interventions in children with comorbid neurodevelopmental disorders, such as ASD, and this will need to be a major focus of clinical research moving forward. With specific regard to ASD, current behavioral interventions seek to improve functioning in multiple domains, including motor functioning. Interventions for children with specific deficits in this area may therefore consist of an increased emphasis on motor skills within an existing framework.

It has also been argued, however, that increased attention to fundamental motor skills among children with ASD generally may help create a context for building and developing social skills though physical play (MacDonald et al. 2013). It may also give them the appropriate foundation for increasing and maintaining physical activity participation. There is a small but growing literature supporting this view. For example, a recent study by Bremer et al. (2014) used a waitlist control study to examine the impact of fundamental motor skill intervention on 4–year-old children with ASD. The intervention itself focused on teaching specific motor skills (e.g., running, kicking, throwing) through single-step skill acquisition strategies, active games, activity stations, and free play in a group setting. Results demonstrated significant group improvements in motor skill proficiency, as well as individual improvements in social skills and behavior, indicating that a group motor skill program can be an effective intervention strategy for young children with ASD.

Conclusion

DCD is a prevalent, neurodevelopmental condition affecting large numbers of children in the general population. While it has for some time been recognized that DCD tends to occur alongside other neurodevelopmental and psychiatric disorders, especially ADHD/ADD and learning disorders, attention to the problem of concurrent motor coordination difficulties in children with ASD is relatively recent. The removal of pervasive developmental delay as an exclusion criterion for DCD in the DSM-V has opened the door not only to clinical diagnosis but also to further scientific investigation. It is axiomatic in pediatrics that children with delays in multiple areas will be at greater risk for negative outcomes related to social, physical, and emotional well-being. Attending to the motor skill deficits in children with ASD holds great promise for improving both participation and overall quality of life. Research on the most appropriate and effective approaches for intervention in this population, however, are needed, as is further research on the health trajectories of children with comorbid ASD and DCD.

References

American Psychiatric Association. (2000). *Diagnostic and statistical manual of mental disorders, text revision (DSM-IV-TR)*. Washington, DC: American Psychiatric Association.

American Psychiatric Association. (2013). *Diagnostic and statistical manual of mental disorders* (5th ed.), Arlington: American Psychiatric Publishing.

Asperger, H. (1944). *Autistic psychopathy in childhood. Translated and annotated by U. Frith (Ed.) in Autism and Asperger syndrome (1991)*. Cambridge: Cambridge University Press.

Ayres, A. J. (1972). *Sensory integration and learning disorders*. Los Angeles: Western Psychological Services.

Ayres, A. J., Robbins, J., & McAtee, S. (1979). *Sensory integration and the child* (Vol. 12). Los Angeles: Western Psychological Services. http://i0.u-mama.ru/fd0/479/02e/Sensory_Integration1.doc.

Berkeley, S. L., & Zittel, L. L. (2010, April 22). Locomotor and object control skills of children diagnosed with autism. http://journals.humankinetics.com.libaccess.lib.mcmaster.ca/apaq-back-issues/apaqvolume18issue4october/locomotorandobjectcontrolskillsofchildrendiagnosedwithautism. Accessed 30 Mar 2015.

Bhat, A. N., Landa, R. J., & Galloway, J. C. C. (2011). Current perspectives on motor functioning in infants, children, and adults with autism spectrum disorders. *Physical Therapy, 91*(7), 1116–1129. http://doi.org/10.2522/ptj.20100294.

Blank, R., Smits-Engelsman, B., Polatajko, H., & Wilson, P. (2012). European academy for childhood disability (EACD): Recommendations on the definition, diagnosis and intervention of developmental coordination disorder (long version)*. *Developmental Medicine & Child Neurology, 54*(1), 54–93.

Bremer, E., Balogh, R., & Lloyd, M. (2014). Effectiveness of a fundamental motor skill intervention for 4-year-old children with autism spectrum disorder: A pilot study. *Autism*, 1362361314557548. http://doi.org/10.1177/1362361314557548.

British Medical Journal. (1962). Clumsy children. *BMJ, 2*(5320), 1665–1666. http://doi.org/10.1136/bmj.2.5320.1665.

Bruininks, R. H., & Bruininks, B. D. (2005). Bruininks-oseretsky test of motor proficiency, (BOT-2). Minneapolis: Pearson. Assessment.

Cairney, J. (2010a). Diagnostic criteria and case ascertainment of DCD in epidemiological studies: Does DSM help? http://pediatrics.aappublications.org/content/123/4/e693.short/reply#pediatrics_el_49177. Accessed 29 March 2015.

Cairney, J., Hay, J. A., Faught, B. E., & Hawes, R. (2005). Developmental coordination disorder and overweight and obesity in children aged 9–14 y. *International Journal of Obesity (2005), 29*(4), 369–372. http://doi.org/10.1038/sj.ijo.0802893.

Cairney, J., Hay, J. A., Faught, B. E., Flouris, A., & Klentrou, P. (2007). Developmental coordination disorder and cardiorespiratory fitness in children. *Pediatric Exercise Science, 19*(1), 20–28.

Cairney, J., Veldhuizen, S., & Szatmari, P. (2010b). Motor coordination and emotional-behavioral problems in children. *Current Opinion in Psychiatry, 23*(4), 324–329.

Cairney, J., Rigoli, D., & Piek, J. (2013). Developmental coordination disorder and internalizing problems in children: The environmental stress hypothesis elaborated. *Developmental Review, 33*(3), 224–238. http://doi.org/10.1016/j.dr.2013.07.002.

Cantell, M. H., Smyth, M. M., & Ahonen, T. P. (2003). Two distinct pathways for developmental coordination disorder: Persistence and resolution. *Human Movement Science, 22*(4), 413–431.

Cermak, S. (1985). Developmental dyspraxia. In E. A. Roy (Ed.), *Advances in psychology* (Vol. 23, pp. 225–248). Oxford: North-Holland. http://www.sciencedirect.com/science/article/pii/S0166411508611437.

Chambers, M., & Sugden, D. (2006). *Early years movement skills: Description, diagnosis and intervention*. London: Wiley.

Clark, J. E. (2005). From the beginning: A developmental perspective on movement and mobility. *Quest, 57*(1), 37–45. http://doi.org/10.1080/00336297.2005.10491841.

Crawford, S. G., Wilson, B. N., & Dewey, D. (2001). Identifying developmental coordination disorder. *Physical & Occupational Therapy in Pediatrics, 20*(2–3), 29–50. http://doi.org/10.1080/J006v20n02_03.

Deloitte. (2010). *Review of school health support services: Final report*. Ministry of Health and Long Term Care. from http://www.peopleforeducation.ca/document/review-of-school-health-support-services/. Accessed 31 March, 2015.

Dewey, D., Kaplan, B. J., Crawford, S. G., & Wilson, B. N. (2002). Developmental coordination disorder: Associated problems in attention, learning, and psychosocial adjustment. *Human Movement Science, 21*(5), 905–918.

Dewey, D., Cantell, M., & Crawford, S. G. (2007). Motor and gestural performance in children with autism spectrum disorders, developmental coordination disorder, and/or attention deficit hyperactivity disorder. *Journal of the International Neuropsychological Society: JINS, 13*(2), 246–256. http://doi.org/10.1017/S1355617707070270.

Diamond, A. (2000). Close interrelation of motor development and cognitive development and of the cerebellum and prefrontal cortex. *Child Development, 71*(1), 44–56. http://doi.org/10.1111/1467-8624.00117.

Dunford, C., Street, E., O'Connell, H., Kelly, J., & Sibert, J. R. (2004). Are referrals to occupational therapy for developmental coordination disorder appropriate? *Archives of Disease in Childhood, 89*(2), 143–147. http://doi.org/10.1136/adc.2002.016303.

Ford, F. R. (1944). *Diseases of the nervous system in infancy, childhood and adolescence*. Springfield: CC Thomas.

Fournier, K. A., Hass, C. J., Naik, S. K., Lodha, N., & Cauraugh, J. H. (2010). Motor coordination in autism spectrum disorders: A synthesis and meta-analysis. *Journal of Autism and Developmental Disorders, 40*(10), 1227–1240. http://doi.org/10.1007/s10803-010-0981-3.

Ghaziuddin, M., & Butler, E. (1998). Clumsiness in autism and asperger syndrome: A further report. *Journal of Intellectual Disability Research, 42*(1), 43–48. http://doi.org/10.1046/j.1365-2788.1998.00065.x.

Gillberg, C., & Kadesjo, B. (2003). Why bother about clumsiness? The implications of having developmental coordination disorder (DCD). *Neural Plasticity, 10*(1–2), 59–68. http://doi.org/10.1155/NP.2003.59.

Goldman, S., Wang, C., Salgado, M. W., Greene, P. E., Kim, M., & Rapin, I. (2009). Motor stereotypies in children with autism and other developmental disorders. *Developmental Medicine & Child Neurology, 51*(1), 30–38. http://doi.org/10.1111/j.1469-8749.2008.03178.x.

Green, D., Baird, G., Barnett, A. L., Henderson, L., Huber, J., & Henderson, S. E. (2002). The severity and nature of motor impairment in Asperger's syndrome: A comparison with specific developmental disorder of motor function. *Journal of Child Psychology and Psychiatry, 43*(5), 655–668. http://doi.org/10.1111/1469-7610.00054.

Green, D., Charman, T., Pickles, A., Chandler, S., Loucas, T., Simonoff, E., et al. (2009). Impairment in movement skills of children with autistic spectrum disorders. *Developmental Medicine & Child Neurology, 51*(4), 311–316. http://doi.org/10.1111/j.1469-8749.2008.03242.x.

Gubbay, S. S. (1975). Clumsy children in normal schools. *The Medical Journal of Australia, 1*(8), 233–236.

Henderson, S. E., Sugden, D. A., & Barnett, A. L. (2007). *Movement assessment battery for children-2: Movement ABC-2: Examiner's manual*. London: Pearson.
Hillier, S. (2007). *Intervention for children with developmental coordination disorder: A systematic review*. Doctoral dissertation, Nova Southeastern University.
Holsti, L. M. A., Grunau, R. V. E., & Whitfield, M. F. M. D. (2002). Developmental coordination disorder in extremely low birth weight children at nine years. *Journal of Developmental, 23*(1), 9–15.
Kadesjo, B., & Gillberg, C. (1999). Developmental coordination disorder in Swedish 7-year-old children. *Journal of the American Academy of Child & Adolescent Psychiatry, 38*(7), 820–828.
Kanner, L. (1943). Autistic disturbances of affective contact. *The Nervous Child, 2*, 217–250. *Autism and Childhood Scbicopbrenia, 4, 131–1, 41.*
Kaplan, B. J., N Wilson, B., Dewey, D., & Crawford, S. G. (1998). DCD may not be a discrete disorder. *Human Movement Science, 17*(4), 471–490.
Kopp, S., Beckung, E., & Gillberg, C. (2010). Developmental coordination disorder and other motor control problems in girls with autism spectrum disorder and/or attention-deficit/hyperactivity disorder. *Research in Developmental Disabilities, 31*(2), 350–361. http://doi.org/10.1016/j.ridd.2009.09.017.
Landa, R., & Garrett-Mayer, E. (2006). Development in infants with autism spectrum disorders: A prospective study. *Journal of Child Psychology and Psychiatry, 47*(6), 629–638. http://doi.org/10.1111/j.1469-7610.2006.01531.x.
Langford, W. S. (1955). Developmental dyspraxia—abnormal clumsiness. *Bulletin of the Orton Society, 5*(1), 3–7. http://doi.org/10.1007/BF02657573.
Laszlo, J. I., & Bairstow, P. J. (1985). *Perceptual-motor behaviour: Developmental assessment and therapy*. London: Holt, Rinehart and Winston.
Laszlo, J. I., Bairstow, P. J., Bartrip, J., & Rolfe, U. T. (1988). Clumsiness or Perceptuo–Motor Dysfunction? In A. M. C. and J. R. Beech (Ed.), *Advances in Psychology* (Vol. 55, pp. 293–310). North-Holland. http://www.sciencedirect.com/science/article/pii/S0166411508606299.
Levac, D., Wishart, L., Missiuna, C., & Wright, V. (2009). The application of motor learning strategies within functionally based interventions for children with neuromotor conditions. *Pediatric Physical Therapy, 21*(4), 345–355. http://doi.org/10.1097/PEP.0b013e3181beb09d.
Lichtenstein, P., Carlström, E., Råstam, M., Gillberg, C., & Anckarsäter, H. (2010). The genetics of autism spectrum disorders and related neuropsychiatric disorders in childhood. *American Journal of Psychiatry, 167*(11), 1357–1363. http://doi.org/10.1176/appi.ajp.2010.10020223.
Lingam, R., Hunt, L., Golding, J., Jongmans, M., & Emond, A. (2009). Prevalence of developmental coordination disorder using the DSM-IV at 7 years of age: A UK population–based study. *Pediatrics, 123*(4), e693–e700. http://doi.org/10.1542/peds.2008-1770.
Lloyd, M., MacDonald, M., & Lord, C. (2013). Motor skills of toddlers with autism spectrum disorders. *Autism: the international journal of research and practice, 17*(2), 133–146. http://doi.org/10.1177/1362361311402230.
Lord, R., & Hulme, C. (1987a). Kinaesthetic sensitivity of normal and clumsy children. *Developmental Medicine & Child Neurology, 29*(6), 720–725. http://doi.org/10.1111/j.1469-8749.1987.tb08816.x.
Lord, R., & Hulme, C. (1987b). Perceptual judgements of normal and clumsy children. *Developmental Medicine & Child Neurology, 29*(2), 250–257. http://doi.org/10.1111/j.1469-8749.1987.tb02143.x.
MacDonald, M., Lord, C., & Ulrich, D. A. (2013). The relationship of motor skills and social communicative skills in school-aged children with autism spectrum disorder. *Adapted Physical Activity Quarterly, 30*(3), 271–282. http://journals.humankinetics.com/apaq. Accessed 20 March 2015.
MacDonald, M., Lord, C., & Ulrich, D. A. (2014). Motor skills and calibrated autism severity in young children with autism spectrum disorder. *Adapted Physical Activity Quarterly: APAQ, 31*(2), 95–105. http://doi.org/10.1123/apaq.2013-0068.

Mandich, A. D., Polatajko, H. J., Macnab, J. J., & Miller, L. T. (2001). Treatment of children with developmental coordination disorder. *Physical & Occupational Therapy in Pediatrics, 20*(2–3), 51–68. http://doi.org/10.1080/J006v20n02_04.

Martin, N. C., Piek, J. P., & Hay, D. (2006). DCD and ADHD: A genetic study of their shared aetiology. *Human Movement Science, 25*(1), 110–124. http://doi.org/10.1016/j.humov.2005.10.006.

McCarron, L. T. (1997). *MAND: McCarron Assessment of Neuromuscular Development, Fine and Gross Motor Abilities*. Dallas: McCarron-Dial Systems, Incorporated.

Missiuna, C., Moll, S., King, G., Stewart, D., & Macdonald, K. (2008). Life experiences of young adults who have coordination difficulties. *Canadian Journal of Occupational Therapy, 75*(3), 157–166. http://doi.org/10.1177/000841740807500307.

Missiuna, C., Cairney, J., Pollock, N., Russell, D., Macdonald, K., Cousins, M., et al. (2011). A staged approach for identifying children with developmental coordination disorder from the population. *Research in Developmental Disabilities, 32*(2), 549–559. http://doi.org/10.1016/j.ridd.2010.12.025.

Missiuna, C., Cairney, J., Pollock, N., Campbell, W., Russell, D. J., Macdonald, K., et al. (2014). Psychological distress in children with developmental coordination disorder and attention-deficit hyperactivity disorder. *Research in Developmental Disabilities, 35*(5), 1198–1207. http://doi.org/10.1016/j.ridd.2014.01.007.

Missiuna, C., Polatajko, H., & Pollock, N. (2015). Strategic management of children with developmental coordination disorder. In J. Cairney (Ed.), Developmental coordination disorder and its consequences (pp. 192–212). Toronto: University of Toronto Press.

Miyahara, M. (1997). Brief report: Motor incoordination in children with asperger syndrome and learning disabilities. *Journal of Autism and Developmental Disorders, 27*(5), 595–603.

Miyahara, M. (2013). Meta review of systematic and meta analytic reviews on movement differences, effect of movement based interventions, and the underlying neural mechanisms in autism spectrum disorder. *Frontiers in Integrative Neuroscience, 7*. http://doi.org/10.3389/fnint.2013.00016.

Mostofsky, S. H., Powell, S. K., Simmonds, D. J., Goldberg, M. C., Caffo, B., & Pekar, J. J. (2009). Decreased connectivity and cerebellar activity in autism during motor task performance. *Brain*, awp088. http://doi.org/10.1093/brain/awp088.

Nicolson, R. I., Fawcett, A. J., & Dean, P. (2001). Developmental dyslexia: The cerebellar deficit hypothesis. *Trends in Neurosciences, 24*(9), 508–511. http://doi.org/10.1016/S0166-2236(00)01896-8.

Niemeijer, A. S., Smits-Engelsman, B. C. M., & Schoemaker, M. M. (2007). Neuromotor task training for children with developmental coordination disorder: A controlled trial. *Developmental Medicine & Child Neurology, 49*(6), 406–411. http://doi.org/10.1111/j.1469-8749.2007.00406.x.

Orton, T. S. (1937). *Reading, writing and speech problems in children*. New York: W W Norton & Co.

Pearsall-Jones, J. G., Piek, J. P., Rigoli, D., Martin, N. C., & Levy, F. (2009). an investigation into etiological pathways of DCD and ADHD using a monozygotic twin design. *Twin Research and Human Genetics, 12*(04), 381–391. http://doi.org/10.1375/twin.12.4.381.

Piek, J. P., & Dyck, M. J. (2004). Sensory-motor deficits in children with developmental coordination disorder, attention deficit hyperactivity disorder and autistic disorder. *Human Movement Science, 23*(3–4), 475–488. http://doi.org/10.1016/j.humov.2004.08.019.

Piek, J. P., Pitcher, T. M., & Hay, D. A. (1999). Motor coordination and kinaesthesis in boys with attention deficit–hyperactivity disorder. *Developmental Medicine & Child Neurology, 41*(3), 159–165. http://doi.org/10.1111/j.1469-8749.1999.tb00575.x.

Pitcher, T. M., Piek, J. P., & Hay, D. A. (2003). Fine and gross motor ability in males with ADHD. *Developmental Medicine & Child Neurology, 45*(8), 525–535.

Polatajko, H. J., & Cantin, N. (2005). Developmental Coordination Disorder (Dyspraxia): An Overview of the State of the Art. *Seminars in Pediatric Neurology, 12*(4), 250–258. http://doi.org/10.1016/j.spen.2005.12.007.

Polatajko, H., Fox, M., & Missiuna, C. (1995). An International Consensus on Children with Developmental Coordination Disorder. *Canadian Journal of Occupational Therapy, 62*(1), 3–6. http://doi.org/10.1177/000841749506200101.

Rivilis, I., Hay, J., Cairney, J., Klentrou, P., Liu, J., & Faught, B. E. (2011). Physical activity and fitness in children with developmental coordination disorder: A systematic review. *Research in Developmental Disabilities, 32*(3), 894–910. http://doi.org/10.1016/j.ridd.2011.01.017.

Schoemaker, M. M., & Smits-Engelsman, B. C. M. (2005). Neuromotor task training: a new approach to treat children with DCD. In D. A. Sugden, M. Chambers (Eds.), *Children with Developmental Coordination Disorder* (pp. 212–227). London: Whurr.

Shores, C., & Bender, W. N. (2007). Response to intervention. In W. N. Bender & C. Shores (Eds.), *Response to intervention: A practical guide for every teacher*. Thousand Oaks: Corwin Press.

Smits-Engelsman, B., & Hill, E. L. (2012). The relationship between motor coordination and intelligence across the IQ range. *Pediatrics, 130*(4), e950–e956. http://doi.org/10.1542/peds.2011-3712.

Spironello, C., Hay, J., Missiuna, C., Faught, B. E., & Cairney, J. (2010). Concurrent and construct validation of the short form of the Bruininks-Oseretsky test of motor proficiency and the movement-ABC when administered under field conditions: Implications for screening. *Child: Care, Health and Development, 36*(4), 499–507. http://doi.org/10.1111/j.1365-2214.2009.01066.x.

Staples, K. L., & Reid, G. (2009). Fundamental movement skills and autism spectrum disorders. *Journal of Autism and Developmental Disorders, 40*(2), 209–217. http://doi.org/10.1007/s10803-009-0854-9.

Strauss, A. A., & Lehtinen, L. E. (1947). *Psychopathology and education of the brain-injured child*. Oxford: Grune & Stratton.

Sugden, D. (2006). *Leeds consensus statement: Developmental coordination disorder as a specific learning difficulty*. Leeds: DCD-UK/Dyscovery Centre.

Sugden, D. (2007). Current approaches to intervention in children with developmental coordination disorder. *Developmental Medicine and Child Neurology, 49*(6), 467–471. http://doi.org/10.1111/j.1469-8749.2007.00467.x.

Sutera, S., Pandey, J., Esser, E. L., Rosenthal, M. A., Wilson, L. B., Barton, M., et al. (2007). Predictors of optimal outcome in toddlers diagnosed with autism spectrum disorders. *Journal of Autism and Developmental Disorders, 37*(1), 98–107. http://doi.org/10.1007/s10803-006-0340-6.

Tan, S. K., Parker, H., & Larkin, D. (2010, April 22). Concurrent Validity of Motor Tests Used to Identify Children With Motor Impairment. http://journals.humankinetics.com/apaq-back-issues/apaqvolume18issue2april/concurrentvalidityofmotortestsusedtoidentifychildrenwithmotorimpairment. Accessed 30 Mar 2015.

Thelen, E. (1995). Motor development: A new synthesis. *American Psychologist, 50*(2), 79–95. http://doi.org/10.1037/0003-066X.50.2.79.

Treuting, J. J., & Hinshaw, S. P. (2001). Depression and self-esteem in boys with attention-deficit/hyperactivity disorder: Associations with comorbid aggression and explanatory attributional mechanisms. *Journal of Abnormal Child Psychology, 29*(1), 23–39. http://doi.org/10.1023/A:1005247412221.

Van Waelvelde, H., Oostra, A., Dewitte, G., Van Den Broeck, C., & Jongmans, M. J. (2010). Stability of motor problems in young children with or at risk of autism spectrum disorders, ADHD, and or developmental coordination disorder. *Developmental Medicine & Child Neurology, 52*(8), e174–e178. http://doi.org/10.1111/j.1469-8749.2009.03606.x.

Veldhuizen, S., & Cairney, J. (2015). Methodological issues in field-based DCD research: Case identification and study design. In J. Cairney (Ed.), *Developmental coordination disorder and its consequences* (pp. 192–212). Toronto: University of Toronto Press.

Visscher, C., Houwen, S., Scherder, E. J. A., Moolenaar, B., & Hartman, E. (2007). Motor profile of children with developmental speech and language disorders. *Pediatrics, 120*(1), e158–e163. http://doi.org/10.1542/peds.2006-2462.

Visser, J. (2003). Developmental coordination disorder: A review of research on subtypes and comorbidities. *Human Movement Science, 22*(4), 479–493.

Whyatt, C. P., & Craig, C. M. (2011). Motor skills in children aged 7–10 years, diagnosed with autism spectrum disorder. *Journal of Autism and Developmental Disorders, 42*(9), 1799–1809. http://doi.org/10.1007/s10803-011-1421-8.

Wilson, S. J., & Lipsey, M. W. (2007). School-based interventions for aggressive and disruptive behavior: Update of a meta-analysis. *American Journal of Preventive Medicine, 33*(2 Suppl.), S130–S143. http://doi.org/10.1016/j.amepre.2007.04.011.

Wilson, P. H., Ruddock, S., Smits-Engelsman, B., Polatajko, H., & Blank, R. (2013). Understanding performance deficits in developmental coordination disorder: A meta-analysis of recent research. *Developmental Medicine & Child Neurology, 55*(3), 217–228. http://doi.org/10.1111/j.1469-8749.2012.04436.x.

Wisdom, S. N., Dyck, M. J., Piek, J. P., Hay, D., & Hallmayer, J. (2007). Can autism, language and coordination disorders be differentiated based on ability profiles? *European Child & Adolescent Psychiatry, 16*(3), 178–186. http://doi.org/10.1007/s00787-006-0586-8.

Zhu, Y.-C., Wu, S. K., & Cairney, J. (2011). Obesity and motor coordination ability in Taiwanese children with and without developmental coordination disorder. *Research in Developmental Disabilities, 32*(2), 801–807. http://doi.org/10.1016/j.ridd.2010.10.020.

Zwicker, J. G., Missiuna, C., Harris, S. R., & Boyd, L. A. (2012). Developmental coordination disorder: A review and update. *European Journal of Paediatric Neurology, 16*(6), 573–581. http://doi.org/10.1016/j.ejpn.2012.05.005.

Appendix

This book presents the similarities and intersections between autism spectrum disorders (ASD) and comorbid conditions in children. It describes the prevalence and magnitude of comorbid conditions occurring in conjunction with ASD that complicate diagnosis and can potentially lead to inappropriate treatment and negative outcomes. It addresses the strengths and limitations of age-appropriate assessment measures as well as activity and motor skill measurement methods. Specific comorbid disorders are examined through the review of core symptoms, prognostic and diagnostic issues, and treatment options for children on the ASD spectrum.

Featured topics include:

- Challenging behaviors in children with ASD.
- Conditions ranging from feeding and gastrointestinal disorders to epilepsy.
- Developmental coordination disorder (DCD).
- Intellectual disability (ID).
- Methods and procedures for measuring comorbid psychological, medical, and motor disorders.

Comorbid Conditions Among Children with Autism Spectrum Disorders is a must-have resource for researchers, clinicians and professionals, and graduate students across such fields as clinical child, school, and developmental psychology, child and adolescent psychiatry, and social work as well as rehabilitation medicine/therapy, behavioral therapy, pediatrics, and educational psychology.

Johnny L. Matson (ed.), *Comorbid Conditions Among Children with Autism Spectrum Disorders,* Autism and Child Psychopathology Series,
DOI 10.1007/978-3-319-19183-6

Index

Johnny L. Matson (ed.), *Comorbid Conditions Among Children with Autism Spectrum Disorders,* Autism and Child Psychopathology Series,
DOI 10.1007/978-3-319-19183-6

www.ingramcontent.com/pod-product-compliance
Lightning Source LLC
Chambersburg PA
CBHW071425230926
51846CB00001B/120
* 9 7 8 3 3 1 9 3 7 1 5 4 2 *